AF531672

CYTOLOGY OF CANCER

ENCYCLOPAEDIA OF CANCER

Vol. III

CYTOLOGY OF CANCER

By

Dr. Amita Sarkar

Dept. of Zoology
Agra College
Agra (U.P.)
(India)

DISCOVERY PUBLISHING HOUSE PVT. LTD.
NEW DELHI-110 002

First Published-2008

ISBN 978-81-8356-356-7 (Set)

Published by:

DISCOVERY PUBLISHING HOUSE PVT. LTD.
4831/24, Ansari Road, Prahlad Street,
Darya Ganj, New Delhi-110002 (India)
Phone: 23279245 • Fax: 91-11-23253475
E-mail: dphbooks@rediffmail.com
dphtemp@indiatimes.com
Website: www.discoverypublishinghouse.com

Printed by : Sachin Printers, Delhi

Preface

Over the past 20 years, technological advances in molecular biology have proven invaluable to the understanding of the pathogenesis of cancer. The application of molecular technology to the study of cancer has not only led to advances in tumor diagnosis, but has also provided markers for the assessment of prognosis and disease progression. The aim of *Encyclopaedia of Cancer* is to provide a comprehensive collection of the most up-to-date techniques for the detection of molecular changes in cancer.

This book is intended to provide a relatively short overview of important concepts and notions on the molecular biology of human cancers, including many facts essential to find one's way in this field. It is, however, not meant to be compreshensive and probably cannot be, as our knowledge is rapidly growing.

The salient feature of this book is that it covers a wide range of molecular techniques and provides a source of information to readers at all levels. Although several books on cancer have been published in the last decade, most of either very shallow or cover few areas in depth. Rarely do they cover the broad spectrum of topics which would provide enough information for understanding the subject or provide simple protocols for execution of molecular change. In my opinion, this book can help the reader to easily understand the subject and also excecute the experiments very efficiently.

There can be no claim to originality except in the manner of treatment and much of the information has been obtained from the books and scientific journals available in the different libraries.

The author expresses his thanks to his friends and colleagues whose continue inspirations have initiated him to bring out this book.

The author is painfully aware of the shortcomings, errors and misprints that have crept in, and shall be greateful to receive suggestion for improvement of the next edition from all the readers.

The author expresses his gratitude to Mr. Wasan and staff of M/s Discovery Publishing House for their whole hearted co-operation in the publication of this book.

Author

CONTENTS

1

INTRODUCTION

Cancer is a complex disease occurring as a result of a progressive accumulation of genetic aberrations and epigenetic changes that enable escape from normal cellular and environmental controls. Neoplastic cells may have numerous acquired genetic abnormalities including aneuploidy, chromosomal rearrangements, amplifications, deletions, gene rearrangements, and loss-of-function or gain-of-function mutations. Recent studies have also highlighted the importance of epigenetic alterations of certain genes that result in the inactivation of their functions in some human cancers. These aberrations lead to the abnormal behavior common to all neoplastic cells: dysregulated growth, lack of contact inhibition, genomic instability, and propensity for metastasis.

The genes affected by mutations in cancer may be divided into two main classes: genes that have gain-of-function (activating) mutations, which are known as *oncogenes*; and genes for which both alleles have loss-of-function (inactivating) mutations, which are known as *tumor suppressor genes*. Close to 100 genes have been shown to play a role in the development or progression of human cancers, some of which have been implicated in a broad spectrum of malignancies, whereas others are unique to a specific type. Cancers can arise via the aberration of different combinations of genes, which in turn may be mutated, overexpressed, or deleted. The order in which these events occur has also proved to be important. For example, in breast cancer it has been proposed that at least 10 distinct gene alterations may be involved in disease initiation and progression. The study of colon cancer has shown that carcinogenesis is a multistage process involving the activation of cellular oncogenes, the deletion of multiple chromosomal regions, and the loss of function of tumor suppressor genes.

Technologic advances in molecular biology over the past 20–25 yr have led to a dramatic increase in the identification of the molecular processes involved in tumorigenesis. Over this period, the molecular basis of cancer no longer holds the mystery that it once did. It is, however, also clear that the knowledge that has been accumulated is insufficient to claim a total understanding of the mechanism of cancer development. This volume has brought together a number of relevant techniques by which genetic abnormalities occurring in cancer can be detected and analyzed. This, in turn, will give rise to other avenues of study, such as: how mutations affect function, how these genes are regulated, and how they interact with each other.

The mutational analysis of oncogenes and tumor suppressor genes can provide evidence for a specific association between these genes and tumor type. These genes can be altered during carcinogenesis by different mechanisms such as point mutations, chromosomal translocations, gene amplification, or deletion. Furthermore, these genes may be analyzed at different levels—DNA, RNA, or expressed proteins.

DNA Analysis

Mutational analysis can be performed using a variety of techniques. The amplification of specific regions of DNA or RNA by the *polymerase chain reaction* (PCR) has opened endless possibilities that can be used for the rapid and efficient detection of alterations, even single nucleotide changes. These PCR-based techniques rely on changes in electrophoretic mobility induced by altered single-stranded secondary structure (single-strand conformation polymorphism), by altered dissociation rates of the DNA fragments (denaturing gradient gel electrophoresis), or by RNase cleavage assays. PCR can also be used for the rapid and quantitative detection of chromosomal rearrangements, such as commonly observed in leukemia. PCR is designed to specifically amplify genomic fragments that are not normally contiguous and are, therefore, unique to that type of gene rearrangement. Converting the RNA to DNA with *reverse transcriptase* (RT) prior to the PCR stage is usually required for this assay. However, in some cases, genomic DNA can be used for the direct amplification of translocation break points. A variation on the PCR theme involves the use of DNA fingerprints to detect genetic rearrangements in cancer. The primers are often arbitrary or repeat (e.g., ALU) sequences, which will give, after electrophoresis, a DNA fingerprint that can be used for the detection of genetic abnormalities. Microsatellite repeats occur throughout the genome and can be used as markers for genetic alterations, usually for the loss of heterozygosity, which will indicate that a deletion has occurred that overlaps that specific marker. For specific genes involved in certain cancers, the mutational analysis can be carried out using a protein truncation assay. This assay involves the identification of abnormal polypeptides synthesized in vitro from RT-PCR products, and the truncating mutations are usually confirmed by sequence analysis.

RNA Expression Analysis

DNA microarray technology, which makes use of high-density two-dimensional oligonucleotide probe arrays containing hundreds or thousands of oligonucleotide probes, represents a powerful new DNA sequence analysis tool to test for a variety of genetic mutations. Hybridization to cDNA microarrays allows the simultaneous parallel expression analysis of thousands of genes. High-throughput gene expression profiling increasingly is becoming a valuable method for identifying genes differentially expressed in tumor vs normal tissues. Gene expression microarrays hold great promise for studies of human tumorigenesis, and the large gene expression data sets produced have the potential to provide novel insights into fundamental cancer biology at the molecular level. Indeed, cDNA microarray technology has already begun to aid in the elucidation of the genetic events underlying the initiation and progression of some human cancers. Differentially expressed genes can also be detected by other techniques such as differential display, which involves a random primed RT-PCR display or fingerprint of subsets of expressed RNA, or subtractive hybridization, which involves the enrichment of genes preferentially expressed in one tissue compared with a second.

Chromosomal Analysis

Fluorescence in situ hybridization (FISH) is one of the techniques with an expanding role in the molecular analysis of cancer. It can be used for the simple detection of numerical and structural chromosomal abnormalities that may occur in cancer cells and is particularly useful as a tool for the diagnosis of nonrandom translocations in leukemia and numerous other cancers. To date, most FISH studies have involved the use of single whole-chromosome or gene probes. This has been taken to new levels by the development of spectral karyotyping, which involves the hybridization of 24 fluorescently labeled chromosome painting probes to metaphase spreads in such a manner that simultaneous visualization of each of the chromosomes in a different color is accomplished. Using this method, it is possible to define all chromosomal rearrangements and identify all of the marker chromosomes in tumor cells. *Comparative genomic hybridization* (CGH) is a FISH-based technique that can detect gains and losses of whole chromosomes and subchromosomal regions. CGH is based on a two-color, competitive FISH of differentially labeled tumor and reference DNA to normal metaphase chromosomes and can scan the whole genome without prior knowledge of specific chromosomal abnormalities.

Analysis of Methylation Status

Some molecular methods will analyze specific changes to the DNA structure or genomic modifications. Changes in the DNA methylation status are one of the most common detectable abnormalities in human cancer. Hypermethylation within the promoters of selected genes is especially common and is usually associated with inactivation of the involved gene or genes and may be an early event in the pathogenesis of some cancers, whereas other genes become methylated during disease progression.

Telomere and Telomerase Activity

Telomeres are repetitive DNA sequences at chromosome ends, which are necessary for maintaining chromosomal integrity. A reduction in telomere length has been described in a wide range of human cancers, including both solid tumors and leukemias. The enzyme telomerase synthesizes *de novo* telomeric repeats and incorporates them onto the DNA 3' ends of chromosomes. Telomere shortening in normal cells is a result of DNA replication events, and reduction beyond a critical length is a signal for cellular senescence. However, the maintenance of telomere length, by the activation of the enzyme telomerase, is thought to be essential for immortalization of human cancer cells to compensate for the loss of DNA from the ends of chromosomes. Therefore, the measurement of telomere length and telomerase enzyme activity levels are important in monitoring disease progression or response to therapy. Recently, the possible manipulation of telomerase has generated some excitement as an anticancer strategy.

Clonal Origin of Cancer

The methods I have described allow the investigator to study the myriad of genetic alterations that can occur during the initiation, development, and progression of cancer. However, it is also possible to provide insight into the transition from somatic cell mutation to neoplasia. The clonal origin of cells can be assessed in patients with X chromosome-linked polymorphisms, taking advantage of the random inactivation of the X chromosome. The inactivation is related to the differentially methylated patterns on the active and inactive X chromosomes.

Human cancers are generally characterized by acquisition of a series of somatic mutations. Molecular techniques, such as those described in this volume, have been used to identify a plethora of chromosomal translocations and mutations associated with carcinogenesis. The analysis and comparison of the array of genetic changes occurring in malignancy will enable a move toward a better understanding of cancer development. This will eventually lead to the development of improved therapies tailored to take into account the cytogenetic and molecular characteristics of specific human cancers.

2

CELL DIVISION

There are two types of organisms-acellular and multicellular. The growth and development of an individual depends exclusively on the growth and multiplication of the cells. It was *Virchow* who first of all adequately stated the cell division. In animal cell the cell division was studied in the form of segmentation division or cleavage by *Prevost* and *Dumas* in 1824. The mechanism of cell division was not precisely investigated until long afterward but *Remak* and *Kolliker* showed that the process involves a division of both the nucleus and the cytoplasm. The term *karyokinesis* was introduced by *Schleicher* (1878) to designate the changes of nucleus during division, and the term *cytokinesis* was introduced by *Whiterman* (1887) to designate the associated changes taking place in the cytoplasm. Cell division is necessarily the avoidance of ageing, and secondly for the segregation of an individual into semi-independent units which leads to efficiency. Thus, we see that cell division is a widespread phenomenon that is essential not only for the maintenance of life but also for the development of the organism itself.

Cell division can be conveniently described as:

(i) *Direct division.* Where the nucleus and cell body undergo a simple mass division into two parts. It is also called *amitosis*.

(ii) *Indirect division.* Here the nucleus undergoes complicated changes before it is divided into two daughter nuclei.

Having seen how the DNA in the nucleus is replicated and repaired, we turn now to the process whereby the two copies of each chromosome that have been generated during the prior S phase are separated from each other and partitioned into daughter cells. These processes are mitosis and cytokinesis.

The Stages of Mitosis

Mitosis has been known and studied for a century, but only in the past 25 years has significant progress been made toward understanding the mitotic process at the molecular level. We will begin by surveying the morphological changes that occur in a cell as it undergoes mitosis; later we will examine the underlying molecular mechanisms.

Morphologically, mitosis can be described as a series of five phases, based primarily on the appearance and behaviour of the chromosomes. As with any dynamic process, we must remember that the division into phase is somewhat arbitrary and that the phase are primarily a convenience for studying and describing the process. The five phases of mitosis are prophase, prometaphase, metaphase, anaphase, and telophase. (An alternative term for prometaphase is simply "late prophase").

Interphase

The period of metabolic activity during which cell division is not in a process, has been called the 'interphase.' This is frequently referred to as the 'resting phase' but this term is not appropriate because the cell is metabolically most active at this stage that is why *Berril* and *Huskins* (1936) referred it as the *energy phases*. The interphase is the period between the telophase of one division and the prophase of the new cell division. During this phase the cell does everything except division. It is during interphase that the genes self-duplicate and carry on their function of supervising synthesis.

The chromatin granules in the nucleus are not readily distinguishable in the living cell, but may be brought out by treatment with chemicals which kill, fix and stain them. They appear at first glance to be scattered throughout the nucleus, but careful study has produced evidence that they are arranged in a definite pattern as long coiled strands and appear as a thread like net work in ordinary stained preparation.

"Nuclear sap" or, "Karyoplasm" fills the interstics between the chromosomes. One of more rounded bodies, the *nucleoli* are usually present. Between the nucleus and the surrounding cytoplasm, is the *nuclear membrane*. In the cytoplasm adjacent to the nucleus, there is a body, the *central body,* which consists of two granules or, after each granule has replicated, of two pairs of granules, the *centrioles*.

A typical cell cycle, including interphase lasts from 20-24 hrs. Interphase in the longest period in the cell cycle, and may last for several days in cells.

Interphase can be further divided into form sub-phases:

1. G_1-phase
2. S-phase
3. G_2-phase
4. M-phase.

G_1-phase includes the synthesis and organization of the substrate and enzyme necessary for DNA synthesis. Therefore, G_1, is marked by the synthesis of RNA and protein.

G_1-phase is followed by the S-phase where the synthesis of DNA occurs.

During G_2-phase, all the metabolic activities are performed. M-phase is the period of chromosomal division.

The relative lengths of these phases differ in different organisms. A human cell in culture at 37°C, completes the mitotic cycle in about 20 hours and the M-phase lasts for only one hour. Temperature and cell environment plays an important role in determining the rate of cell division. Even the non-meristematic cells can sometimes be made to divide by changing the environmental conditions. Those cells which are not going to divide any more, have the mitotic cycle at the G_1 phase and start differentiating.

The cells shows following changes:

1. The cell, as a whole, attains the maximum growth and possesses synthesized proteins for energy for various divisions and processes.
2. The nuclear membrane is intact and the chromosomes are found in the form of more or less loosely coiled threads, somewhat closely appressed to the membrane. In this condition of chromosomes, most of the cytologists regard them to be duplicated, while some workers are of the opinion that they are multipartite.
3. The two centrioles, which are found at right angles to each other replicate into two each. *Mazia* (1961) has described that, if the replication is checked, then division will not take place.
4. For the future spindle condensation of protoplasm into a coherent area of jelly-like consistency also takes place. The spindle also starts growing and pushes the centrioles apart.
5. DNA synthesis occurs during autosynthetic interphase, when the chromosomes and dispersed.
6. Chromocentre are also conspicuous during the interphase.

Duration of Cell Division

The time required for completion of mitosis varies from cell type to cell type and is related to the length of the G_1 phase. Temperature, within certain limits, also affects the duration of the process. In general the metaphase and anaphase stages are of short duration; most of the time of cell division is spent in prophase and telophase stages. It must be remembered that the period between cell division, interphase, is usually long. For instance, in some mammalian cell cultures 16 to 20 hours between cell divisions is a common occurrence.

Many cells of both plants and animals studied in tissue culture show the following durations in the cell cycle.

G_1	10–20 hours (usually less than 50 percent of the total)
S	6–8 hours
G_2	1–4 or more hours (usually less than 20 percent of the total)
M	1 hour
Total	18–33 hours

Formation of Mitotic Apparatus: Prophase

Toward the end of G_2, the chromosomes start to condense from the extended, highly diffuse form of interphase chromatin to the dense, coiled structures characteristic of mitosis. Although the transition from interphase to mitotic prophase is not sharply defined, a cell is considered to be in *prophase* when the chromosomes have condensed to the point of being visible as threads in the light microscope. Each chromosome has duplicated during the preceding S phase and now consists of two sister chromatids. Sister chromatids are tightly attached to each other at a constricted region, the *centromere*, which corresponds to a particular stretch of the chromosome's DNA. As the chromosomes condense, the nucleolus (or nucleoli) gradually disappears.

Meanwhile, outside the nucleus, another important organelle has sprung into action. This is the *centrosome*, an amorphous cloud of material that, in most animal cells, surrounds a pair of *centrioles*. Because they are lacking in some mitotic cells, including all plant cells and fungal cells, centrioles cannot be essential for mitosis, and their function in the centrosome remains a mystery. However, the centriole structure—a cylinder made of microtubules—is related to the centrosome's role in the cell. The centrosome is a cellular organizing center for microtubules. During interphase, the microtubules of the cytoskeleton originate there. During prophase, the cytoskeletal microtubules disassemble, and their tubulin subunits start to reassemble to form the *mitotic spindle*, the apparatus that will distribute chromosomes to the daughter cells. The centrosome, including its two centrioles, has duplicated during interphase, and in prophase the two

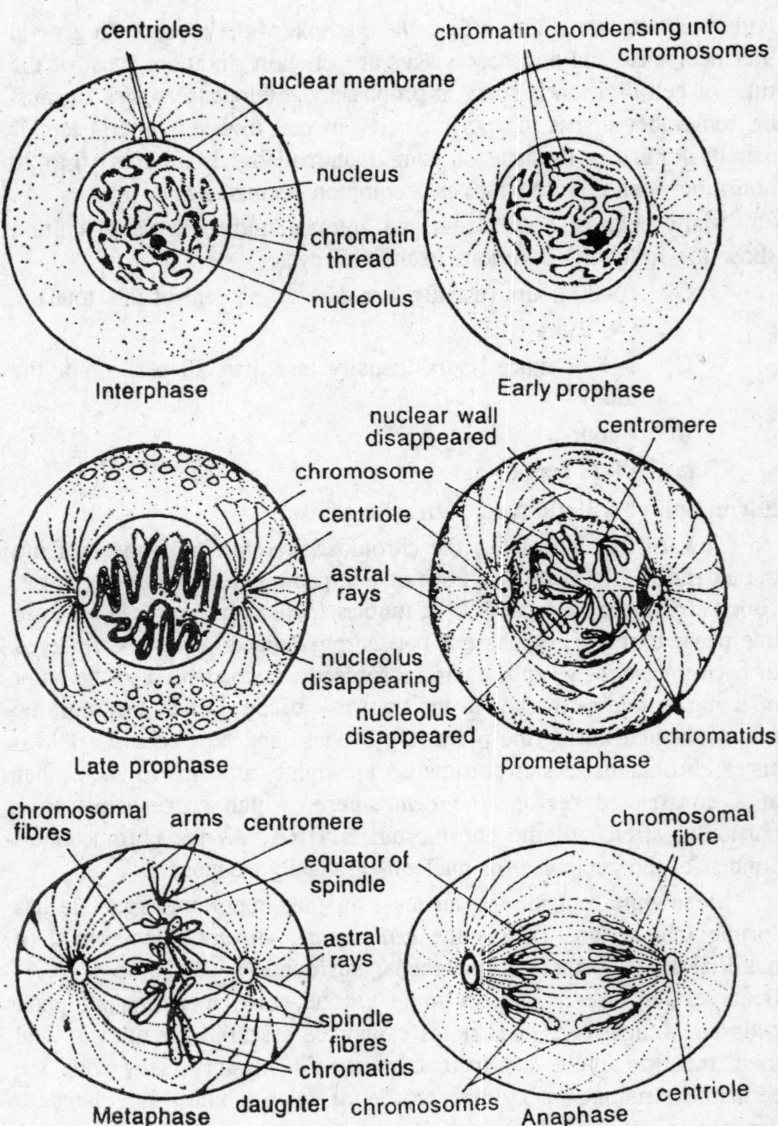

Fig. 2.1. Mitotic cell division in animal cells.

centrosomes are seen to be moving apart from each other. Radiating from them are microtubules that are growing to form the mitotic spindle. The starburst of microtubules in the immediate vicinity of a centrosome is called an aster. The terms centrosome and aster were first used for animal cells but are now used more broadly.

Prometaphase

The start of *prometaphase* is marked by the fragmentation of the nuclear envelope into membranous vesicles, allowing the mitotic spindle to enter the nuclear area. Eventually the two centrosomes are at opposite poles of the cell. On each chromosomal centromere, proteins assemble to form a protein-DNA complex called a *kinetochore*; thus there are two kinetochores on each chromosome, one on each chromatid. The two kinetochores face in opposite directions, as the diagram shows. Some of the spindle microtubules "capture" (attach to) kinetochores; others interact with microtubules coming from the other centrosome. Forces exerted within the assembly of microtubules throw the chromosomes into agitated motion and gradually move them toward the center of the cell.

Division of the Centromeres: Metaphase

The second stage of mitosis, *metaphase*, begins when the pairs of sister chromatids align in the center of the cell. When viewed with a light microscope, the chromosomes appear to be lined up in a circle along the inter circumference of the cell, as the equator girdles the earth. An imaginary plane perpendicular to the axis of the spindle that passes through this circle is called the *metaphase plate*. The metaphase plate is not an actual structures but rather an indication of where the future axis of cell division will occur. Positioned by the microtubules attached to the kinetochores of their centromeres, all of the chromosomes line up on the metaphase plate, their centromeres neatly arrayed in a circle, each equidistant from the two poles of the cell.

At the end of metaphase, the centromeres divide. Each centromere splits in two, freeing the two sister chromatids from their attachment to one another. Centromere separation is synchronous for all the

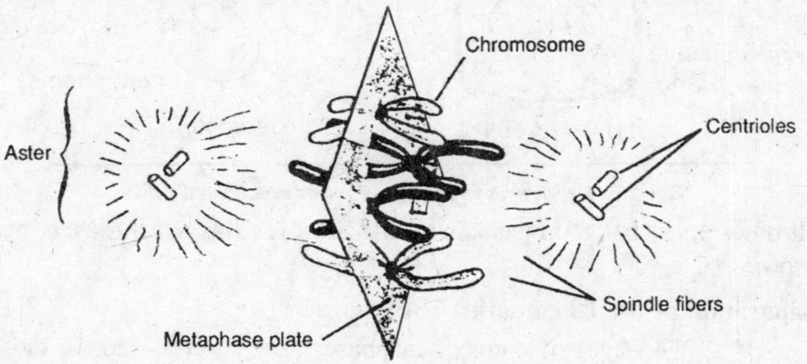

Fig. 2.2. The metaphase plate

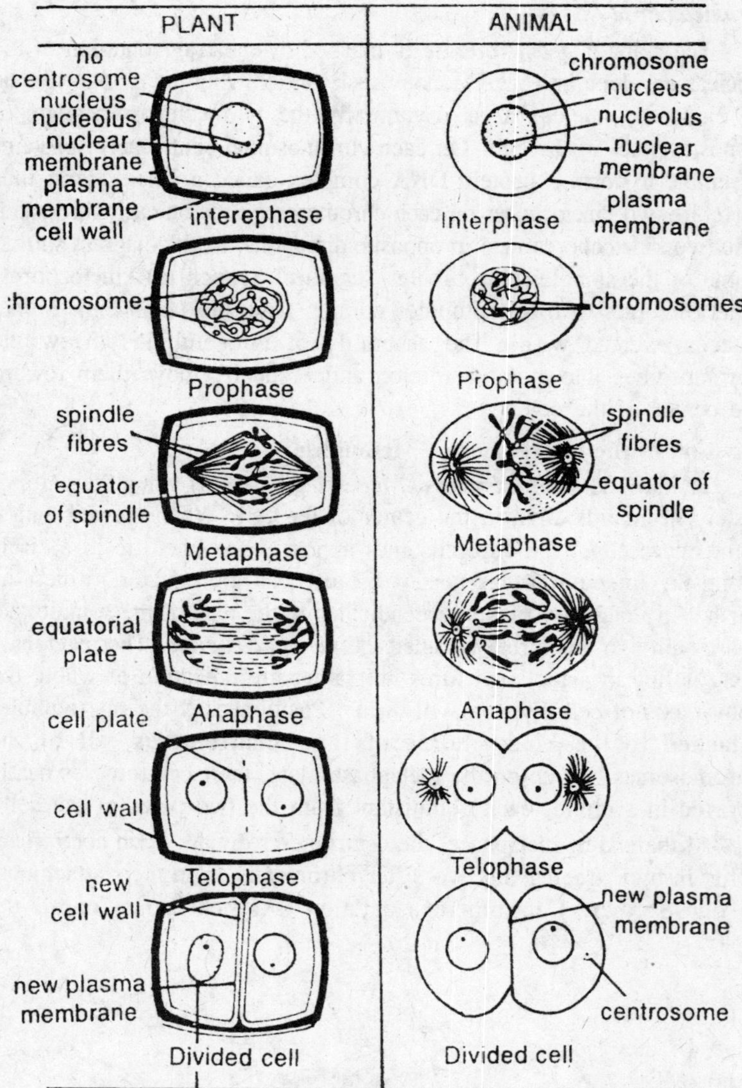

Fig. 2.3. Differences in mitosis in plants and animal cells.

chromosomes, but the mechanism that achieves this synchrony is not known.

Separation of the Chromatids : Anaphase

Of all the stages of mitosis, anaphase is the shortest and the most beautiful to watch. Freed from each other, the sister chromatids are pulled rapidly toward the poles to which their kinetochores are attached. In the process, two forms of movement take place simultaneously, each driven by microbutules.

First, *the poles move apart*, as microtubular spindle fibers that are physically anchored to opposite poles slide past each other, away from the center of the cell. Because the chromosomes are attached to the poles by another group of microtubules, they move apart, too. If the cell is bounded by a flexible membrane, is becomes visibly elongated. This part of the anaphase is called *Anaphase B*.

Second, *the centromeres move toward the poles*, as the microtubules that connect them to the poles shorten. This shortening process is not a contraction, since the microtubules do not get any thicker. Instead, tubulin subunits are removed from the kinetochore ends of the microtubules by the organizing center. As more subunits are removed, the chromatid-bearing microtubules are progressively disassembled, and the chromatids are pulled ever closer to the poles of the cell at the rate of about 1 μm/min. This part of anaphase is called *Anaphase A*.

Reformation of Nuclei: Telophase

The separation of sister chromatids achieved in anaphase completes the accurate partitioning of the replicated genome, the essential element of mitosis. In *telophase*, the spindle apparatus is disassembled, as the microtubules are broken down into tubulin monomers that can be used to construct the cytoskeleton of the daughter cells. A nuclear envelope forms around each set of sister chromatids, which can now be called chromosomes, since each has its own centromere. The chromosomes soon begin to uncoil into the more extended form that permits gene expression. An early group of genes to be expressed are the rRNA genes, resulting in the reappearance of the nucleolus.

Cytokinesis

Mitosis is complete at the end of telophase. The eukaryotic cell has partitioned its replicated genome into two nuclei, which are positioned at opposite ends of the cell. While mitosis has been going on, the cytoplasmic organelles, including mitochondria and chloroplasts (if they are present), have also been reassorted to the areas that will separate and become the daughter cells. The replication of organelles takes place before cytokinesis, often in the S or G_2 phase. The process of cell division is still not complete at the end of mitosis, however, because the division of the cell proper has not yet begun. The phase of the cell cycle at which cell division occurs is called *cytokinesis*. It generally involves the cleavage of the cell into roughly equal halves.

In the cells of animals and all other eukaryotes that lack cell walls, cytokinesis is achieved by means of a constricting belt of actin filaments. The sliding of these filaments past one another decreases the diameter of the belt and pinches the cell, creating a *cleavage furrow* around the circumference of the cell. As constriction proceeds, the furrow deepens until it eventually extends all the way into the center of the cell, at which point the cell is divided in two.

Plant cells possess a cell wall that is far too rigid to be deformed by actin filament sliding. Instead, they assemble membrane components in their interior, at right angles to the spindle apparatus. This expanding membrane partition is called a *cell plate*. It continues to grow outward until it reaches the interior surface of the plasma membrane and fuses with it, effectively dividing the cell in the two. Cellulose is then laid down on the new membranes, creating two new cell walls. The space between the daughter cells becomes impregnated with pectins and is called a *middle lamella*.

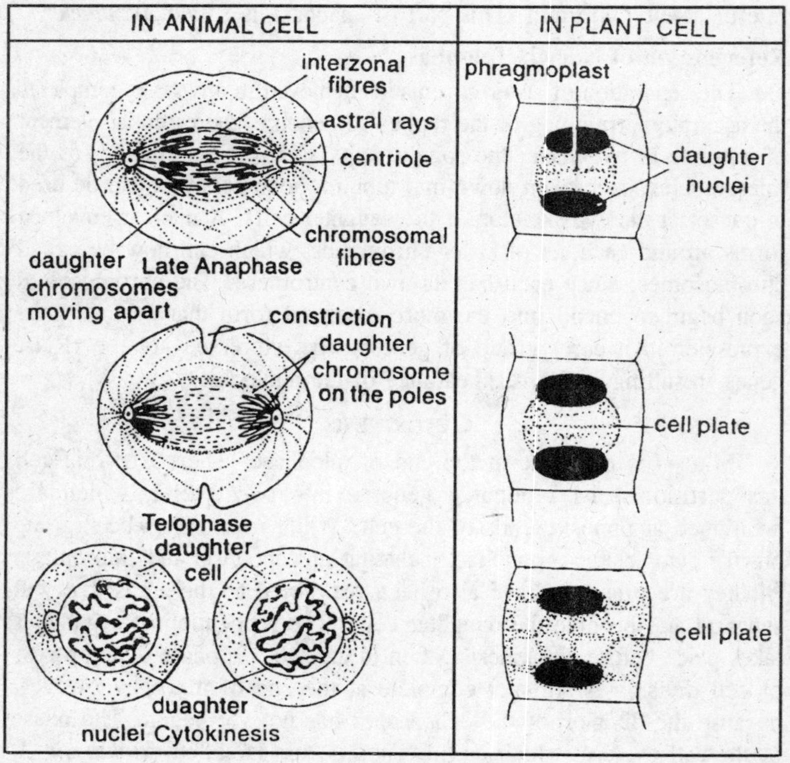

Fig. 2.4. Division of cell cytoplasm in animal and plant cell.

In fungi and some groups of protists, the nuclear membrane does not dissolve and mitosis is confined to the nucleus. When mitosis is complete in these organisms, the nucleus divides into two daughter nuclei, one of which goes to each daughter cell during cytokinesis. This separate nuclear division phase of the cell cycle does not occur in plants, animals, or in most protists.

Control of the Cell Cycle

Research of the cell cycle has tended to focus traditionally on the events of mitosis, at least in part because the segregating chromosomes are readily visible in the light microscope. This attention to the movements of the chromosomes led biologists to conclude that the cell cycle was dissimilar in different organisms, and even in different tissues, because the chromosomes they were studying often seemed dissimilar in appearance and arrangement. The advent of sophisticated immunological and genetic engineering techniques over the last decade has led to a radical change in that conclusion. It now seems clear that the events of the cell cycle are coordinated in much the same way in all eukaryotes. The control system that human cells utilize first evolved among the protists over a billion years ago, and today it operates in essentially the same way in fungi as it does in humans. The proteins that regulate the cell cycle have been conserved so carefully that many of them function just as well when transferred from a human cell into a yeast cell.

General Strategy of Cell Cycle Control

The goal of controlling any cyclic process is to adjust the duration of the cycle so that there is sufficient time for all events to occur, without expending any more time than is necessary. In principle, there are a variety of ways to achieve this goal. An internal clock can be employed to allow adequate time for each phase of the cycle to be completed. That is how many organisms control their daily activity cycles. The disadvantage of using such a clock as a control strategy for the cell cycle is that it is not very flexible. The time required for growth or DNA replication can vary greatly, depending upon changes in the local environment of a cell. One way to achieve a more flexible and sensitive regulation of a cycle is simply to let the completion of each phase of the cycle trigger the beginning of the next phase, like a runner passing a baton to start the next leg in a relay race. Until recently, this is how biologists thought the cell division cycle was controlled. However, we now know that eukaryotic cells employ a separate centralized controller to regulate the process: at critical points in the cell cycle, further progress is dependent upon a central set of "go/no-go" switches that are regulated by feedback from the cell.

This mechanism is the same one that engineers use to control many processes. The furnace that heats a home in the winter typically goes through a daily heating cycle, as the thermostat is turned to a lower setting at night to conserve energy while we are sleeping, and then to a higher setting during the day to warm the house while we are active. When the daily cycle reaches the morning "turn on" check point, sensors report whether the house temperature is below the set point (e.g., 70°F). If it is, the thermostat triggers the furnace, which warms the house. If the house is already at least that warm, the thermostat does not start up the furnace, as no added heat is necessary. Similarly in the cell cycle, there are key check points where feedback signals from the cell about how big it is and the condition of its chromosomes can either trigger subsequent phases of the cycle or delay them to allow more time for completion of the current phase.

The cell cycle is eukaryotes is controlled at three principal check points:

Cell growth is assessed at the G_1 check point

Located near the end of G_1, just before entry into S phase, this check point makes the key decision of whether the cell will divide or not. In yeasts, where it was first studied, it is called START. If conditions are favourable for division, the cell begins to copy its DNA, initiating S phase. The G_1 check point is where more complex eukaryotes typically arrest the cell cycle if environmental conditions make cell division impossible, or if the cell passes into G_0 for an extended period.

DNA replication is assessed at the G_2 check point

The second check point occurs at the G_2 and triggers the start of M phase. If this check point is passed, the cell initiates the many molecular processes that are involved in mitosis.

Mitosis is assessed at the M check point

Occurring at metaphase, the third check point triggers the exit from mitosis and the beginning of G_1, the major growth period of the cell cycle.

Molecular Mechanism of Cell Cycle Control

How does central control of the cell cycle work? The basic mechanism is quite simple and is similar to gene control mechanisms. A set of proteins interact at the check point to trigger the next events in the cycle, and their activity is sensitive to the condition of the cell. There are two key types of proteins that participate in this interaction: cyclin-dependent protein kinases and cyclins.

Cyclin-dependent protein kinases (*Cdk's*) are enzymes that phosphorylate (that is, add phosphate groups to) the serine and threonine amino acids of important cellular enzymes and other proteins. At the G_2 check point, for example, Cdk's phosphorylate histones, nuclear membrane filaments, and the microtubule-associated proteins that form mitotic spindle. Phosphorylation of these components of the cell division machinery causes them to initiate activities that carry the cycle past the check point and into mitosis. All three check points appear to use the same Cdk molecules in yeasts; in mammals, there is a unique Cdk for each check point.

Cyclins are proteins that bind to Cdk's enabling the Cdk's to function as enzymes. Cyclins are so named because they are destroyed and resynthesized during each turn of the cell cycle. Different cyclins regulate the three check points.

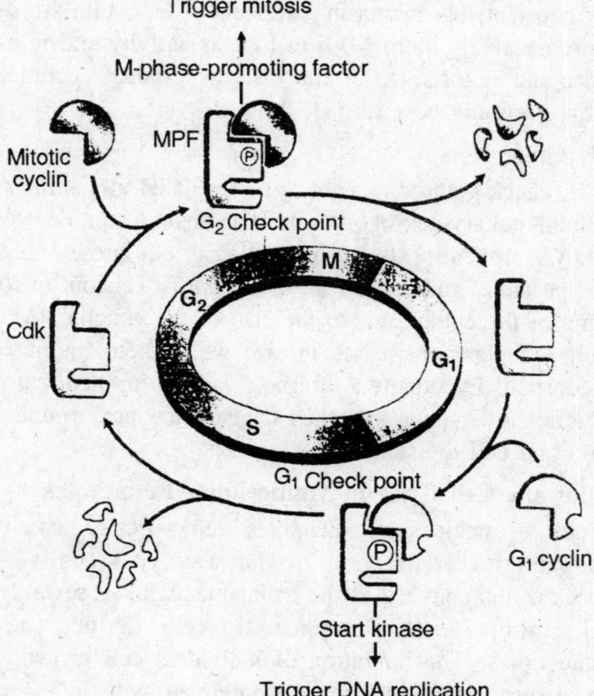

Fig. 2.5. Control of cell cycle.

Let us take a closer look at how cyclins and Cdk's interact to control the G_2 and G_1 check points of the cell cycle.

G_2 check point

During G_2, the cell gradually accumulates G_2 cyclin (also called mitotic cyclin), which binds to Cdk to form a complex called MPF (mitosis promoting factor). At first, MPF is not active in carrying the cycle past the G_2 check point, but eventually a few molecules of MPF are phosphorylated and activated by other cellular enzymes. These activated MPF's in turn increase the activity of the enzymes that phosphorylate. MPF, setting up a positive feedback that leads to a very rapid increase in the cellular concentration of activated MPF. When the level of activated MPF exceeds the threshold necessary to trigger mitosis, G_2 phase ends.

MPF sows the seeds of its own destruction. The length of time the cell spends in M Phase is determined by the activity of MPF, for one of its many functions is to activate proteins that destroy cyclin. As mitosis proceeds to the end of metaphase, levels of Cdk stay relatively constant, but increasing amounts of G_2 cyclin are degraded, causing progressively more MPF to lose its activity and initiating the events that end mitosis. After mitosis, the gradual accumulation of new cyclin starts the next turn of the cell cycle.

G_1 check point

The G_1 check point is thought to be regulated in a similar fashion. In unicellular eukaryotes like yeasts, the main factor controlling the start of DNA replication is cell size. Yeast cells grow and divide as rapidly as possible, and they make the START decision by comparing the volume of the cytoplasm to the size of the genome. As the cells grow their cytoplasm increases in size while their amount of DNA remains constant. Eventually a threshold ratio is reached that promotes the production of cyclins and thus triggers the next round of DNA replication and cell division.

Controlling the Cell Cycle in Multicellular Eukaryotes

The cells of multicellular eukaryotes are not free to make individual decisions about cell division in the way yeast cells are. The organization of the body cannot be maintained without severely limiting cell proliferation, so that only certain cells divide, and only at appropriate times. The inhibition of individual cell growth by other cells can be seen readily in mammalian cells growing in tissue culture: a single layer of cell expands over a culture plate until the growing border of cells comes into contact with neighbouring cells, and then the cells stop dividing. If a sector of cells is cleared away, neighbouring cells rapidly refill it and then stop dividing again. How are the cells able to sense the density of the cell culture around them? Each growing cell apparently takes up minute amounts of positive regulatory signals called growth factors (such as MPF;) that stimulate cell division. When neighbouring cells have taken up what little of the growth factor is present, there is not enough left to trigger cell division in any one cell.

Growth Factors and the Cell Cycle

It has already been observed a cell-cell interactions, growth factors work by triggering intracellular signaling systems. Fibroblasts, for example, possess numerous receptors on their plasma membranes for one of the first growth factors to be identified, platelet-derived growth factor (PDGF). Binding of PDGF to a membrane receptor initiates an amplifying chain of internal cell signals that stimulates cell division. PDGF was discovered when investigators found that fibroblasts would grow and divide in tissue culture only if the growth medium was provided with blood serum (the liquid that remains after blood clots); blood plasma (blood from which the cells have been removed without clotting) would not work. The researchers hypothesized that platelets in the blood clot were releasing into the serum one or more factors required for growth. Eventually, they isolated such a factor and named if PDGF. Growth factors like PDGF act to override cellular controls that otherwise inhibit cell division. When a tissue is injured, release of PDGF by platelets triggers neighbouring cells to divide, helping to heal the wound. Only a tiny amount of PDGF (approximately 10^{-10} M) is required to stimulate cell division.

Over 50 different proteins that function as growth factors have been isolated and more undoubtedly exist. Each is recognized by a specific cell surface receptor that has a shape into which the growth factor fits precisely. Binding of the growth factor to the receptor triggers events within the cell. The cellular selectivity of a particular growth factor depends upon which target cells bear its unique receptor. Some growth factors, like PDGF and epidermal growth factor (EGF), affect a broad range of cell types, while others affect only specific cell types. For example, nerve growth factor (NGF) promotes the growth of certain classes of neurons, and erythropoietin triggers cell division in red blood cell precursors. Most animal cell require a combination of several different growth factors in order to overcome the various controls that inhibit cell division. If cells are deprived of

Table 2.1. Growth factors of mammalian cells

Factor	*Range of Specificity*	*Effects*
Epidermal growth factor (EGF)	Broad	Stimulates cell proliferation in many tissues; plays a key role in regulating embryonic development.
Erythropoietin	Narrow	Required for proliferation of red blood cell precursors and their maturation into erythrocytes
Fibroblast growth factor (FGF)	Broad	Initiates the proliferation of many types of stem cells; acts as a signal in embryonic development
Insulin-like growth factor	Broad	Stimulates metabolism of many cell types; potentiates the effects of other growth factors in promoting cell proliferation
Interleukin-2	Narrow	Triggers the division of activated T lymphocytes during the immune response
Mitosis-promoting factor (MPF)	Broad	Regulates entrance of the cell cycle into the M phase.
Nerve growth factor (NGF)	Narrow	Stimulates the growth of neuron processes during neural development
Platelet-derived growth factor (PDGF)	Broad	Promotes the proliferation of many connective tissues and some neurological cells
Transforming growth factor β (TGF-β)	Broad	Accentuates or inhibits the responses of many cell types to other growth factors; often plays an important role in cell differentiation

appropriate growth factors, they stop at the G_1 check point of the cell cycle. With their growth and division arrested, they are said to be in the G_0 phase we discussed earlier. Cells like liver cells that divide only once every year or two spend most of their time in G_0 phase, and mature neurons and muscle cells usually never leave it.

Cancer and the Control of Cell Proliferation

How do growth factors influence the cell cycle? As you have seen, there are two different approaches, one positive and the other negative. PDGF and many other growth factors utilize the positive approach. They trigger passage through the G_1 check point by aiding the formation of cyclins and activating genes that promote cell division. Genes that normally stimulates cell division are sometimes called *proto-oncogenes* because mutations that cause them to be overexpressed or hyperactive convert them into oncogenes (Greek *onco*, "cancer"), leading to the excessive cell proliferation that is characteristic of cancer. Even a single such mutation (creating a heterozygote) can lead to cancer, if the other cancer-preventing genes are nonfunctional. In Mendelian terms, such mutations are said to be dominant.

Some 30 different proto-oncogenes are known. Some act very quickly after stimulation by growth factors. Among the most intensively studied of these are *myc*, *fos*, and *jun*, all of which cause unrestrained cell growth and division when overexpressed. In a normal cell, the *myc* proto-oncogene appears to be important in regulating the G_1 check point because cells in which *myc* expression is prevented will not divide even in the presence of growth factors. A critical activity of *myc* and other genes in this group of immediately responding proto-oncogenes is to stimulate a second group of "delayed response" genes, including those that produce cyclins and Cdk proteins.

Growth factors that utilize a negative approach to cell cycle control block passage through the G_1 check point by preventing the binding of cyclins to Cdk, thus inhibiting cell division. Genes that normally inhibit cell division are called *tumor-suppressor genes*. When mutated, they can also lead to unrestrained cell division, but only if both copies of the gene are mutant. Hence, these cancer-causing mutations are recessive.

The most thoroughly understood of the tumor-suppressor genes is the retinoblastoma (Rb) gene. This gene was originally cloned from children with a rare form of eye cancer that was inherited as a recessive trait, implying that the normal gene product was a "cancer suppressor" that helped keep cell division in check. The Rb gene encodes a protein that is present in ample amounts within the nucleus. This protein interacts with many key regulatory proteins of the cell cycle, but how it does so depends upon its state of phosphorylation. In G_0 phase, the Rb protein is dephosphorylated. In this state, it binds to and ties up a set of regulatory proteins like myc and fos that are needed for cell proliferation, blocking their action and so inhibiting cell division. When phosphorylated, the Rb protein releases its captive regulatory proteins, freeing them to act and so promoting cell division. Growth factors lessen the inhibition imposed by the Rb protein by activating kinases that phosphorylate it. Free of Rb protein inhibition, cells begin to produce cyclins and Cdk, pass the G_1 check point, and proceed through the cell cycle.

VARIATIONS IN THE CELL CYCLE

As mentioned already that, eukaryotic cells do not always proceed continuously through predictable cycles of growth and division, with G_1, S, G_2 and M following one another in uninterrupted progression and with every nuclear division accompanied by cytokinesis. Such is often the case, of course, particularly in growing organisms or cultured cells that have not run out of nutrients or space. But many variations are also possible, especially in terms of the relative length of time spent in various phases of the cycle and in the immediately with which mitosis and cytokinesis are coupled.

Variations in Cell Cycle Length

Some of the most common variations in the cell cycle in vivo involve difference in generation time between different cell types. Within the same organism, some cells divide at approximately the same rate as cells in culture, but others differ greatly, depending on their role in organism. Some cells divide rapidly and continuously throughout the life of the organisms as a means of replacing cells that are lost or destroyed during the normal functioning of the organism. Included in this category are the cells that lead to sperm formation and the precursor cells, called *stem cells*, that give rise to blood cells, skin cells, and the epithelial cells that line the inner surfaces of body organs such as the lungs and intestines. Human stem cells may have generations times as short as 8 hours.

Cells of slow-growing tissues, on the other hand, may have generations times of several days or more, and some cells, such as those of nerve or muscle tissue, do not divide at all. Still other cell types do not divide under normal conditions but can be induced to begin dividing again by an appropriate stimulus. Liver cells are in this category; they do not normally proliferate in the mature liver but can be induced to do so if a portion of the liver is removed surgically. Lymphocytes (white blood cells) are another example; when exposed to a foreign protein, they begin dividing as part of the immune response.

Most of these variations in generation time involve differences in G_1, although S and G_2 can also vary somewhat. Cells that divide very slowly can spend days, months, or even years in the offshoot of G_1 called G_0, whereas cells that divide very rapidly have almost no G_1

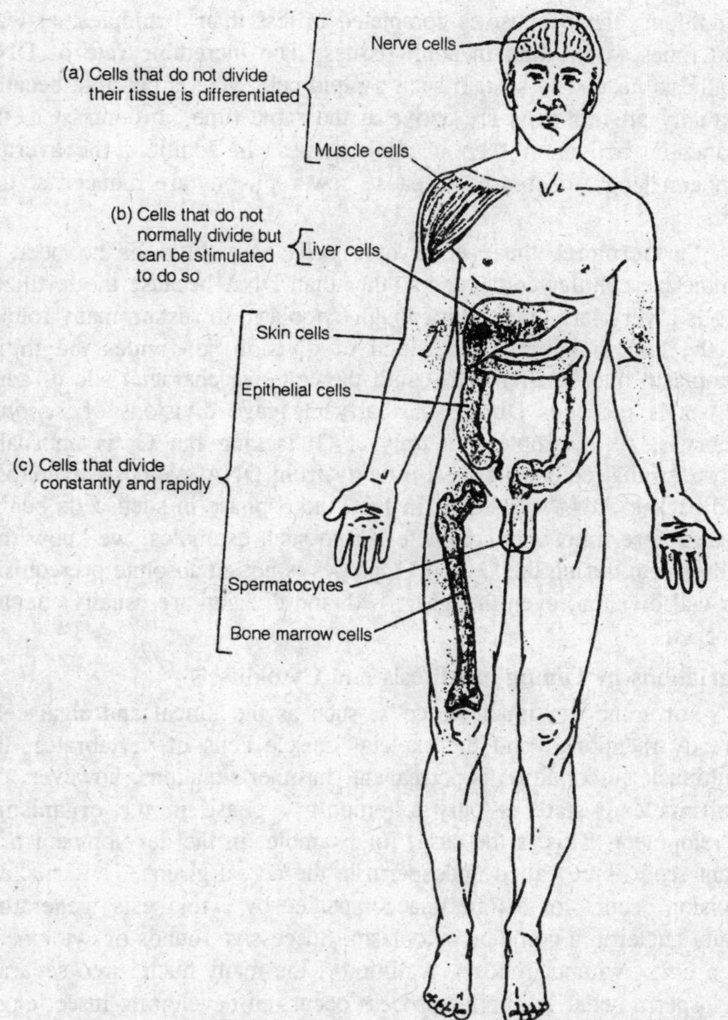

Fig. 2.6. Variation of generation time for cells of different tissue.

phase at all. In fact, some cells even begin DNA synthesis before mitosis is complete, eliminating G_1 entirely.

The embroys of insects, amphibians, and certain other non-mammalian animals are dramatic examples of very short cell cycles, with no G_1 phase and a very short S phase. During early embryonic development in amphibians such as the frog *Xenopus laevis*, for instance, cell division can take less than 30 minutes, even though the normal length of the cell cycle in adult tissues is about 20 hours. Under these conditions, the S phase is completed in less than 3 minutes, at least 100 times faster than in adult tissues. The incredible rate of DNA synthesis needed to sustain such a rapid cell cycle is possible because virtually all replicons are active at the same time, in contrast to the sequential activation seen in adult tissues. In addition, the average replicon length decreases, because new replicons are induced at this time.

Furthermore, these embryonic cells have little or no need to synthesize cellular components other than DNA because the fertilized egg is a very large cell with enough cytoplasm to sustain many rounds of the cell division. Each round of division subdivides the initial cytoplasm into smaller cells, until the cell size characteristic of adult tissues is reached. During the early cleavage divisions of *Xenopus* embryos, for example, not only is G_1 lacking but G_2 is unusually short, so that cells go almost directly from DNA synthesis to mitosis and back to DNA synthesis. In fact, the S phase in such cells begins even before mitosis is complete. From such examples, we know that cell growth during the G_1 and G_2 phases is not an absolute prerequisite for cell division, even though growth and division are usually coupled process.

Variations in Timing of Mitosis and Cytokinesis

For some multinucleate cells, such as the fungal and algal cells already mentioned and the skeletal muscle cells of vertebrates, the multinucleate condition is permanent. In other situations, however, the multinucleate state is only a temporary phase in the organism's development. This is the case, for example, in the development of a plant seed tissue called endosperm in the cereal grains. Here nuclear division occurs for a time unaccompanied by cytokinesis, generating many nuclei in a common cytoplasm. Successive rounds of cytokinesis then occur without mitosis, walling off the many nuclei into separate endosperm cells. A similar process occurs in developing insect eggs. The fertilized egg undergoes mitosis but not cytokinesis and soon consists of hundreds of nuclei in the same cytoplasm; later, cytokinesis catches up.

Regulation of the Cell Cycle

The variability in generation time for cells of the same organism tells us that the cell cycle must somehow be regulated. The molecular basis of this regulation is a subject of intense interest, not only for understanding the life cycles of normal cells but also for understanding how cancer cells manage to escape normal control mechanisms. Now one of the hottest areas of biological research, cell cycle regulation is beginning to reveal its underlying molecular mechanisms. We will begin our discussion with a look at the general concept of cell-cycle checkpoints and some of the early experimental evidence for the nature of their control.

Cell Cycle Checkpoints

Evidence acquired decades ago pointed to a particular point in G_1 as critical for regulation of the mammalian cell cycle. We have already seen that G_1 is the phase that varies most among cell types. Moreover, mammalian cells that have stopped dividing are almost arrested during the G_1 phase. For example, we can stop or slow down the process of cell division in cultured cells by allowing the cells to run out of either nutrients or space or by adding inhibitors of vital processes such as protein synthesis. In all such cases, the cells are arrested in G_1.

These findings suggest that when a cell leaves G_1 and enters the S phase, it is committed to completing the cycle. Therefore, the release of cells from G_1 appears to be a critical control mechanism. More specifically, early researchers identified a point of no return in late G_1, which they called the *restriction point*. Cells that have passed this point are committed to division, whereas those that have not passed this point can remain in G_1 indefinitely, in the resting state called the G_0 state. As the previously mentioned experiments demonstrated, the

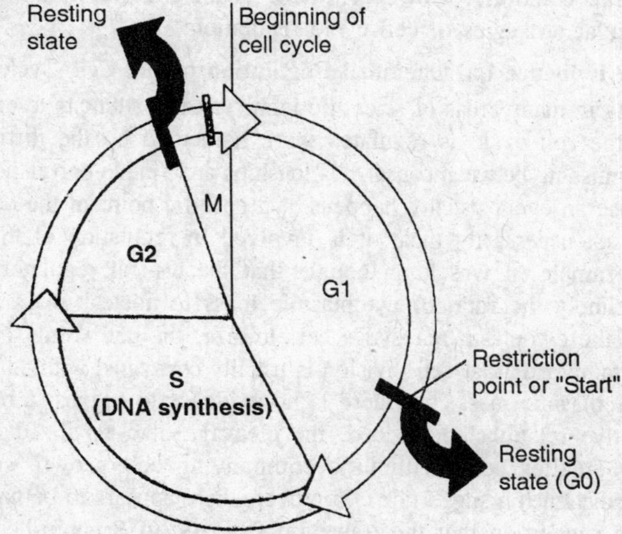

Fig. 2.7. Cell-cycle checkpoints.

ability to pass the restriction point can be heavily influenced by factors in the cell's environment.

Later, research with other types of cells revealed two other points of no return, and all three are now generally termed *cell cycle checkpoints*. At the end of G_2 is a major checkpoint that controls the cell's entry into mitosis (M phase). At the G_2 checkpoint, certain kinds of cells can enter a resting state analogous to G_0. Within M phase, at metaphase, is a third checkpoint, which somehow determines whether all the chromosomes are properly attached to the spindle before allowing anaphase to begin. The relative importance of the G_1 and G_2 checkpoints varies with the organism and cell type. For example, the G_1 checkpoint is the more important checkpoint in the budding yeast *Saccharomyces cerevisiae* (where it is called "Start"), as it is in most cells of multicellular organisms. However, the G_2 checkpoint is the more important one in, for example, the mitotic divisions of a fertilized frog egg and in the yeast *Schizosaccharomyces pombe* (called a *fission yeast* because it reproduces by dividing evenly in two, rather than by budding). A cell's behaviour at a checkpoint is influenced both by preceding events in the cell cycle (such as DNA replication) and by factors in the cell's environment (such as nutrients or hormones). Whatever the influence, its effects are mediated by cellular proteins, activating or inhibiting one another in chains of interactions that can be quite elaborate. However, there is an underlying unity in the molecular strategies of cell cycle regulation.

Early Evidence for Chemical Regulation of the Cell Cycle

As in many areas of scientific inquiry, early attempts to determine how the cell cycle is regulated were hampered by the difficulty of distinguishing between causal relationships and simple correlations. Just because an event usually happens at a specific point in the cell cycle does not necessarily mean it is involved in regulation of the cycle. For example, it was long thought that the critical regulatory factor was simply the ratio of cytoplasmic mass to nuclear mass and that when the cytoplasm reached a certain size, the cell would divide. It is certainly true that cell division is usually correlated with an increase in cytoplasmic mass, but there is no evidence to suggest a necessary causative relationship. Indeed, the cleavage of a fertilized egg into many smaller cells without accompanying cell growth seems to contradict such a suggestion. Moreover, there appears to be no validity to the suggestion that the transition from G_1 to S controlled by the availability of the DNA replication enzymes.

Between 1970 and 1975, it became clear that specific chemical signals present in the cytoplasm were responsible for moving the cell cycle past the G_1 and G_2 checkpoints—that is, for triggering DNA replication (S phase) and mitosis (M phase). Some of the first strong evidence for this came from experiments in which two cultured mammalian cells in different phases of the cell cycle were fused to form a single cell with two nuclei, a *heterokaryon*. If one of the original cells is in S phase and the other is in G_1, the G_1 nucleus in the heterokaryon immediately enters S phase, as though a signal present in the cytoplasm of the first cell triggers the S phase events. Similarly, if a cell undergoing mitosis is fused with another cell in any stage of its cell cycle, even G_1, the second nucleus is immediately driven into the preparatory steps for mitosis, including condensation of dispersed interphase chromatin into visible chromosomes, spindle formation, and fragmentation of the nuclear envelope. If the second cell was in G_1, the condensed chromosomes will be unduplicated.

More direct evidence for a mitosis-including chemical signal came from experiments with frog eggs. In the frog, the oocyte, an egg cell precursor, is arrested in G_2 until hormones stimulate meiosis. (Meiosis is the variation of mitosis that halves the number of chromosomes in egg or sperm production). The oocyte proceeds through most of the phase of meiosis but is arrested in M phase—in metaphase of the second of two meiotic divisions. It is now a "mature" egg cell, capable of being fertilized. Because frog oocytes and eggs are very large, about 1 mm in diameter, it is easy to transfer cytoplasm between them with a fine pipette. In a crucial experiment, it was shown that if cytoplasm taken from a mature egg cell is injected into the cytoplasm of an oocyte, the oocyte immediately begins meiosis. The hypothetical cytoplasmic chemical that induces this oocyte "maturation" was *dubbed maturation-promoting factor* (MPF). It was quickly established that MPF also induces mitosis of fertilized frog eggs (cleavage).

MPF-like activities have since been found in the cytoplasms of a broad range of eukaryotes, including yeasts, marine invertebrates, and mammals. Furthermore, the mitosis inducing factors have proven to be very similar in all these organisms. For example, in yeast cells with a defective or missing MPF gene, the human version of the gene can substitute perfectly well, despite the fact that the last ancestor common to yeasts and humans probably lived about 3 billion years ago! Through these and other kinds of experiments, investigators learned a lot about the MPF activity even before the MPF protein was purified in 1988.

Molecular Basis of Cell Cycle Regulation

The study of cell cycle regulation entered a molecular era in 1988. This new era was brought about by the merging of results from two main lines of research, the physiological/biochemical study of developing frog eggs and the genetic study of yeasts. Their status as single-celled microbes makes yeasts particularly useful model organisms for studying many aspects of eukaryotic cell biology. Intensive research on the genetics of yeast cell cycles had begun in the late 1960s, just a few years before MPF was discovered.

Working with *S. cerevisiae*, geneticist Leland Hartwell undertook a search for mutants that were "stuck" at some point in the cell cycle. Most such mutants would be difficult or impossible to work with, because their blocked cell cycle would prevent them from reproducing. But Hartwell was able to use a powerful strategy of microbial genetics, focusing his search on *conditional mutants*. These are mutants whose defect is apparent only under certain conditions–in this case, at temperatures above the normal range for the organism. A yeast cell with such a *temperature-sensitive mutation* in a gene required for cell cycle operation reproduces normally at 20–30°C but poorly or not at all at 35–37°C. The mutant can thus be grown at the lower ("permissive") temperature for genetic and biochemical study. How can the mutant behave normally under permissive conditions? Presumably the protein encoded by the mutated gene is close enough to the normal gene product to function at the lower temperature, while the increased thermal energy at higher temperatures disrupts its active conformation (the molecular shape needed for function) more readily than that of the normal protein.

In this way, Hartwell and his colleagues identified many genes involved in the cell cycle of *S. cerevisiae* and established the points in the cell cycle at which their products functioned. Predictably, some of these genes turned out to encode DNA replication proteins, but others seemed to function in cell cycle regulation. A breakthrough discovery was made by Paul Nurse and his colleagues, who carried out similar research with the fission yeast *Schizosaccharomyces pombe*. They identified a gene called *cdc2* whose activity was essential for the initiation of mitosis—that is, for passing the G_2 checkpoint. The acronym *cdc* stands for cell division cycle. The *cdc2* gene turned out to be essentially identical to a *S. cerevisiae* gene that Hartwell's group had called *CDC28* and to have counterparts in all eukaryotic cells. (It was Nurse who showed that the human version of the gene could "rescue" mutant yeast cells.) In tribute to the importance of Nurse's discovery, the protein encoded by such a gene is often called a *Cdc2protein*, regardless of the organism where it is found.

This yeast research came together with the frog egg research when it was established that Cdc2 protein was one of two proteins making up MPF. Researchers were now primed to unravel the mysteries of the G2 checkpoint.

Cdc2 protein, a protein kinase

The Cdc2 protein is a protein kinase, an enzyme that catalyzes the transfer of a phosphate group from ATP to certain other proteins. Phosphorylation by ATP is a major theme in cell biochemistry and is the usual mechanism by which ATP functions to activate molecules,

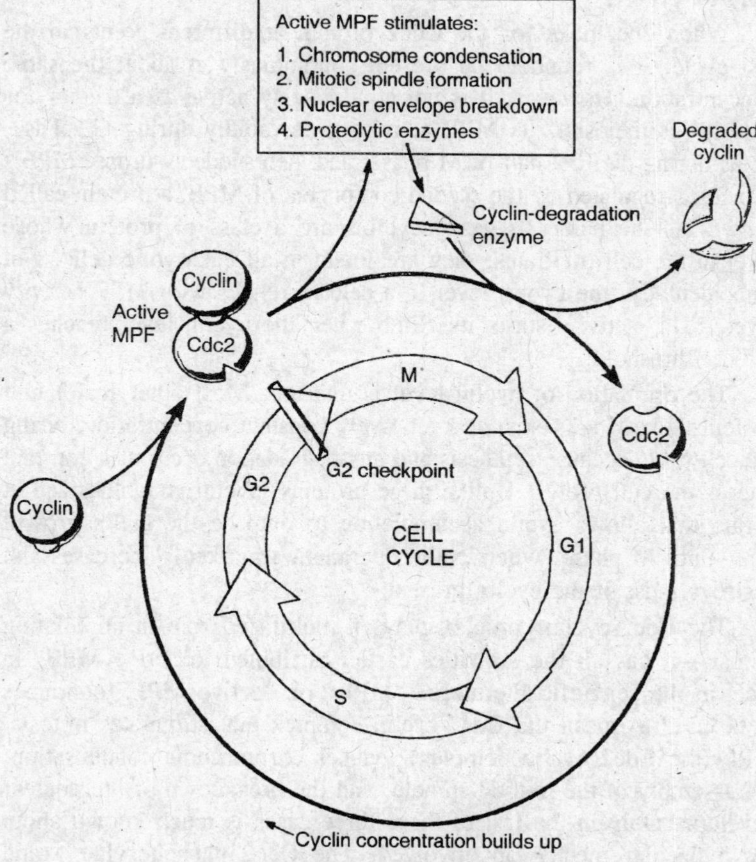

Fig. 2.8. The Cdc2 activity cycle.

both large and small. In earlier chapters, you have seen that phosphorylation of glucose activates it for glycolysis and that phosphorylation and dephosphorylation of the protein of the sodium-potassium pump causes the shape change that allows Na^+ and K^+ to cross the plasma membrane. The sodium potassium pump protein has its own innate ability to hydrolyze ATP. However, in many other cases the phosphorylation of a protein is catalyzed by a separate protein—that is, a protein kinase. The phosphorylation of proteins by kinases, and their dephosphorylation by enzymes called *phosphatases*, is turning out to be a common cellular mechanism for regulating protein activity. And it is a mechanism that is used many times over in regulating the cell cycle.

Role of cyclins

When one looks for the Cdc2 protein at different points in the cell cycle, it is found to be present continuously at about the same concentration. However, it is not continuously active as a trigger for mitosis (or meiosis). Its MPF activity rises rapidly during G_2 phase, peaks during the first half of M phase, and then suddenly drops. MPF's activity is regulated by the second component of MPF, a protein called *cyclin*. As the name suggests, cyclins are a class of protein whose level in the cell oscillates; they are found in all eukaryotic cells. Not coincidentally, the cyclin level in a cell correlates with MPF activity level. MPF activity starts its climb when the cyclin level reaches a critical threshold.

The oscillation of cyclin level is unusual. Most other major cell proteins, like Cdc2, exist at a relatively constant concentration during the cell cycle because synthesis and any degradation occur at a constant rate as the cell grows. Unlike these proteins, cyclin is synthesized at a rate that allows cyclin accumulation to outpace the cell's growth rate—until M phase, when cyclin degradation markedly increases and destroys most of the cyclin present.

The Cdc2-cyclin complex plays a multifaced role in stimulating mitosis—it has all the activities earlier attributed to active MPF. In fact, in the scientific literature. "MPF" or "active MPF" continues to be used to mean the Cdc2-cyclin complex that stimulates mitosis. MPF (the Cdc2 cyclin complex) induces chromosome condensation, the assembly of the mitotic spindle, and the breakdown of the nuclear envelope. Only in the last of these three cases is much known about the molecular mechanism involved: The Cdc2 phosphorylates (and stimulates other kinases to phsophorylate) the *lamin* proteins of the *nuclear lamina*, to which the inner nuclear membrane is attached. phosphorylation causes the lamins to dissociate from each other, and pieces of the nuclear envelope follow suit. By the time mitosis is well under way, yet another activity of the Cdc2-cyclin complex becomes important: It activates proteolytic enzymes that cause its own demise by degrading cyclin, including both cyclin bound to Cdc2 and free cyclin. The Cdc2 protein is recycled.

What about the G_1 checkpoint, the restriction point identified decades ago in mammalian cells? In yeast, in which the G_1 checkpoint is called Start, the go-ahead signal is also given by a Cdc2-cyclin complex, although the cyclin is a different one. In cells of vertebrates, including both frogs and humans, there is a whole family of different cyclins and also a family of proteins more or less similar to the Cdc2 protein. The generic term for a member of the Cdc2 protein family is *cyclin-dependent protein kinase* (Cdk). The various types of Cdk and cyclins act in different combinations at different stages of the animal cell cycle. The details are still begins determined, but current evidence supports the involvement of the animal cell's Cdc2 along with cyclins B and A at the G_2 checkpoint, and Cdk proteins called Cdk2, Cdk4 and Cdk5, along with cyclins E and D (several kinds), at the G_1 checkpoint. Cdk2-cyclin A seems to be important during S phase. The different cyclins are made during different phases of the cell cycle.

You may be wondering about the third checkpoint mentioned earlier, the M-phase checkpoint where the decision is made whether or not to separate the metaphase chromatids and initiate anaphase. Here neither a new cyclin nor a new Cdk seems to be involved. Instead, the onset of anaphase appears to be triggered by proteolytic enzymes activated by the Cdc2-cyclin complex. However, cyclin breakdown (and the concomitant inactivation of the Cdc2-cyclin complex itself) is, surprisingly, not the anaphase-triggering event. In an experiment using an in vitro system based on from egg extracts a nondegradable from of cyclin B was added, creating a nondegradable, continuously active Cdc2-cyclin complex. Although this complex prevented mitosis from proceeding to completion, sister chromatid separation did occur. This result suggests that the proteolytic enzymes that normally attack cyclin must also attack other key proteins, perhaps including proteins required for holding sister chromatids together.

Regulation of Cdk-cyclin complexes by other kinases

Unfortunately for students of this subject, there are additional levels of complexity in the regulation of the cell cycle–making up, along with Cdk proteins and cyclins, the chains of activating and inactivating proteins we mentioned earlier. Fortunately, the reactions catalyzed by these proteins have a common theme: phosphorylation and dephosphorylation. To put it another way, most of these other proteins are protein kinases and phosphatases.

Figure indicates the main proteins and the four main reactions involved in the formation of active MPF during G_2, starting with the Cdc2 protein. This scheme is probably similar to what happens at the G1 checkpoint, also. The initial complex formed by the joining of the Cdc2 protein and the MPF (mitotic) cyclin is inactive in the cell; to trigger mitosis, the complex requires the addition of a phosphate group on a particular amino acid of Cdc2 (Thr-161). In the figure, this phosphate is highlighted with yellow. It is added by a specific kinase, which the figure calls "activating kinase." But before that enzyme acts, another *inhibiting* kinase phosphorylates the protein in two other places. (Thr-14 and Tyr-15), such a that its active site is blocked. So the last set pin the activation sequence is actually the removal of the inhibiting phosphates by a phosphatase enzyme. The extra phosphorylations and dephosphorylation steps provide other points in the pathway where the process is subject to control by other factors. In addition, a positive feedback loop is involved: The active form of Cdc2-cyclin activates more and more phosphatase.

At either checkpoint, the Cdk protein and/or the cyclin protein may need to be further modified by additional sequences of reactions before the final Cdk2-cyclin complex is fully active. The details of these process may vary with the organism and, in a multicellular organism, with the cell type. Furthermore, various environmental influences, such as nutrients and hormones, may help determine which cyclins accumulate and at what rate. Most cells have many layers of cell cycle control.

Putting it all together: the cell cycle regulation machine

Figure is a generalized and simplified summary of the operation of the molecular machine that regulates the eukaryotic cell cycle, as currently understood. Although much of what we know to date comes from research on the G_2 checkpoint in frogs and yeasts, most cell cycle decisions are probably controlled in a similar way, with the key molecules being protein kinases and cyclins.

The cell cycle machine can be described in terms of two fundamental, interacting mechanisms. One mechanism is an autonomous clock, which on its own goes through a fixed cycle over and over

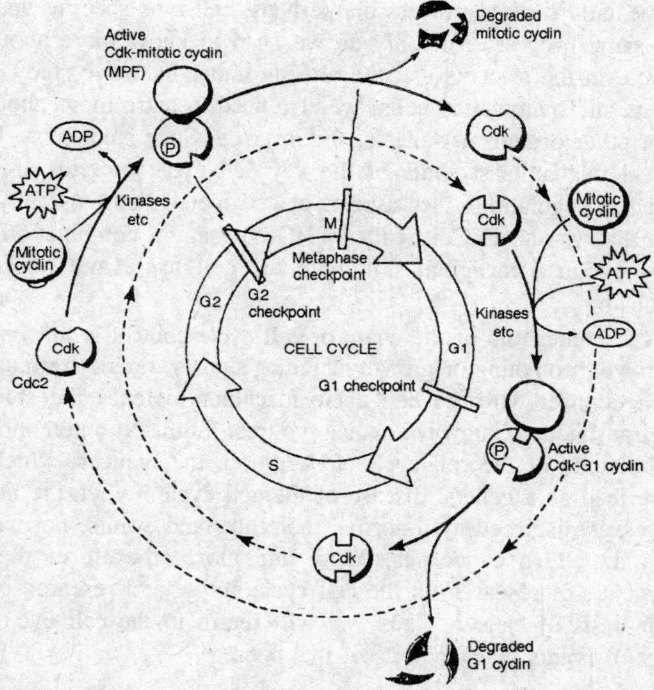

Fig. 2.9. A general model for cell cycle regulation.

again. The molecular basis of this clock is the synthesis and degradation of cyclins, which occur in a rhythmic fashion. The other mechanism adjusts the clock as needed, by providing feedback from the cell's internal and external environments. This mechanism makes use of cyclin-dependent kinases and additional proteins that, directly or indirectly, interact with cyclins. Many of the additional proteins are themselves protein kinases or phosphatases. It is this part of the cell cycle machine that transmits information about the state of the cell's metabolism–including DNA replication–and about conditions outside the cell. Energy required to activate the machine is supplied by ATP.

Even though the Cdk-cyclin core of the cell cycle regulatory machine has been identified, we are still in the dark about many aspects of the cell cycle regulation. How exactly do the Cdk-cyclin complexes influence cell cycle events? That is, what are the actual substrates in vivo for Cdk-cyclin kinase activity? Researchers have a number of candidates, but only lamins have thus far been proven to qualify. Only with more information about substrates will we be able to determine to what extent the different Cdk-cyclins control fundamentally distinct process or, perhaps, cell-type specific versions of the same process. Not only do we need to know more about the cell cycle in the systems that are already under intensive study, such as yeasts and mammalian cells; we also need to learn more about the cells of other organisms—plants, for instance. Such studies are likely to reveal that at least some of the key cell cycle proteins are also involved in regulating other aspects of cell metabolism. Already it is known that yeast has Cdk (called PHO85) that, in combination with various cyclins, participates in both the cell cycle and phosphate metabolism.

At the other end of the chain of cell cycle control is the issue of how growth-promoting or growth-inhibiting signals coming from outside the cell connect with the cell cycle machinery. Hence the study of signal transduction pathways, which we treat intimately interconnected with the study of the cell cycle. In addition, the cancer, which can be described as a genetic disease of the cell cycle. When the normal cell cycle is disturbed by a normal molecules and events, normal cell growth may turn cancerous. More and more, therefore, there is convergence of research on the cell cycle per se and research on the cellular basis of cancer. Thus, we will return to the cell cycle at a number of points in later parts of this book.

What are the Functions of Mitotic Cell Division?

Mitotic cell division plays several roles in the lives of multicellular eukaryotic organisms. First, in conjuction with the differential expression of genes in different cells, it allows a fertilized egg eventually to become an adult consisting of perhaps trillions of individual cells.

Mitotic cell division also allows an organism to maintain its tissues, many of which require frequent replacement. For example, your skin cells live for only about 2 weeks. As dead skin flakes off imperceptibly but constantly, skin cells are continuously replaced by cell division. Your red blood cells become worn out after about 4 months. Through cell division, specialized cells in bone marrow give rise to new red blood cells, which enter the bloodstream at the rate of 3 million per second! Cells of your stomach lining, exposed to acid and digestive enzymes, survive only about 3 days before they must be replaced through the division of underlying cells.

Mitotic Cell Division Forms the Basis of Asexual Reproduction

Mitotic cell division provides the basis of asexual reproduction, in which offspring are formed from a single parent without the uniting of male and female gametes. This mode of reproduction is normal fot many unicellular organisms, such as *Tetrahymena*, and yeasts. Many multicellular organisms can also reproduce asexually. Small replicas of the parent grow by means of cell division. Like its relative the sea anemone, a *Hydra* can reproduce by growing a miniature replica of itself as a bud. Eventually the bud separates from its parent, going off to live independently. Because mitosis produces genetically identical cells, these offspring are genetically identical to their parents; they are called clones.

Many plants reproduce both asexually and sexually. The beautiful aspen grooves of Colorado, Utah, and New Mexico develop asexually from shoots growing up from the root system of a single parent tree. The entire groove, although seeming to be a population of separate trees to the admiring visitor, may actually be considered to be a single individual, with its multiple trunks interconnected by a common root system. Recently, biologists at the University of Colorado reported that one of the single largest organisms yet discovered on Earth is a huge aspen groove in Utah, covering 106 acres and including about 47,000 trunks with a total mass of up to 6 million kilograms (13 million pounds). Although individual trunks age and die, the groove lives on; some grooves are thought to be hundreds of thousands of years old. If you plant an aspen tree in your backyard, who knows what you may be starting! Mitosis also gave rise to the nucleus that produced Dolly. As you will learn in "Scientific Inquiry" Much Ado About Dolly, researchers removed the nucleus of a cell from the udder of a sheep and used it to produce a whole new lamb. This type of asexual reproduction in mammals can occur only in the laboratory!

Autoradiographic Studies on Chromosomal Duplication

Autoradiography is useful technique for cell studies that involve small amounts of materials. Radioactively labeled compounds are used. After the experiment has been performed, the radioactive atoms are localized, by putting a photographic film against the fixed (chemically killed and immobilized) cells. The β rays (electrons) emitted by the radioactive atoms expose the silver grains in the photographic emulsion. Thus by looking at the dark spots on the developed film, one can see the pattern of radioactive compounds in the biological material.

J. Herbert Taylor and his associates studied the transfer of atoms of DNA in the chromosomes of the English broad bean (*Vicia faba*) during mitosis. DNA in the root tips of the broad bean was labeled with tritium (^{3}H), the radioactive isotope of hydrogen, by exposing the growing tips to a solution containing ^{3}H-labeled thymidine. After about one third of a division cycle the seedling were transferred to a growth medium without labeled thymidine but containing colchicine. After periods equal to one or two division cycles, the root tips were fixed and pressed against the photographic film. The electrons emitted by the incorporated tritium are of such low energy that they do not penetrate deeply into the film, and they therefore produce images only at their point of entry into the film emulsion. The chromosomes and their autoradiorgrams can be viewed simultaneously with the light microscope.

The broad bean contains 12 chromosomes (2n =12, n =6). Some nuclei treated in this experiment contained 12 chromosomes, some contained 24, and some contained 48. The chromosomes in cells with 12 metaphase chromosomes have not duplicated following labeling. The chromosomes in cells with 24 and 48 metaphase chromosomes have duplicated once and twice, respectively. The chromosomes in the nuclei containing 12 chromosomes were equally radioactive in the two chromatids. Those chromosomes that had experienced a division and were in the second metaphase after labeling (24 chromosome nuclei) were labeled in one chromatid only. In those cells with 48 chromosomes, two sets of chromosomes were completely unlabeled and the other two sets were labeled like those that had undergone only one division. Although the actual arrangement of DNA in chromosomes is yet unknown, the transmission of atoms to daughter chromosomes supports the idea that a DNA double helix runs the entire length of the chromosome. For simplicity of presentation the metaphase chromatids in Figure 2.10 have been represented as containing two linear DNA molecules rather than a double helix.

Abnormalities in Mitosis

Under unfavourable conditions the mitotic divisions become defective and thus various abnormalities are formed when exposed to physical and chemical agents like temperature, radiations, necrotics and enzyme inhibitors etc. Some abnormal mitotic divisions are given under the following heads:

1. C-Mitosis (Abnormal Spindle Formation)

Brachet (1975) has described that colchicine inhibits mitosis by disorganizing spindle formation. The results are the formation of polyploid cells, and reduplication of chromosomes. Besides, during mitosis, sometimes cell nucleus is either deformed into a single spheriod compact mass (pycnosis) or becomes broken down (karyorrhexis).

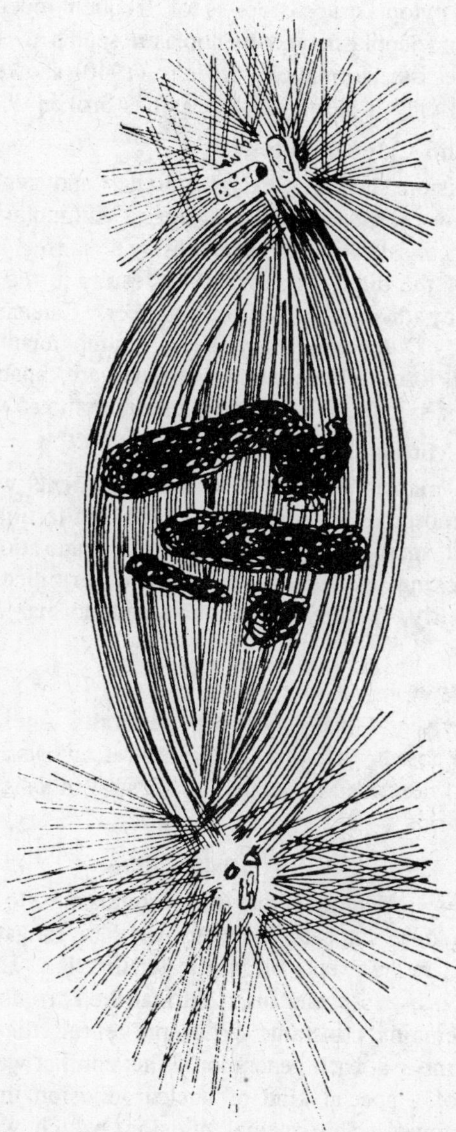

Fig. 2.10. Showing achromatic figure.

2. Cytasteral Mitosis

Wilson (1901) noticed the formation of numerous asters in the cytoplasm of unfertilized eggs called cytasters by placing them in hypertonic sea water. In the eggs of marine invertebrates, production of many small cytoplasmic asters is of frequent occurrence. The intermixing of nucleoplasm and hyaloplasm seems to be neccesary condition for the aster formation. *Costello* (1940) showed that asters can be produced only if germinal vesicles has broken down.

3. Multipolar and Catenar Mitosis

Mitotic division showing several spindles and centrosomes are common in many protozoans and fish eggs. Multipolarity is usually caused by uneven division of centrosomes as well as irregular distribution of chromatids of the different spindles. It results in the formation of cells as aneuploidy (uneven chromosome number). Catenar mitosis have been described by *Dalcq* and *Simon* (1932) in amphibian eggs. During this, dividing cell forms a large number of asters are capable of dividing in the absence of spindle or nucleus in an autonomous way.

4. Achrosomal Mitosis

Sometimes, mitosis in induced by various agents without use of nucleus or chromosomes. *Briggs et. al.* (1951), in fertilized eggs with heavily X-rayed sperms, removed the egg's maturation spindle by pricking and sucking. In this way, he obained very nice non-nucleate blastulae. Similarly, *Stauffer* (1945) obtained normal non-nucleated Axolotl blastula.

5. Anastral Mitosis

In plant cells and many oocytes, generally asters around the centromeres are absent, thus producing anastral mitosis. *Bataillon and Tchou Su* (1933) described in details the anastral mitosis in amphibian interspecific hybrids.

MEIOSIS

Since it was evident that the job of mitosis is to maintain the chromo-some number in each nucleus, early investigators noted an apparent conflict in the events of gamete fertilization. They knew that during this process, two nuclei fuse, but that the chromosome number nevertheless remains constant. What prevented the doubling of chromosome number at each generation? This conflict was resolved by the prediction of a special kind of nuclear division that halved the chromosome number. This special division, which was eventually discovered in the gamete-producing tissues of plants and animals, was called meiosis.

Meiosis is also preceded by a premeiotic S phase, during which the bulk of DNA synthesis for meiosis occurs. (Some DNA synthesis also occurs during the first prophase of meiosis.) Since meiosis consists of two cell divisions, they are distinguished as meiosis I and meiosis II. The events of meiosis I are quite different from those of meiosis II, and both differ significantly from those of meiosis. Each meiotic division is formally divided into prophase, metaphase, anaphase, and telophase. Of these, the most complex and lenghty is prophase I, which has its own subdivisions: leptotene, zygotene, pachytene, diplotene, and diakinesis. Once again, try to imagine those processes as dynamic, merging into each other with no clear borders.

Prophase I

The prophase I differ from mitotic prophase in two aspects. Firstly, it is of longer duration than the mitotic prophase and secondly, most cytogenetical events such as synapsis, crossing over, etc. occur during prophase first. For the sake of convenience, the prophase first has been subdivided into five consecutive stages: leptonema, zygonema, pchynema, diplonema and diakinesis. The name of these substages of prophase first have been derived from the specific morphology or behaviour of the chromosomes within the nuclear membrane at each substage of prophase. Thus leptotene means thin thread, zygotene means yolked thread, pachytene means thick thread, diplotene means double thread and diakinesis is essentially the end of both diplotene and prophase I.

Leptotene

The chromosomes become visible at this stage as long, thin threads. No longitudinal doubleness is apparent. The process of chromosome contraction continues in leptotene and throughout the entire prophase. One other feature of leptotene is the development of small areas of

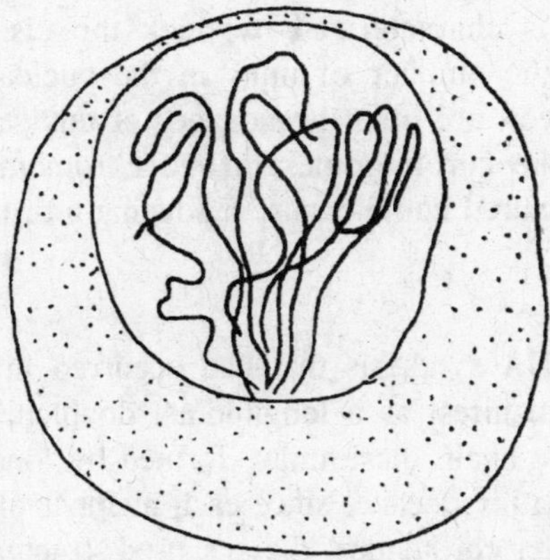

Fig. 2.11. Leptotene chromosomes arranged in a 'bouquet'.

thickening, called chromomeres, along the chromosome, which give it the appearance of a bead necklace.

Zygotene

This is time of active pairing at which it becomes apparent that the chromosome complement of the meiocyte is in fact two complete chromosome sets. Thus, each chromosome has a pairing partner, and the two become progressively paired, or synapsed, side by side in zipper fashion. Each pair is called a homologous pair, and the two members of a pair are called *homologous*. We see that meiocytes always contain two homologous chromosome sets, or genomes. A cell with two homologous genomes is called diploid. One genome is said to have a haploid chromosome number, usually designated *n*. Hence diploid cells are 2*n*. It should be noted that the occurrence of pairing represents a striking difference from mitosis, in which there is not such process.

What is mechanism whereby two homologous can pair so precisely along their length? First, how do they find each other in the first place? The probable answer to this is that the ends of the chromosomes, the telomeres, are anchored in the nuclear membrane, and it is likely that homologous telomeres are close, so that the zippering-up process can begin there. Second, how does the zippering-up work? Although the mechanism involved is not precisely understood, one important factor is an elaborate structure composed of protein and DNA, called a synaptonemal complex, that is always found sandwiched between homologous during synapsis.

Pachytene

This stage is characterized by thick threads representing full synapsis. Thus the number of units in the nucleus is equal to the number *n*. Nucleoli are often pronounced at this stage. The beadlike thickenings of the chromosomes, called chromomeres, are aligned precisely in the paired homologous, producing a distinctive pattern for each pair.

Diplotene

Here the DNA synthesis that had occurred in the premeiotic S phase becomes manifest as a longitudinal doubleness of each paired homologue. Once again these units, formed by longitudinal division, are called chromatids. Hence, since each member of homologous pair produces two sister chromatids, the synapsed structure now consists of a bundle of four homologous chromatids. At diplotene the pairing between homologs becomes less tight; in fact, they appear to repel each other, and as they separate slightly, cross-shaped structures called chiasmata (singular, chiasma) appear between two nonsister chromatids. One or more chiasmata are found on each chromosome pair. Chiasmata are visible manifestations of events, called crossovers, that occurred earlier, probably during zygotene or pachytene, when there is some DNA synthesis. Crossovers represent one major way in which meiosis differs from mitosis (where they occur only rarely). A crossover is a precise breakage-and-reunion event occurring between two nonsister chromatids. Studies performed on abnormal lines of organisms that undergo crossing-over very inefficiently, or not at all, show severe disruption of the orderly events that partition chromosomes into daughter cells at meiosis. Thus, crossing-over obviously plays a key role in determining the behaviour of paired homologs, and the occurrence of at least one cross-over per pair is usually essential for proper segregation. Crossovers have another interesting role, which is to promote genetic variation by making new gene combinations.

Diakinesis

This stage does not differ appreciably from diplotene except for further chromosome contraction. By this time, the long filamentous chromosome threads of interphase are replaced by compact units far more maneuverable in the movements of the meiotic division.

Metaphase I

During the first meiotic metaphase, the bivalents orient themselves at random on the equatorial plate. The centromere of each chromosome of a terminalized tetrad is directed towards the opposite poles. The chromosomal microtubular spindle fibres remain attached with the centromeres and homologous chromosomes become ready to separate.

Anaphase I

In contrast to mitotic anaphase in which separation of sister chromatids occurs, the meiotic anaphase I is characterized by the separation of whole chromosomes of each homologous pair (tetrad), so that each pole of the dividing cell receives either a paternal or maternal longitudinally double chromosome of each tetrad. This ensures a change in chromosome number from diploid to monoploid or haploid in the resultant reorganized daughter nuclei.

Telophase I

The arrival of chromosomes at the poles of the spindle signals the end of anaphase I and the beginning of telophase I. During telophase I,

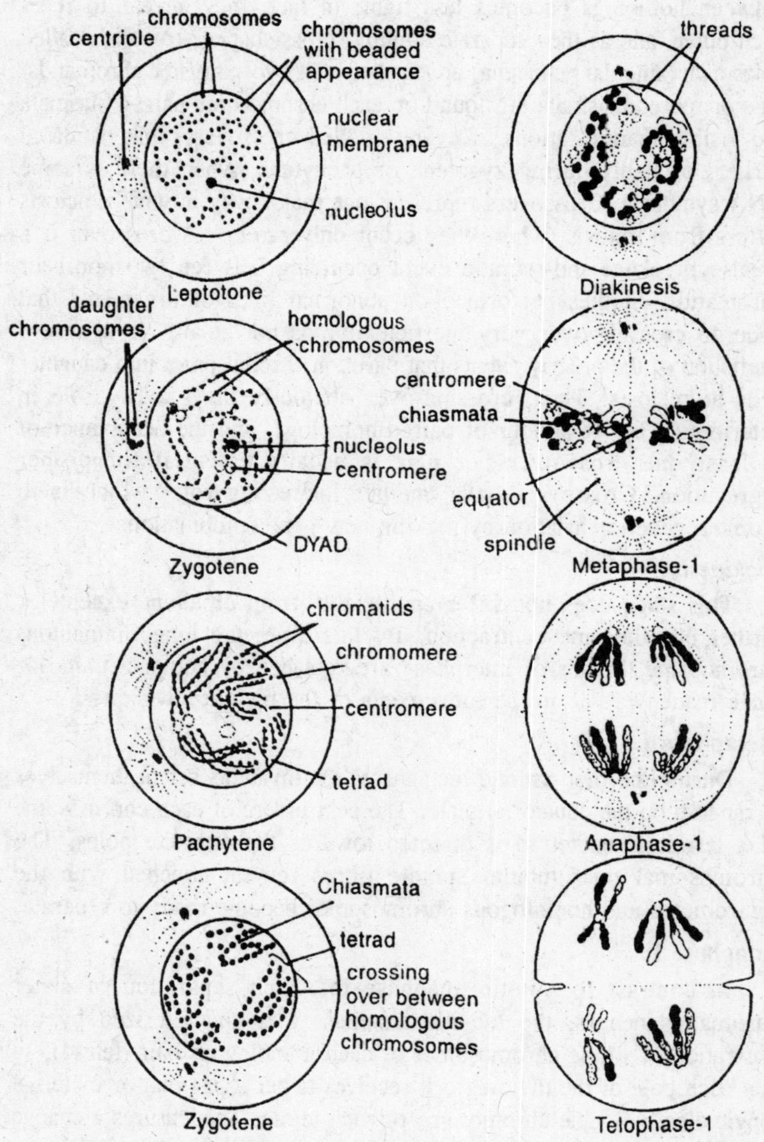

Fig. 2.12. Diagrammatic representation of different stages in the first meiotic division.

the chromosomes may persist for a time in the condensed state, the nucleolus and nuclear membrane may be reconstituted and cytokinesis may also occur to produce two haploid cells. In Trillium meiocytes are reported to progress directly from anaphase I to prophase II.

II. Homotypic or 2nd Meiotic Division

Before the start of this division, most of the activities of heterotypic division cease for sometime. This resting stage is termed as the interkinesis. 2nd meiotic division involves following steps:

Prophase II

This stage superficially resembles that of the mitosis prophase with following exceptions:

At the early prophase II, the two chromatids of each dyad looks like X, since they are conjoined by a common centromere. The four arms are widely separated. There is no rational coiling. The X-shaped dyads are quite longer than at telophase. The chromonemata are still not completely coiled. The genetic constitution of the two chromatids of each dyad depends upon the kind and number of cross overs which took place in the phase I. If there is no crossing over, the dyads would consist of two identical sister chromatids of either paternal or maternal origin. At the end of the prophase II the nucleolus disappears. The nuclear membrane disappears and the acromatic figure is developed.

Metaphase II

As usual, all the chromosomes arrange themselves on the equator for a short duration. The centromeres touch the equator but their arms radiate out in different directions. Later on the centromere in each dyad divides into two sister centromeres.

Anaphase II

Sister centromeres separate to the poles, pulling with them the chromatids to which they are attached. The chromatids, however, become much thick and stout.

Telophase II

The chromosomes at each pole uncoil and thin out to form the nuclear net. Each group gets surrounded by a nuclear membrane. Nucleolus reappears. Thus two nuclei are recognised in each cell. This is soon followed by cytokinesis and two cells are formed from each haploid daughter cell. Thus as a result of meiosis four cells are produced, each with a haploid set of chromosomes, i.e., each contains just one members of each homologous pair.

Cytokinesis

Sometimes meiosis I is followed by cytokinesis and sometimes it is deferred until the end of meiosis II. The details of the process are same as during mitosis. Cell plate formation results into a tetrad of

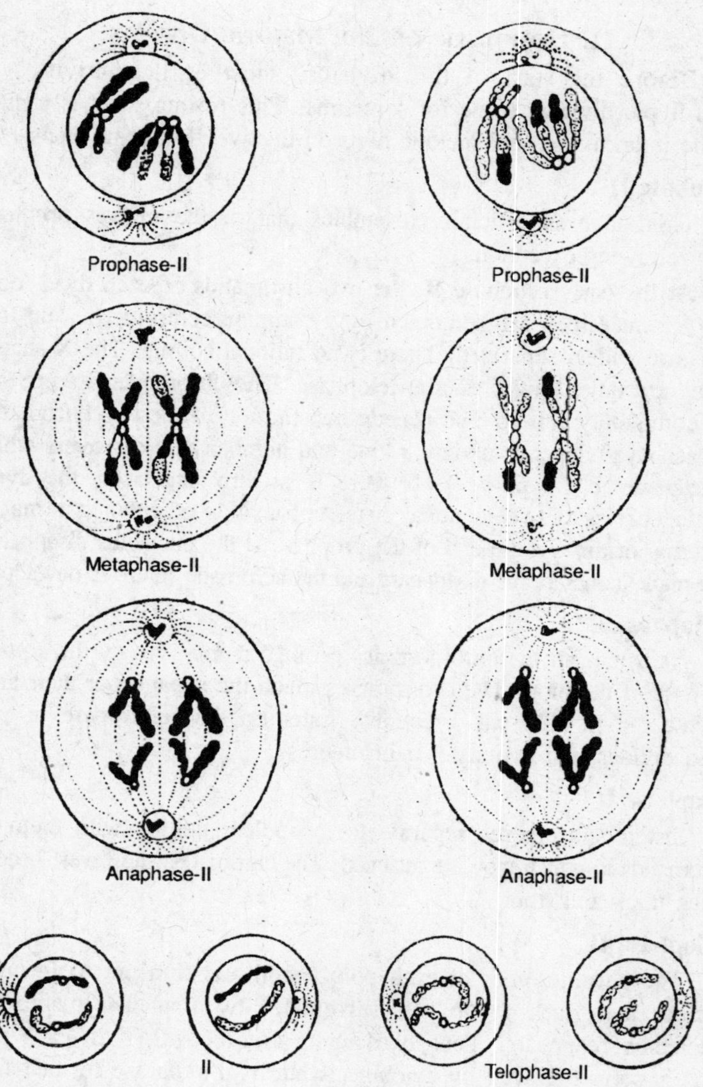

Fig. 2.13. Diagrammatic representation of homeotypic division of meiosis.

cells with reduced chromosome numbers. The arrangement of cells in a tetrad is different in different organisms, but is characteristic of the species.

Like mitosis, meiosis too is a dynamic process and its different stages merge into subsequent ones. There is no sharp demarcation between different stages. DNA synthesis takes place during interphase,

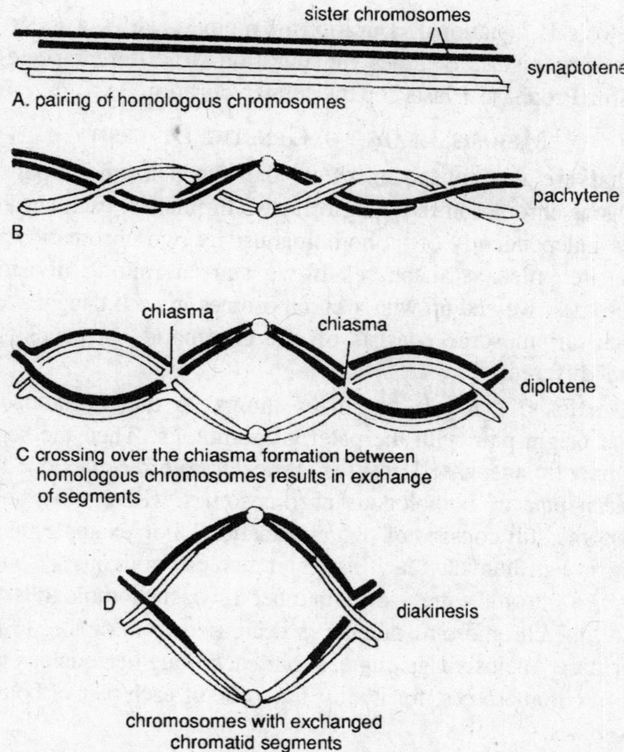

Fig. 2.14. Mechanism of chiasmata formation and crossing over.

prior to prophase I. Duplication of chromosomes takes place during interphase itself and the chromosomes that appear during leptotene are double and not single. Number of chromosomes is reduced during meiosis I. If the reduction process is examined more closely, it becomes clear that there is qualitative reduction during meiosis I of those part of chromosomes which are not involved in exchange. The homologous chromosomes or the maternal and paternal chromosomes segregate or undergo qualitative reduction during meiosis I. Their quantitative reduction takes place during meiosis II, when their centromeres divide and the sister chromatids separate. But the reverse is true of those parts of chromatids which are exchange due to the formation of chiasmata. For these parts quantitative reduction takes place during meiosis I and qualitative reduction during meiosis II. Thus, complete of both qualitative and quantitative reduction takes place as a result of meiosis I and II and none of them alone can bring about complete reduction. It is, therefore, not proper to say that meiosis I is reductional and meiosis II equational. Duration of meiosis varies a great deal in different organisms. So does the duration of different stages in an organism. Prophase I lasts for the longer duration.

Meiosis Leads to Genetic Diversity

What are the consequences of the synapsis and separation of homologous chromosomes during meiosis? In mitosis, each chromosome behaves independently of its homologous; its two chromatids are sent to opposite poles at anaphase. If we start a mitotic division with chromosomes, we end up with x chromosomes in each daughter nucleus, and each chromosome consists of one chromatid. In meiosis, things are very different.

In meiosis, synapsis organizes things so that chromosomes of maternal origin pair with the paternal homologs. Then the separation during meiotic anaphase I ensures that each pole receives one member from each pair of homologous chromosomes. (Remember that each chromosome still consists of two chromatids.) For example, at the end of meiosis I in humans, each daughter nucleus contains 23 out of the original 46 chromosomes–one member of each homologous pair. In this way, the chromosome number is decreased from diploid to haploid. Furthermore, meiosis I guarantees that each daughter nucleus gets one full set of chromosomes; for it must have one of each pair of homologous chromosomes.

The products of meiosis I are genetically diverse for two reasons. First, synapsis during prophase I allows the maternal chromosome to interact with the paternal one; if there is crossing over, the recombinant chromatids contain some genetic material from each chromosome. Second, which member of a pair of chromosomes goes to which daughter cell at anaphase I is a matter of pure chance. If there are two pairs of chromosomes in the diploid parent nucleus, a particular daughter nucleus could get paternal chromosome 1 and maternal chromosome 2, or paternal 2 and maternal 1, or both maternals, or both paternals. It all depends on the random way in which the homologous pairs line up at metaphase I.

Note that of the four possible chromosome combinations just described, two produce daughter nuclei that are the same as one of the parental types (except for any material exchanged by crossing over). The greater the number of chromosomes, the less probable that the original parental combinations will be reestablished. Most species of diploid organisms do, indeed, have more than two pairs. In humans, with 23 chromosome pairs, 2^{23} different combinations can be produced.

MEIOTIC ERRORS

Source of Chromosomal Disorders

A pair of homologous chromosomes may fail to separate during meiosis I, or sister chromatids may fail to separate during meiosis II or during mitosis. This phenomenon is called nondisjunction, and it results in the production of aneuploid cells. Aneuploidy is a condition in which one or more chromosomes or pieces of chromosomes are either lacking or are present in excess.

If, for example, the chromosome 21 pairs fails to separate during the formation of a human egg (and thus both members of the pair go to one pole during anaphase I), the resulting egg contains either two copies of chromosome 21 or none at all. If an egg with two of these chromosomes is fertilized by a normal sperm, the resulting zygote and infant has three copies of the chromosome: He or she is trisomic for chromosome 21. As a result of carrying an extra chromosome 21, such a child demonstrates the symptoms of Down syndrome: impaired intelligence; characteristic abnormalities of the hands, tongue, and eyelids; and an increased susceptibility to cardiac abnormalities and diseases such as leukemia.

Other abnormal events can also lead to aneuploidy. In a process called translocation, a piece of a chromosome may break away and become attached to another chromosome. For example, a particular large part of one chromosome. For example, a particular large part of one chromosome 21 may be translocated to another chromosome. Individuals who inherit this translocated piece along with two normal chromosomes 21 have Down syndromed.

Other human disorders result from particular chromosomal abnormalities. Sex chromosome aneuploidy causes disorders such as Turner syndrome and Klinefelter syndrome, discussed in Chapter 10 in connection with sex determination. Deletion of a portion of chromosome 5 results in cri du chat (French for "cat's cry") syndrome, so named because an afflicted infant's cry sounds like that of a cat. Symptoms of this syndrome include severe mental retardation.

Trisomies (and the corresponding monosomies) are surprisingly common in human zygotes, but most of the embryos that develop from such zygotes do not survive to birth. Trisomies for chromosomes 13, 15, and 18 greatly reduce the probability that an embryo will survive to birth, and virtually all infants who are born with such trisomies die before the age of 1 year.

Trisomies and monosomies for other chromosomes are lethal to the embryo. At least one-fifth of all recognized pregnancies spontaneously terminate during the first two months, largely because of such trisomies and monosomies. (The actual proportion of spontaneously terminated pregnancies is certainly higher, because the earliest ones often go unrecognized).

Polyploids can have Difficulty in Cell Division

Both diploid and haploid nuclei divide by mitosis. Multicellular diploid and multicellular haploid individuals develop from single-celled beginnings by mitotic divisions. Mitosis may proceed in diploid organisms even when a chromosome from one of the haploid sets is missing or when there is an extra copy of one of the chromosomes (as in Down syndrome).

Under some circumstances triploid ($3n$), tetraploid ($4n$), and higher-order polyploid nuclei from. Each of these ploidy levels represents an increase in the number of complete sets of chromosomes present. If, through accident, the nucleus has one or more extra full sets of chromosomes—that is, if it is triploid, tetraploid, or of still higher ploidy—this abnormally high ploidy in itself does not prevent mitosis. In mitosis, each chromosome behaves independently of the others.

In meiosis, by contrast, chromosomes synapse to begin division. If even one chromosome has no homologous, anaphase I cannot send representatives of that chromosome to both poles. A diploid nucleus can undergo normal meiosis; a haploid one cannot. A tetraploid nucleus has an even number of each kind of chromosome, so each chromosome can pair with its homolog. But a triploid nucleus cannot undergo normal meiosis, because one-third of the chromosomes would lack partners.

This limitation has important consequences for the fertility of triploid, tetraploid, and other chromosomally unusual organisms that may be produced by plant breeding or by natural accidents. Modern bread wheat plants are hexaploids, the result of the accidental crossing of three different grasses, each having its own diploid set of 14 chromosomes.

Cell Death

As we mentioned at the start of the chapter, an essential role of cell division in complex eukaryotes is to replace cells that die. In humans, billions of cells die each day, mainly in blood and epithelia lining organs such as the intestine. Cells die in one of two ways. The first, necrosis, occurs when cells either are damaged by poisons or are starved of essential nutrients. The scab that forms around a wound is a familiar example of necrotic tissue. More typical in an organism is apoptosis, a series of events that constitute genetically programmed cell death. Why would a cell initiate apoptosis, which is essentially "cell suicide"? One reason is that the cell in question is no longer needed by the organism. For example, before birth a human fetus has weblike hands, with connective tissue between the fingers. As development proceeds, this unneeded tissue disappears as the cells undergo apoptosis. A second reason for apoptosis is that the longer cells live, the more prone they are to damage that could lead to cancer. This is especially true of cells in the blood and intestine, which are exposed to high levels of toxic substances. In these cases, cells sacrifice their lives to the good of the organism.

Like the cell cycle, the events of apoptosis are very similar in most organisms. The cell becomes isolated from its neighbours, chops up its chromatin into nucleosome-sized pieces, and then fragments itself. In a remarkable example of the economy of nature, the surrounding living cells ingest the remains of the dead cell. The genetic signals that lead to apoptosis are common to many organisms.

Senescence of Dividing Somatic Cells

The senescence of normal diploid cells was first revealed in detailed studies of cultured human fibroblasts. Fibroblasts are connective tissue cells that have a characteristic morphology and synthesize collagen. After a long period of normal growth, the yield of cells per flask began to decrease, and finally reached a very low level, with no further proliferation. These investigators referred to the establishment of a primary culture of normal cells as Phase I, the long period of normal growth as Phase II, and the senescent period as Phase III. Previously, it had been generally assumed that cultured mammalian cells grew indefinitely, but this was based on the growth of neoplastic or transformed cells, and such cell populations are generally known as permanent lines. Saksela and Moorhead (1963) were the first to show that human fibroblasts retain a diploid karyotype during the long period of normal growth, but chromosome abnormalities appear with increasing frequency as cells enter senescence.

There is some controversy about the relationship between senescence, aging, and cell death. If the cells are cultured to a stage where they remain subconfluent, abnormalities in cell morphology are clearly visible. The cells vary in size and shape; the cytoplasm is granular, with many cell inclusions; and debris is formed in the medium. Some of the cells detach to form debris, whereas others remain attached to the substrate. At an earlier stage when the cells still become confluent, these abnormalities are less apparent. However, the cells do not form the "*whorls*" of growth that are characteristic of younger cultures, and the monolayer of cells is distinctly grainy in appearance. With regular changes of medium, these confluent cells remain attached to the substrate for long periods and continue metabolism with occasional celi division. Innumerable studies of cellular senescence have depended on the use of such cell populations, in comparison to early-passage cells. These studies have documented a large number of changes in physiological, biochemical, or molecular parameters that occur during the aging of human fibroblasts. Hayflick lists 167 parameters that have been examined; of these, 117 change during senescence. More recently, a single "*biomarker*" of aging has been extensively used. This is the formation of β galactosidase, but the reason for its appearance is not known; nor is it clear why this particular biomarker is usually preferred to many others that are available. The actual age of a culture is normally recorded in *population doublings* (PDs), and, typically, human fibroblasts reach 50–70 PDs. In some studies, PDs are broadly equivalent to passages, provided a 1:4 split is recorded as two passages and a 1:8 split as three. However, in many studies, passages are simply the number of subcultures, and they may not correspond at all to PDs.

Following the demonstration of the limited growth potential of human fibroblasts, the same or similar limited life span has been demonstrated in many other cultured somatic cells. With the exception of T lymphocytes, the cells listed typically have a shorter in vitro life span than fibroblasts. Studies of other species also demonstrate the limited growth potential of normal diploid cells, and there is a rather clear relationship between the longevity of the donor species and the growth potential of its fibroblasts in culture. From all these studies, the strong conclusion can be drawn that specialized dividing cells eventually become senescent and cease growth in culture. Whereas human cells do not transform to permanent cell lines (with the exception of lymphoblastoid cells from lymphocytes previously infected with Epstein-Barr virus), cells from short-lived animals, such as rodents, do commonly give rise to permanent lines with abnormal karyotypes.

Variability in Growth Potential of Human Fibroblasts

Human fibroblasts are usually stored at early passage in liquid nitrogen. It is evident that cultures obtained from different ampoules of the same cell strain have very different life spans in PDs. The ranges for the well-known strains WI-38 and MRC-5 are 38–60 PDs and 55–75 PDs, respectively. It should be noted that a difference of 10 PDs represents a thousand-fold difference in cell mass (if all the cells were grown to senescence), so the range demonstrated is a very substantial variability in growth potential. The studies of clones of cells also demonstrate a very substantial variability in growth potential, and even the daughters of individual cells have different longevities. It is evident that stochastic events have an important role in determining the life span of somatic cells. The variability in the growth potential of populations and clones of cells can complicate the interpretation of experiments designed to uncover possible causes of senescence.

Theories of Cellular Senescence

The key feature of the senescence of dividing cells is the fact that a long period of normal growth is followed by cessation of growth. Therefore, events must be occurring and accumulating through a life span that culminate in senescence. This immediately gives rise to the concept of a molecular clock. At present, most attention has been directed to the loss of telomeric DNA. In the absence of the enzyme telomerase, telomeres gradually get shorter as cell division proceeds, and shortening of telomeres throughout the life span is well documented. The consequence may be the inactivation of genes closest to the telomere sequences, either directly, or indirectly by a position effect, perhaps involving the formation of heterochromatin. This would happen at the ends of all 46 chromosomes.

Since the lengths of telomeric DNAs could vary, as well as could the loss of the number of DNA base pairs per cell division, this interpretation of cell senescence could probably accommodate the observed variability in life spans. A prediction of the theory is that the introduction of DNA coding for telomerase should immortalize the cell population. This prediction has been verified, although a number of questions about the generality of the loss-of-telomerase theory of cellular senescence remain unanswered and are discussed below.

A second general type of theory proposes that during the normal cell division in Phase II, molecular defects gradually accumulate. This is most easy to envisage at the DNA level, but it is also possible that defects could occur in proteins, membranes, or organelles, provided that their natural dilution by growth and cell division is not sufficient to produce a steady-state level of defects. This theory, in its most general form, is broadly supported by the finding that a large number of genetic, biochemical, or physiological parameters are affected during aging.

With time, some indispensable cellular component or function may fail, but a more attractive possibility is that a given level of defects triggers a checkpoint control mechanism. This could block DNA synthesis or introduce some irreversible inhibition of cell division. This was first suggested by Rosenberger et al. (1991), and in the last few years has been confirmed by the discovery of checkpoint controls. Thus, there are many studies of genes and proteins involved in one way or another in the regulation of the cell cycle in senescent cells, including the tumor suppressor genes, p53, Rb, and p16, and the p21 cell cycle regulator gene. It is generally agreed that senescent cells are irreversibly blocked in cell division, but they are still capable of many other cell functions. According to the telomere theory of cellular senescence, the shortening of chromosome ends would itself trigger a cell cycle block.

The commitment theory of cellular aging dealt with the population dynamics of senescence and did not depend on any specific molecular mechanism. It proposed that in the founder population of human fibroblasts there are cells that have unlimited division potential; that is, they are potentially immortal. These cells give rise during division, at probability P, to cells that become committed to eventual senescence after M cell divisions. Provided P is sufficiently high (in the range 0.25–0.275) and M sufficiently long, the immortal cells are gradually lost during routine subculture. The final loss of all uncommitted or immortal cells is a stochastic process, which determines the final life span of the whole culture.

The model predicts that the population size, N, is an important parameter and, in particular, that an extremely large population (unfortunately too large to handle in a laboratory) would grow indefinitely. It also predicts that reducing population size at critical times during the life span would have significant life-shortening effects, and this was confirmed by experiment. The commitment theory also receives support from the study of immuno-globulin molecules in populations of T lymphocytes. As the cells approach the end of their life span, the population can often be shown to be clonal, suggesting that all these cells are derived from the last remaining uncommitted cell, many cell generations earlier. It should be noted that the conversion of uncommitted or immortal cells, at rate P, to committed mortal cells could be due to the loss of telomerase activity.

Senescence of Somatic Cells In Vivo

There is indirect evidence that somatic cells in their normal environment use up some of their proliferative potential, although they may not actually reach the senescent state. It was shown that the growth potential of human fibroblasts was inversely related to donor age, although a contrary result has recently appeared. The results of Martin et al. (1970) suggested that the cells, on average, underwent 0.2 PDs per year of chronological life. Moreover, cells from the premature aging syndrome, Werner's syndrome, have a very short in vitro life span. The gene has now been cloned and been shown to belong to a family of DNA helicases. The most clear-cut evidence that cell life span is inversely related to donor age comes from studies of Syrian hamster dermal fibroblasts. Fetal cells, at 13 days gestation, grew for 30 PDs, whereas cells for a 24-month adult grew for only 9 PDs. Those from a 3-day-old animal had a life span of 19 PDs, and those from a 6-month young adult, 14 PDs. These results strongly suggest that dermal fibroblasts continually turn over in vivo, and that cells from old animals have "*used up*" most of their growth potential. Tissue transplantation experiments also indicate that in vivo aging is a reality. For example, mouse mammary tissue can be transplanted between isogenic animals but eventually becomes senescent and is unable to proliferate further.

It is widely believed that somatic stem cells have unlimited growth potential. Although this may be so, it is hard to prove experimentally. The population of stem cells may be structured in such a way that a relatively small pool of cells can give rise to a very large number of descendants. Alternatively, there could be a pool of potentially immortal cells that give rise to stem cells with finite growth. Telomerase is present in hematopoietic stem cells, suggesting they are immortal, but a discussion of the growth potential of the various components of this stem cell system is outside the scope of this chapter.

Environmental Influences on Population Life Spans

In addition to the intrinsic variability of culture life spans, there are also well-documented examples of an induced decrease or increase in longevity of human fibroblasts. In one of the earliest experiments, the incubation temperature was varied. Interestingly, a reduction of the normal temperature of 37°C to 34°C had no effect on growth potential. However, an increase to 40°C appeared to have a severe life-shortening effect, which could not be reversed by returning the cultures to 37°C. The antibiotic paramycin reduces the fidelity of ribosomal translation in eukaryotes. At concentrations that did not affect growth rate, the life span of human fibroblasts was significantly reduced, provided treatment was continuous. A more dramatic result was obtained with the pyrimidine analogs 5-aza-cytidine (5- aza-C) or 5-aza-deoxycytidine (5-aza-dC). These are both incorporated into DNA and are known to inhibit DNA methyl transferase activity. It is well known that a single treatment with either analog will significantly reduce the total level of 5-methylcytosine in the genome. It is also well established that the level of DNA methylation declines during serial passaging. The striking result is that a single treatment of 5-aza-C or 5-aza-dC to young cells, followed by full growth recovery, produces a population of cells with a greatly reduced life span in comparison to untreated controls.

The significance of this result is that the single treatment is "*remembered*" by the cells, and the final effect is seen only many generations later. The results suggest that artificially reducing the level of 5-methyl-cytosine in DNA, followed by further natural decline, leads to the critical level seen in senescent cells. This in turn suggests that the gradually decreasing level of DNA methylation may be an important molecular clock in its own right, which induces senescence. Other studies with primary mouse, hamster, and human fibroblasts support this view. Wilson and Jones (1983) found that mouse primary cells lose DNA methylation at a very high rate, and they have a short life span.

Syrian hamster cells lose DNA methylation at a rate intermediate between mouse and human, and their life span is intermediate as well. In the same and other studies, it was shown that two permanent lines maintain DNA methylation at a constant level, which is what one might expect. Additionally, when 5-aza-C was used to repeatedly drive down the level of DNA methylation in the mouse permanent line, C3H 10T1/2, it was found that it could not be reduced to zero (0.45% was the lowest achieved), so presumably some DNA methylation is essential for viability of these cells.

Many years ago, it was discovered that hydrocortisone significantly increases the growth potential of normal human fibroblasts, but the mechanism remains unknown. More recently, it was found that physiological concentrations of the natural dipeptide L-carnosine (β-alanyl-L-histidine) also increases culture life span. Moreover, when division finally ceases, the cells have a normal rather than a senescent morphology. Switching senescent cells to a high concentration of carnosine produces a rejuvenated phenotype, and removal of the dipeptide causes the cells to revert to senescence. Again, the specific mechanism of action of carnosine is not known, but it has been suggested that it may have an important role in cell maintenance in vivo.

Some Problems with the Telomere Theory of Senescence

Comparative studies strongly indicate that somatic cells from different species have a limited life span in culture, and it is reasonable to suppose that all these cells have the same or similar mechanism of senescence. It is therefore a surprise to find that Syrian hamster cells, which have very clear-cut senescence, have long telomeres, an active telomerase, and maintain their telomere lengths. Furthermore, mouse cells also have very long telomeres, and yet they only divide about 10 times before becoming senescent.

The fact that environmental treatments can significantly increase or reduce culture life span suggests that telomeres can be lost at different rates under different conditions. This need not be a serious problem for the theory, but a study of the effect of increased oxygen is harder to explain. It was found that cells incubated in 40% oxygen soon stopped growing and, at the same time, had shortened telomeric DNA. This shows that telomeric DNA can be lost without cell division, perhaps by the introduction of single-strand breaks in DNA.

DNA methylation poses another problem. What happens in diploid cells immortalized by the introduction of telomerase activity? Presumably, the DNA methylation does not decline to zero, so one must suppose that the DNA methylation is stabilized at a constant level. If this is so, it implies that DNA methylation is in some way coupled to telomere maintenance. In normal cells, both DNA methylation and telomere length decline in concert. When normal human fibroblasts are infected by SV40, the large-T antigen transforms these cells so that they lose contact inhibition and have an abnormal karyotype and an extended life span.

These cells eventually enter a non-proliferative phase known as crisis. SV40-infected cells maintain their DNA methylation level, but they do not maintain their telomeres, which continue to shorten until crisis is reached. It is well established that crisis occurs later than senescence and is distinct from it. Immortalized cells that emerge from crisis either have telomerase or maintain telomeres by another mechanism known as *alternative lengthening of telomeres* (ALT). These observations suggest that it may be the loss of telomeres that precipitates crisis, and this is later than the senescence of normal

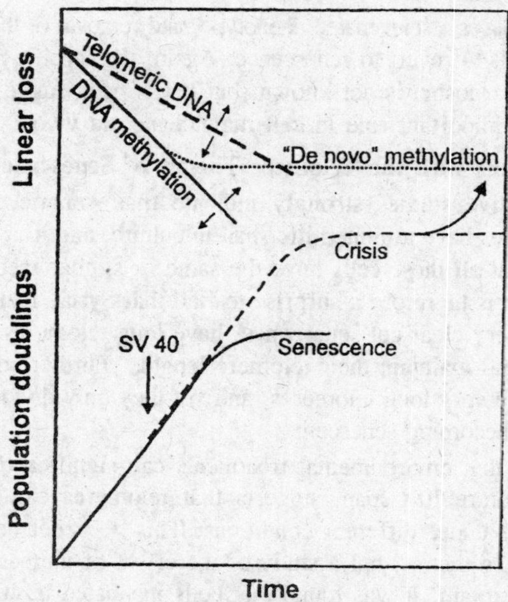

Fig. 2.15. During serial passaging of human diploid fibroblasts, telomeric DNA and DNA methylation are lost linearly with time.

cells. The interesting observation is that senescent cells have telomere lengths which are significantly longer than those of cells entering crisis. Perhaps, then, it is the loss of DNA methylation that precipitates senescence. How then should one explain the results of Bodnar et al. (1998) and Vaziri and Benchimol (1998), namely, that normal cells are immortalized by telomerase? One could conclude they are in a steady state both with regard to telomere length and DNA methylation and, furthermore, that telomerase in some way restores maintenance of DNA methylation. However, the reverse could not be true, at least in pre-crisis cells, because they maintain DNA methylation but continue to lose telomeric DNA.

Is Cell Senescence a Barrier to the Emergence of Malignant Tumor Cells In Vivo?

Tumor cell lines are immortal, so it has often been asserted that the senescence of normal diploid cells is a barrier, or defense mechanism, to the emergence of neoplastic cells. In other words, overcoming this barrier is an essential step in tumor progression. This hypothesis is not as simple and straightforward as it may seem. It is probably rare for somatic cells to reach senescence in vivo. Skin fibroblasts from 90-year-old individuals are capable of 20–40 PDs in vitro, and much the same residual growth is probably true for other types of dividing cells. Therefore, the initiation of early steps in carcinogenesis is occurring in cells with considerable remaining growth potential. Let us assume that these cells proliferate with a transformed, or perhaps partially transformed, phenotype.

It is probable that they already have abnormal karyotypes and may also be mutator strains. Thus, while growing, these cells are generating considerable genetic diversity, and it is generally agreed that cell selection is very important during tumor progression. This leads to the formation of a primary tumor (note that a tumor of 1 gm contains about 10^9 cells, after about 30 PDs from a single cell). These cells would not be expected to enter senescence, in the normal sense, but they may enter the period of growth arrest known as *crisis*. In transformation experiments in vitro, crisis is demonstrably different from senescence. For example, cells in crisis have a high mitotic index, and the cells regularly detach from the substrate. Nevertheless, it is quite possible that crisis is due to the loss of telomeric DNA, and the emergence of permanent lines depends on the acquisition of the means to maintain telomeres.

With regard to primary tumors in vivo, it is well known that tissue biopsies from them rarely give rise to permanent cell lines. However, by the time secondary tumors have appeared, it is somewhat easier to obtain such cell lines. Thus, this scenario suggests that many small primary tumors consist of transformed pre-crisis cells. This crisis could be a barrier to the emergence of metastatic malignant cells, but it is not clear that senescence, in the normal sense, is involved. Primary tumors in many, but not all, cases can give rise to immortalized cells, following rare mutations or epigenetic events. These cells are fully transformed and malignant.

It should be noted that cultured human diploid cells do not spontaneously give rise to transformed pre-crisis cells. They are very resistant to transformation, irrespective of senescence. It is possible to regard the senescence that is regularly seen in vitro as simply a result of imperfect cell maintenance. It benefits the organism to down-regulate or turn off maintenance mechanisms that are not required during the lifetime of the individual. Thus, many human somatic cells no longer synthesize telomerase if their telomeres are long enough for many sequential divisions. They also presumably reduce DNA methyl transferase activity, which results in a continual decline in total DNA methylation. They may turn off other activities, such as DNA repair mechanisms, which may be only fully maintained in germ-line cells. It is now well recognized that the efficiency of cell maintenance mechanisms is related to the longevity of mammalian species, and the resources invested must be at some optimum value for each species. It is also well known that the incidence of tumorigenesis per cell in short-lived animals such as rodents is enormously higher than in humans, and also that rodent cells spontaneously transform in vitro. The rare emergence of human tumors may have nothing to do with cell senescence, but may instead be related to an intrinsic resistance to transformation.

Concluding Remark

Specialized mammalian cells that are capable of division normally have a finite life span in vitro, and there is evidence that the extent of proliferation is related to the longevity of the donor species. Cells from long-lived species do not become transformed in vitro, but instead enter an irreversible non-proliferative state known as senescence. Senescence of human cells can be bypassed if certain tumor suppressor genes are inactivated, or if appropriate oncogenes are present. These cells characteristically proliferate to a higher PD level than senescence and then enter a period of growth arrest known as *crisis*.

The emergence of immortalized transformed cell lines depends on the ability to maintain telomeres either by telomerase activity or by an alternative mechanism known as ALT. It is reported that the introduction into normal cells of a gene coding for the catalytic subunit of telomerase known as hTERT results in a greatly extended life span. These cells have reachedat least 400 PDs and can be regarded as immortal. However, there is no published information about their karyotypes, cell morphology, or other phenotypic characteristics, such as contact inhibition. It is possible that events other than the acquisition of telomerase are necessary to establish immortalization. This is known to be the case in immortalized keratinocytes where loss of the Rb/ $p16^{INK4a}$ cell cycle control mechanism is also necessary.

Normal human diploid fibroblasts have at least two molecular clocks, and possibly there are others. The loss of telomeric DNA has received the most attention, but it is also well established that total DNA methylation steadily declines during the serial passaging of human fibroblasts. In contrast, immortalized cells maintain both telomeres and DNA methylation. Therefore, if maintenance of telomeres is the essential vent, it mst also be linked to maintenance of DNA methylation. Little is known about the regulatory mechanism that silences the gene(s) for telomerases in many normal somatic cells, or about the events that have activated it in many immortalized cells. Similarly, nothing is known about the conrol or maintenance of total DNA methylation.

Normal Syrian hamster fibroblasts have a very clear-cut senescence in vitro, from which transformed lines emerge rather rarely. These cells have telomerase actvity and maintain their telomeres. In contrast, they steadily lose DNA methylation during serial subculture. This suggests that the molecular clock for senescence may be loss of DNA methylation. In addiion, it is known that artificially reducing the level of DNA methylation in young human fibroblasts significantly reduces their final life span. These results indicate that senescence may be triggered by the loss of methylation. Oncogenes, or the loss of tumor suppressors, can lead to the bypass of senescence, and de novo methylation to maintain a constant level. These cells continue to lose telomeric DNA, and it may well be that this precipitates crisis, at a greater PD level than senescence. Many more studies are necessary to unravel the respective roles of different molecular clocks for senescence, or to discover whether an accumulation of cellular defects is responsible. Whatever precipitates senescence, it is widely agreed that this is related to an interference with normal cell cycle controls that results in an irreversible block in cell division.

3

MUTATION

Mendel's work in 1900. In 1901 he published his accumulated data in a book entitle. The Mutation Theory. De Varies was careful to distinguish between hereditary and environmental variations, but his mutations are now known to have included several kinds of changes in the hereditary material. It took nearly half a century to clarify the situation in Oenothera and discover the causes of the variations that he observed. Chromosome changes, both structural and numerical, were eventually found to cause the phenotypic variation that de Vries had grouped under the heading of mutations. One complex alteration is described later on in this chapter in connection with the discussion of permanent heterozygotes. It was de Vries' concept of discontinuous variation rather than his precise observations and example that became significant. None of his examples would now be classified as gene mutations.

MUTATIONS AND PHENOTYPIC CHANGE

Because genes are chemical entities that cannot be observed and compared directly, some phenotypic alteration must be associated with the gene change (mutation) or it will go unrecognized. Minor changes presumably occur in genes as a matter of course without producing any phenotypic alterations. Some gene changes are known to be associated with only slight effects on the fertility or viability of the organism. These alterations ordinarily go undetected unless critical comparisons are made. They may, however, influence natural selection and thus represent a factor in evolution.

Mutations also represent in evolution, by which the presence of particular wild-type genes can be postulated. Normal development of any organism is influenced by numerous genes. An observable characteristic of the adult may be altered by an individual gene substitution, but because the entire organism develops as a unit, the action of individual wild-type genes is not always apparent. The existence of mutant and wild-type genes is substantiated when a gene is changed so that its influence on developmental reactions causes a visible difference from that exerted by the unmutated gene. Mutations thus provide the basis for postulating wild-type genes.

Mutated as well unmutated genes tend to give rise to other genes exactly like themselves. Once established, a mutated gene is as stable as the original gene from which the mutation occurred. This process of duplication is associated with mitotic cell division and occurs repeatedly as the number of cells increases. Duplication among genes has a crude parallel in the procedure of printing. After type is set and placed on the printing press; similar copies can be made repeatedly. If the type is changed slightly with an altered template replacing the original, the new pattern reproduces itself faithfully. Instead of a physical change, such as the substitution of one piece of metal for another, the gene in the process of mutation undergoes a chemical change. A part of the gene unit is altered by the chemical modification in such a way that it henceforth behaves differently from its unmutated ancestral gene.

Not all mutations are immediately detectable because many, perhaps the great majority, are recessive and must become homozygous before they can express themselves. Because the phenotypic effect is the only readily observable evidence of mutations, however, a sudden phenotypic change that subsequently proves to be heritable is an accepted indication that mutation has occurred in an organism. In everyday language, the phenotypic change is synomous with the gene change or actual mutation. This is quite natural because the term"mutation" was coined and used before the present gene concept was established. Historically, therefore, the word has been used to describe the perceptible change alteration. It is now known that most mutations that are not detectable by visible phenotypic change influence the viability of the organism in some indirect way.

Classification for Mutations

Dominance and recessiveness provided convenient, although perhaps superficial, criteria for early classifications of mutations. Mutations also may occur in either the autosomes or the X chromosomes, and thus may be classified as autosomal or sex-linked. Viability mutations have also been classified on the basis of their effect on the organism.

Various mutations of this nature in Drosophila have been expressed in the egg, larva, pupa, or adult. When disadvantageous, the mutations are called deleterious; when disastrous to the individual, they are called lethals. Relatively few mutations occur as dominants and even fewer are advantageous in the environments where they occur. The great majority of changes are recessive and detrimental under usual environmental conditions. In a changing environment, a mutation may happen to coincide with new environmental situations and be favourable.

Pleiotropy

A given mutation may alter the organism severely or have such slight effect that it can be detected only when associated with other genes, through cumulative action. The name and gene symbol associated with a mutation are usually taken from the most conspicuous phenotypic alteration that the mutation produces. Thus, white eye (w) is used in contrast to the wild type, red; and ebony (e) body designates the deviation of dark from wild type, gray body colour. This method of designation perpetuates an overly simplified concept of the effects of mutations. Because they exert their influence on basic chemical reactions in the developmental period, single mutant genes affect more than a single trait and may modify in some way every trait of the organism.

The term *pleiotropy* refers to the situation in which a gene is known to influence more than a single trait. For example, in the presence of the white-eye mutation in *Drosphila melanogaster*, the ocelli, malpighian tubules, and testicular envelopes are colourless, whereas these structures in wild flies are coloured. The balancers and wing muscles are altered and the general viability and fertility of the flies are changed. Sheldon Reed has demonstrated a discrimination against white-eyed flies in mating. Such discrimination indicates that the gene causes some effect on the cuticle that influences the mating stimulus. White eye is thus only one several effects of the single mutant gene (w). Many examples of genes with more than single effect have been discovered. All genes (mutants and nonmutants) may be pleiotropic, even though their various effects are not recognized at present. Even though a gene may have many end effects, probably it influences only one primary function in the chemistry of the developing individual.

Congenital hydrocephalus in the mouse, cited by Gruneberg, illustrates the manifold effects of a single gene, ch, on the developing mouse. The gene occurred as a spontaneous mutation and was found by preliminary studies to influence cartilage formation in early development of the mouse. Mice that carried the gene in homozygous condition were born alive but died immediately after birth because the lungs did not inflate properly. Other conspicuous abnormalities also occurred: the skull, forehead, and face were out of proportion; large protuberances filled with fluid extended out from the cerebral hemispheres because the skull bones were abnormal and only skin covered the forehead; eyelids were always open; sensory hairs of the face were abnormal; and the sternum was abnormal with little or no bone formation. Developmental studies showed that abnormalities occurred as early as the thirteenth day in the embryo. The manifold effects were traced back to a single cause, the abnormal cartilage formation. Various skeletal abnormalities were involved directly; physiological disturbances occurred secondarily. A single primary reaction concerned with cartilage formation was controlled by the mutant gene.

Somatic and Germinal Mutation

Mutations may occur in any cell and at any stage in the cell cycle. The immediate effect of the mutation and its ability to produce phenotypic change is determined by its dominance, the type of cell in which it occurs, and the stage in the cycle of the cell. If the mutation occurs in a somatic cell that can reproduce other cells like itself but not the whole organism, the mutant change would be perpetuated only in somatic cells that descended from the original cell in which the mutation occurred.

The "Delicious" apple and the naval orange have resulted from mutations that occurred in somatic tissues. Changes that gave these two fruits their desirable qualities apparently followed spontaneous mutation in single cells, which constituted only a very small part of the body of the individual apple and orange trees that were involved. In each case, the cell carrying the mutant gene gave rise to more of its own kind, eventually producing an entire branch on its respective tree which had the charactristics of the mutant type. Fortunately, it is possible to propagate desirable types of many plants by vegetative methods such as budding and grafting. Vegetative propagation was feasible for both the delicious apple and the navel orange, and today numerous progeny from grafts and buds have perpetuated the original mutation. Descendants of the mutant types are now widespread in apple orchards and orange groves.

Results of somatic mutations have been detected in animals as well as in plants. In Drosophila, white sectors are infrequently observed in an otherwise red eye. Sectors in some male flies have been demonstrated to be composed of descendants from a single cell in which a mutation had occurred (at the w locus in the X chromosome). If the same change had occurred in a germ cell, a white-eyed male might have been produced.

If dominant mutant genes occur in germ cells, their effects may be expressed immediately in the progeny. If they are recessive or hypostatic, their effects may be obscured by other genes. Germinal mutations, like somatic mutations, may occur at any stage in the cycle of the organism but they are more common in some stages, particularly during the gene replication process preceding gametogenesis. If the mutation arises in one of the gametes produced by an individual, a single member of the progeny may receive the mutatant gene. If, on the other hand, a mutation occurs during an earlier stage of gametogenesis, several gametes may receive the mutant gene and therefore several individuals could perpetuate it. In any case, the dominance of the gene and the stage in the cycle when the mutation occurs are major factors in determining the extent of any expression that follows.

Wright noticed a peculiar male lamb with unusually short legs in this flock of sheep. It occurred to him that it would be an advantage to have a whole flock of these short-legged sheep, which could not get over the low stonefences in his New England neighbourhood. Wright used the new short-legged ram for breeding his 15 ewes in the next season. Two of the 15 lambs produced were short-legged. Short-legged sheep were then bred together and a line was developed in which the new trait was expressed in all individuals. The mutation that gave rise to the short-legged sheep was obviously of the germinal type because the cell carrying the mutation had the capacity to reproduce the entire organism. Other examples of germinal mutations have since been described in a wide variety of animals and plants.

Mutation by Deletion or Insertion of Nucleotide Bases

Consider the sequences of bases written in the RNA code shown in Figure 3.1. Now suppose that a base is deleted or an additional base is inserted. The net effect of either a deletion or an insertions that the reading frame is shifted, because different triplets are now read after the mutation site. These are called frameshift mutations. Their net effect is that the amino acids inserted after the deletion or insertion will be different from those in the unmutated cell, and hence the polypeptide will contain a grossly abnormal amino acid sequence

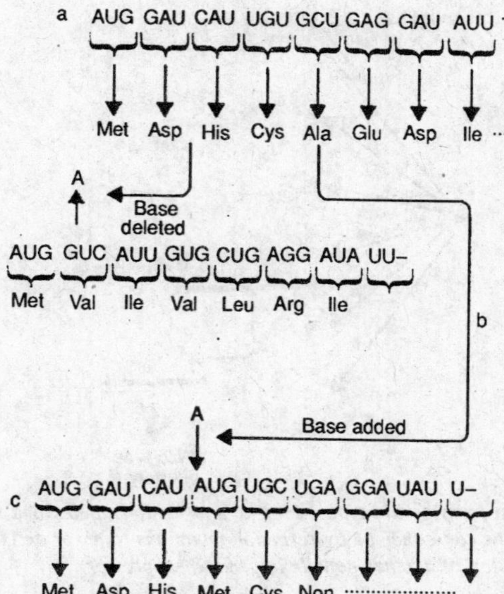

Fig. 3.1. Base deletion and base addition resulting in frameshift mutations. Translation is from left to right.

and be nonfunctional. In addition, somewhere along the line it is possible for a nonsense codon to be produced and the "nonsense" chain will be terminated.

Note that the addition or deletion of two bases will have essentially the same effect as a single base addition or deletion because the reading frame will shift. A three-base change will not shift the reading frame if three immediately adjacent nucleotides are added or deleted, but simply add or delete an amino acid. This is also true for duplication or insertion of adjacent bases in multiples of three. Two or more amino acids will be affected instead of one.

Like nonsense mutations, frameshift mutations can be expected to have drastic effects on the phenotype, unless they occur in multiples of three or cause a change at a nonessential end of a protein. In the latter case, the effect may be great or hardly noticeable, depending again on the position of the deleted or added amino acid(s) in the polypeptide chain. Frameshift mutations can be suppressed by other mutations.

The Reversal of the Mutant Phenotype

So far in this chapter we have been looking at mutation in a somewhat restricted way. It has been tacitly assumed that there is a

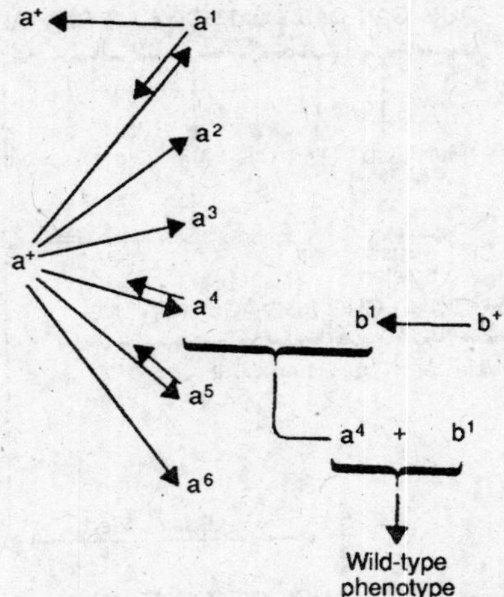

Fig. 3.2. Mutation from a wild-type allele (a^+) to mutant alleles and reversions. The reversions can either be by reversion mutations to a^+ or an isoallele ($a^{+\prime}$) or by mutation of another nonallelic gene (a suppressor).

wild-type allele (or group of wild-type alleles called *isoalleles*, which all produce a wild-type phenotype) for each gene that mutates to produce mutant alleles in an unidirectional way. However, mutation can occur either way. The mutant phenotype observed is a result of a forward mutation, and the change back to the original genotypic state is a reverse mutation, by definition. In addition, reversal of phenotype to the original situation, or almost so, may occur without a reversal of genotype but rather by a further mutation in the same gene or in another nonallelic gene. We consider these two situations in this section.

Reverse Mutation

If a missense mutation occurs by substitution of a nucleotide base, it should be expected that it can be reversed by a second substitution in the same codon so as to change it back to the condition in which it will code for the original amino acid, or one which will again give a wild-type phenotype. This has been demonstrated in a most convincing fashion by the use of the chemical mutagens about whose action we have some knowledge. Consider the action of 5-bromouracil, which, pointed out previously, causes transitions of the A:T–G:C type, if 5-bromouracil is able in its enol state to pair with guanine it should also be able to pair with adenine when not in the enol state, as the new chain is forming in the mutant. The net effect is another transition, G:C – A:T, the reverse of the first situation. Therefore, mutations

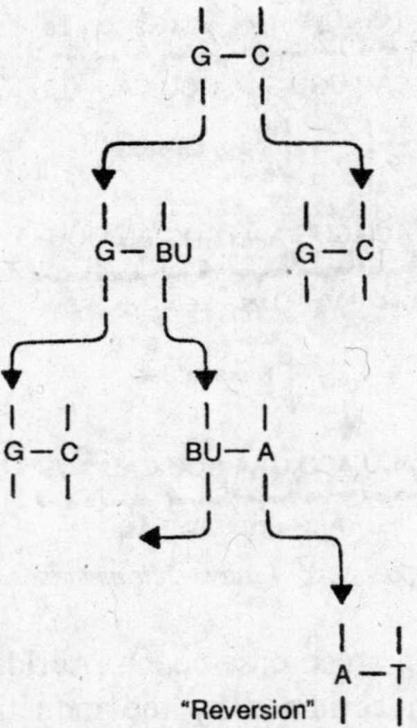

Fig. 3.3. The reversion of a mutation initially caused by 5-bromouracil.

caused by 5-bromouracil should be reversible by 5-bromouracil, and this turns out to be the case. 2-Aminopurine and nitrous acid will also cause reversion of 5-bromouracil-induced mutations.

Hydroxylamine is somewhat different from 5-bromouracil, 2-aminopurine, an nitrous, acid; mutations caused by it are not truly reverted by it. All these results agree with the theory that 5-bromouracil, 2-aminopurine, and nitrous acid should cause transitions in both direction (A:T G:C). Hydroxylamine should cause transitions in only one direction (G:C A:T).

Ethyl ethanesulfonate (EES) apparently causes transitions in the G:C—A:T direction and also transversions such as G:C T:A and G:C C:G. Some, but not all, EES-induced mutants are reverted by base analogues and nitrous acid. The reading frame mutations caused by acridines do not revert in the presence of base analogues or compounds that later bases. And this, of course, is precisely what is to be expected, because acridines cause the deletion and duplication of bases. On the other hand, mutations caused by acridines are for the most part revertible by acridines. In this fact there resides another interesting story; revertants of reading frame mutations may occur in several ways as related in the next several paragraphs.

Intragenic Supressors

An acridine-induced mutant will usually (if not always) result in a gene deficient or duplicated for bases. This shifts the reading frame

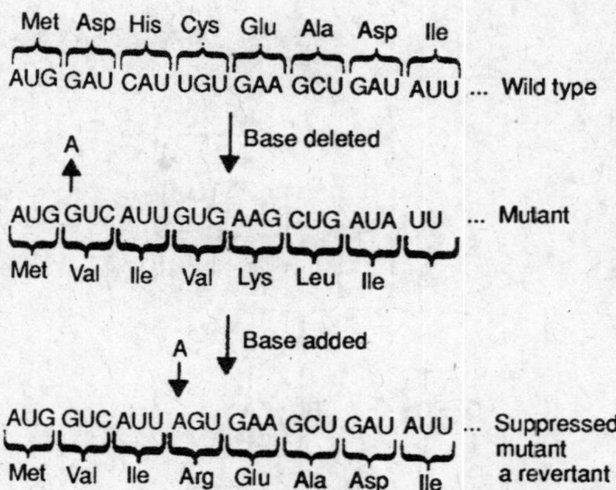

Fig. 3.4. How intragenic suppressors of frame-shift mutations act to produce a functional polypeptide.

and generally results in a nonsense codon, Acridine-induced mutations can be reverted with acridines by the induction of an intragenic suppressor. If the original mutation is a deletion of a base, the suppressor will be an insertion of a base occurring nearby in the DNA. As a result, the reading frame would be brought back to the state in which the proper amino acids are now coded, except for that region between the two mutations. In an analogous way an insertion initially caused by acridine can be suppressed by a deletion. If the amino acids coded for in this region do not form a segment that is important to the protein's ability to function, a true suppression of the mutant phenotype will occur.

A second type of intragenic suppressor involves missense mutations. As stated before, a single amino acid substitution caused by a missense mutation may so disrupt a polypeptide's tertiary conformation that is inactive as a protein. It has been shown that such a mutation may be rectified by a second missense mutation in the same gene. The second amino acid substitution in some way erases the "lethal" change in tertiary conformation caused by the first. This has been demonstrated in the tryptophan synthetase of E. coli and is probably a fairly common even in all organisms.

Extragenic Suppressors

When a nonsense codon is formed either by missense or frameshifts mutation, a drastic phenotypic change is expected because the polypeptide encoded by the affected gene will be incompletely synthesized during translation. Such mutants can be restored to approximately the wild-type phenotype by the occurrence of another mutation in a gene at another locus. Five such suppressors have been described in E. coli. They all suppress one or the other of the two nonsense codons: UAG and UAA or both. It has been shown that in the presence of a suppressor mutation amino acids are actually inserted during translation at points where nonsense codons exist. Hence the polypeptide chains are completed, although the completed chains may not function as well as the polypeptide chains coded in the wild type.

As might be expected, it has been found that the biochemical basis for the action of these suppressor genes is that they code for tRNA's. The sup D gene codes for serine tRNA. In its mutant condition, it produces an altered serine tRNA that introduces serine where a UAG occurs in the messenger. Similar explanations apply for the other suppressor genes, which presumably code for other tRNA's.

These kinds of suppressors have been *supersuppressors*. They are so named because they are capable of suppressing nonsense mutations in a wide range of different genes with quite different and unrelated functions. Theoretically, any gene can mutate by the formation of a nonsense codon. Hence, a single suppressor may effectively suppress specific alleles of a large number of different genes, provided the amino acid it introduces through its altered tRNA results in functional polypeptides. Suppressors have been reported in yeast, *Neurospora*, and perhaps barley. They probably also occur in *Drosophila*. The suppressor of Hairy Wing in *D. melanogaster* suppresses at least 10 other mutant genes, all of which are at different loci and have seemingly unrelated functions.

Suppressors in diploid organisms theoretically should always be dominant, because only one dose of altered tRNA gene should be necessary to produce the tRNA necessary to recognize a nonsense codon. However, suppressors do exist that are expressed only when homozygous. The suppressor of Hairy Wing is one example. Another example in Drosophila is the suppressor of vermilion su(s). It suppresses the mutant condition, sable(s). The action of this type of suppressor, other examples of which are known in *Drosophila*, is not clear.

Missense, Nonsense, and Frameshift Mutations

Various types of mutations can conveniently be discussed in relation to the b-globin gene. It has already been described that the human b-globin gene is split into three coding regions interrupted by two intervening sequences. The nucleotide sequence of the beginning of the first coding region, the sense strand is at the top, and transcription occurs from left to right (from the 3' end of the sense strand to the 5' end). The spaces that separate adjacent triplets of bases do not exist in the actual molecule. It shows the corresponding portion of the b-globin mRNA produced after transcription and RNA processing. Although it is not shown in the figure, the next upstream codon from GUG is the AUG initiation codon, which codes for methionine. Figure shows the first eight amino acids at the amino terminal end of normal b-globin; the initial methionine with which translation begins is not represented in the finished polypeptide because it is enzymatically removed from the chain. The underlined nucleotides represent the restriction site for the restriction enzyme *Mst*II, which cleaves the DNA at this position.

As noted in the previous section, a *base substitution* mutation is one in which a base pair in a DNA duplex is replaced with a different base pair. A base substitution that leads to an amino acid substitution in the corresponding polypeptide is called a missense mutation, and there are two principal types of missense mutations. Part (*a*) again shows a portion of the first coding region of the b-globin gene, and part (B) shows the result of a base substitution in which the normal TA pair indicated is replaced with an AT pair. In this substitution, a pyrimidine base in the sense strant (T) is replaced with a purine base (A), and a purine base in the antisense sense strant (A) is replaced with a pyrimidine base (T). Any base substitution in which a purine (A or G) is replaced with a pyrimidine (T or C), or in which a pyrimidine is replaced with a purine, is called a *transversion*. Transcription and RNA processing of the mutant DNA lead to the mRNA shown in Figure; note that the sixth codon, which normally reads GAG, now reads GUG. Tranlation of this mRNA leads to a substitution of valine for glutamic acid at the sixth position in the polypeptide (black arrow). The transversion mutation is indeed the actual molecular change responsible for b^s hemoglobin. The b^s mutation also obliterates the *MSt* II restriction site, so *MSt* II will not cleave the b^s DNA at this position. This molecular difference provides a rapid and convenient method for *in vitro* diagnosis of sickle cell anemia.

There is another type of missense mutation, which is called a *transition* mutation because it involves the replacement of one purine (in this case G) with another purine (in this case A) or one pyrimidine (in this case C) with another pyrimidine (in this case T). In the transition mutation a CG base pair in the original molecule is replaced with a TA base pair. The corresponding portion of the mRNA is shown in part (C), and in this case the original GAG codon in position 6 is altered to AAG. Translation of the mutant mRNA produces a β-globin polypeptide in which the normal glutamic acid at position 6 is replaced with a lysine. This particular mutation is known as the β^c mutation. Sine the b^c mutation is relatively common in areas of the world where malaria is prevalent, it is thought that heterozygotes for β^c may have some protection against malaria, as is certainly the case with β^c.

Not all base substations are missense mutation. There is also another type of mutation called a nonsense mutation. A nonsense mutation is one that creates a chain-terminating codon [i.e., uAA (orchre), UAG (amber), or UGA (opal)] in a coding region. The name nonsense mutation may seem odd, but it comes from the fact that chain-terminating codons are times referred to as nonsense codons. The transvertion to leads to a UAG terminating codon at the sixth position in the mRNA. Thus, translation of this mRNA leads to a truncated polypeptide because translation terminates at the UAG codon.

In prokaryotes such as *E. coli* and in lower eukaryotes such as yeast, certain mutations have the ability to suppress nonsense mutations. These nonsense-suppressing mutations are called nonsense suppressors, and they involve mutations in genes for transfer RNA (tRNA) that reduce the faithfulness of translation so that chain-terminating codons are sometimes misread.

Such a mutant tRNA will correctly translate serine codons, but, on occasion, will misread a chain-terminating codon (in this case UAG) as a serine codon. Consequently, in some fraction of attempts at translation of the mutant mRNA, the UAG codon will be misread as serine (stipulated arrow), and translation will be able to produce normally beyond this point. If the serine-containing polypeptide is able to function, the phenotypic effects of the original nonsense mutation will have been suppressed by the nonsense suppressor.

Of course, nonsense suppressors can occur in tRNA genes other than serine tRNA. For example, if a UAG suppressor occurs in a gene for glycine tRNA, a UGA codon will sometimes be misread as a glycine codon, and glycine will be inserted into the polypeptide at this position. It should also be emphasized that a particular nonsense suppressor will suppress only one of the chain-terminating codons; that is, an *amber suppressor* will suppress only the UAG (amber) terminator, or *ochre suppressor* will suppress only the UAA (ochre) terminator, and an *opal suppressor* will suppress only the UGA (opal) terminator. Of course, a nonsense suppressor will occasionally misread normal termination codons, too; for example, an amber suppressor will occasionally misread a UAG codon at the end of a normal gene and the result is an abnormally long polypeptide. However, organisms that carry nonsense suppressor are able to survive in spite of the occasional misreading of normal genes.

Not all base-substitution mutations lead to missense or nonsense codons. Because the genetic code contains many synonymous codons, some base substitutions leave the amino acid sequence of the corresponding polypeptide unaltered. Such mutations are said to be silent. In this case a C/G-to-T/A transition at the third position in codon 6 of the β-globin gene leads to an mRNA that has GAA as its sixth codon. However, GAA is a synonymous codon for glutamic acid, so the amino acid sequence of the resulting polypeptide will be completely normal. As a brief inspection of the genetic code will reveal most silent substitutions in coding regions would be expected to involve transitions in the third position of a code. The situation may be very different for intervening sequence, however. Since a particular length and base sequence of an intervening sequence does not seem to be essential for proper gene function, many mutations in intervening sequences—transitions, transversions, even inversions, deletions, or insertions–may be silent.

A final example of a type of mutation that has relatively simple molecular basis is known as a *frameshift* mutation. A frameshift mutation alters the reading frame of an mRNA during translation and thereby greatly alters the amino acid sequence of the corresponding polypeptide. Frameshift mutations are caused by deletions of additions of a small number of nucleotides in a coding region; since the genetic code consists of triplets of nucleotides, any deletion or addition of a number of nucleotides other than an exact multiple of three will cause a shift in reading frame. An example of a frameshift mutation associated with a single nucleotide deletion is Part (a) is again a portion of the first coding region of the human β-globin gene, and the left side of the figure illustrates the normal course of transcription and translation of this sequence. As in previous figure involving this gene, small gaps are introduce in part (c) to show the normal triplet reading frame. The right side of the figure shows the consequence of a deletion of the indicated A/T nucleotide pair. When this deletion-bearing sequence is examined in terms of its triplet reading frame, it can be seen that all triplets beyond the second one are different from those in normal sequence. This lack of correspondence occurs, of course, because the

Table 3.1. Disorders of human hemoglobin

Type of hemoglobin	*Signs and cause*
S	Hemozygosity for β^S mutation (sickle cell anemia)
C	Homozygosity for β^C mutation
Lepore	δ-β chain fusion caused by unequal crossing-over in misaligned δ-β region
Anti-Lepore	Triplication consisting of normal δ gene-δ-β fusion gene-normal β gene; reciprocal crossover product of the unequal crossover leading to Lepore hemoglobin
Constant Spring	Elongated α chain due to missense mutation in terminator codon
Gun Hill	Shortened β chain due to deletion eliminating amio acids 91-95
Unstable hemoglobin	Increased blood destruction; associated with at least 70 mutations, most affecting β chain
Methemoglobulinemia	Reduced ability to transport oxygen; associated with several mutations, some affecting α, others β
Hemoglobin-induced erythrocytosis	Anemia due to increased oxygen affinity of hemoglobin causing stimulation of red blood cell production and consequent increased destruction; associated with at least 20 mutations
α-thalassemia	Reduced synthesis of α chain; principal cause is deletion of one or more α-gene copies; *hydrops fetalis* is a lethal disorder associated with absence of α chain
β-thalassemia	Reduced synthesis (β^+ form) or no synthesis (β^0 form) of β chain; some patients have β deletions; at least one β^0 form involves a mutation at the splice junction at the downstream end of the second intron.
Hereditary persistence of fetal hemoglobin	Continued synthesis of γ chains; postulated detection of DNA sequence responsible for γ→β switch

single-nucleotide deletion causes the triplet reading frame beyond the deletion to be shifted one nucleotide to the left. The extensive lack of correspondence due to the frameshift mutation is also evident in the mRNA, and the resulting amino acid sequence in the polypeptide is hardly recognizable as a β-globin sequence. Such out-of-frame translation will continue along the mutant mRNA until a termination codon is encountered.

Mutations Resulting from Unequal Crossing-Over

It has been stated that unequal crossing-over involving duplications can lead to an increase or decrease in the number of copies of the region. When this process occurs at the molecular level, it creates new types of DNA sequences that qualify as mutations. An example of unequal crossing-over creating new mutations is found in the human β-globin gene. Part (a) shows part of the DNA sequence coding for amino acids 83 through 98, which is 18 nucleotides upstream from the second intervening sequence. The boxes indicate two nearby regions that have a perfect eight-nucleotide homology that can act as a duplication. Part (b) shows the coding sequence for amino acids 88 through 103; it has been shifted to the left relative to part (a) to show how the regions of homology can mispair (shaded boxes). As before, the gaps in the DNA sequence indicate the translational reading frame.

Sequence (c) combines the left part of (a) with the right part of (b). This sequence is deleted for the nucleotides that code for amino acids 91 through 95, and it is of some interest that this deletion, called the *Gun Hill deletion*, is found in certain rare individuals. Sequence (d) is the complementary crossover product to sequence (c); this sequence carries a duplication of the nucleotides that code for amino acids 91 through 95.

Mutagenic agents and the Mechanisms of Mutation

Mutations occur in the somatic and germ cell of all organisms. In organisms like Drosophila, mutations are detected for specific loci in one in about 10^5 to 10^6 gametes. Therefore the spontaneous mutation rate for most genes is about 10^{-5} to 10^{-6} mutations per locus per generation. First, agents that increase the mutation rate above the spontaneous level will be discussed because they help explain the spontaneous rate. The two basic kinds of mutagenic agents are (1) physical ones including radiation (s) and (2) chemical ones, consisting of both "natural" and "unnatural" substances.

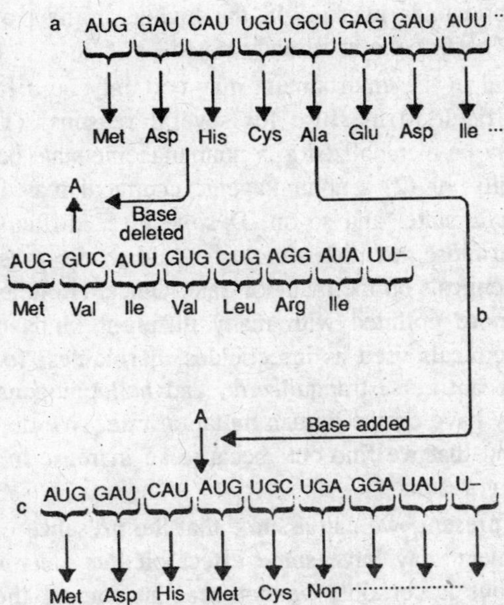

Fig. 3.5. Base deletion and base addition resulting in frameshift mutation.

The Spontaneous Mutation Rate

An organism carefully protected from known mutagenic chemicals and from known artificially made radioactive sources will still produce gametes or cells with new gene mutations, What causes these spontaneous mutations? A number of factors can be enumerated and may be divided into two categories: environmental and genetic.

Environmental Factors

Background radiation comes to mind as a factor almost immediately, because we have been sensitized since the 1950s to the hazards of ionizing radiation from atomic bombs, industrial and medical applications of nuclear energy, and so forth. However, the average background measured in roentgens per generation is insufficient to account for more than a small fraction of spontaneously occurring sex-linked recessive lethals in Drosophila. But, course, if the background radiation is raised, this could cause additional mutations that might become an important factor in the future of humans and all other organisms.

Ultraviolet light may not be of much significance in the production of mutations since the ultraviolet in sunlight that reaches the surface of the earth has wavelengths only above 300 nm. This range of wavelengths is not effective in inducing mutations to any marked extent except somatic ones in skin. In the higher animals overlying tissue protects the germ cells as already noted.

Chemical in the environment may certainly be a factor, but their effect is difficult to measure for several reasons: (1) a mutagenic chemical may be metabolized to a nonmutagenic state before it reaches the germ cells, or (2) a nonmutagenic chemical may be metabolized to a mutagenic state, and so on. Despite these difficulties, it is now apparent that close attention should be paid to the present and future effects of chemicals on the mutation rate. Our environment is becoming more and more polluted with many different kinds of natural and synthetic chemicals used as insecticides, herbicides, food preservers, medicines, beautifiers, tranquilizers, and hallucinogens. What effect do these how have on the human mutation rate? We do not know, but it is important that we find out, because an increase in the rate could have diastrous results.

For the present, we can assume that the presence of chemicals in the environment may have some effect on the mutation rate of all organisms, but it certainly cannot account for all the spontaneous mutation rate. Metabolic products, such as formaldehyde and hydrogen peroxide produced within cells, may also be involved, but here again it is doubtful that their effects are highly significant.

Genetic Factors

Organisms evolved in a changing environment to which they had to continually adapt as they evolved. Mutations were necessary for this evolution to occur, just as they are necessary for future evolution. But the mutation rate must not be so high that it results in the production of many deleterious mutation that would act as "genetic load" on the population.

It is highly probable that the main component of the spontaneous mutation rate is genetically controlled. As we have described in previous pages, enzymes are involved in the replication of DNA. Mistakes of different types may occur during replication that may lead to mutation, especially if the replicating enzymes themselves are deficient. These mistakes may be replicated or they may be repaired by the repair systems that we known to exist. Thus, two opposing systems, genetically controlled, may be postulated to exist: the replicative synthetic one and the repair system. The spontaneous rate of mutation may be determined by an equilibrium point between them.

It has long been known that different populations of *Drosophila melanogaster* collection from widely scattered areas in different part of the world show significantly different mutation rates. Furthermore, genes have been identified that have an influence on the mutation rate A second chromosome gene, *hi*, and a third chromosome gene, *mu*, have been located in *melangoaster*. Both of these increase the "spontaneous" mutation rate when homozygous, although *mu* appears to act in this way only in females. Extensive work has been done in E. coli with mutant strains that show a high rate of A:T → C:G transversions. The result is that the mutation rates as specific loci are raised several thousand fold!

Table 3.2. Spontaneous mutation rates found in different populations of *D. melanogaster*, sex-linked and second chromosome recessive lethals

	X chromosome			*Second chromosome*		
Stock	*Number tested*	*Number lethals*	*Percent lethals*	*Number tested*	*Number lethals*	*Percent lethals*
Florida inbred	2108	23	1.09	—	—	—
Wooster	1266	8	0.63	—	—	—
Oregon R	3049	2	0.07	—	—	—
Florida No. 10	916	10	1.09	516	9	1.74
Lausanne	955	2	0.21	436	3	0.69
Leningrad	8614	14	0.16	—	—	—
Sukhami	2309	24	1.04	—	—	—

Genes that raise the mutation rate are called *mutator* genes. A number of these have been identified in yeast, *Drsosophia*, and E. coli. They have yet to be directly implicated in the DNA replicative and repair processes, but it is difficult to believe that they are not.

In addition to mutator genes, there are also numerous examples of mutable loci in a variety of organisms. Certain alleles of some genes exhibit an unstable condition, so that they mutate from the wild type to mutant condition at a high rate in either the germ cells, or somatic cells, or both.

Phenotypic Effects of Mutations

Mutations must normally cause some detectable *phenotypic change* for their presence to be recognized. The effects of mutations on phenotype range from alterations so minor that they can be detected only by special genetic or biochemical techniques to gross modifications of morphology to lethals. A gene is a specific sequence of nucleotide pairs coding for a particular polypeptide. Any mutation occurring within a given gene will thus produce a new form or *new allele* of that gene. Because of the degeneracy of the genetic code, some base pair changes do not change the protein products coded for by the genes in any way. Genes containing mutations with small effects that can be recognized only by special techniques are called "isoalleles." Other mutations result in total loss of gene-product activity. If mutations of the latter type occur in essential genes (genes required for viability), they will, of course, be lethal.

Mutations may be either recessive or dominant. In haploid (or, more accurately, monoploid) organisms like viruses and bacteria, both recessive and dominant mutations can be recognized by their effects on the phenotype of the organism in which they originated. The dominance or recessiveness of mutations in bacteria can be determined only by studying partial diploids. In diploid (or polyploid) organisms, recessive mutations will be recognized only when present in the homozygous condition. Most recessive mutations in diploids will not be recognized at the time of their occurrence, since they will be present in the heterozygous state. Sex-linked recessive mutations are an exception, since they will be expressed in the hemizygous state in the heterogametic sex (males in humans and fruit flies; females in birds). Sex-linked recessive lethal mutations will alter the sex ratio, since hemizygous individuals carrying the lethal will not survive.

The most useful mutations for the genetic analyses of many biological processes are conditional lethal mutations. These are mutations that are (1) lethal in one environment, the so-called restrictive conditions, but are (2) viable in a second environment, the permissive conditions. Such mutations allow geneticists to identify and study mutations in essential genes that result in complete loss of gene-product activity even in haploid organisms. Mutants carrying conditional lethal can be propagated under permissive conditions, and information about the functions of the gene products can be deduced by studying the consequences of their absence under the restrictive conditions. Conditional lethal mutations also provide valuable selective mutations also provide valuable selective sieve for genetic fine structure analysis.

The three major classes of mutants with conditional lethal mutations are (1) *auxotrophic mutants*, (2) *temperature-sensitive mutants*, and (3) *suppressor-sensitive mutants*. Auxotrophic mutants (as opposed to prototrophic "wild-types") are mutants that are unable to synthesize an essential metabolite (amino acid, purine, pyrimidine, vitamin, etc.) That is synthesized de novo by wild-type individuals of the species.

Such auxotrophic mutants will grow and reproduce when the metabolite is supplied in the medium (the permissive condition); they will not grow when the essential metabolite is absent (the restrictive condition). Temperature-sensitive mutants will grow at one temperature but not at another temperature. Most temperature-sensitive mutants are heat-sensitive some, however, are cold-sensitive. The temperature sensitivity usually results from increases heat or cold lability of the mutant gene product, for example, an enzyme which is active at low temperature but partially or totally inactive at higher temperatures. Occasionally, only the synthesis of the gene product is sensitive to temperature, and once synthesized, the mutant gene product may be as stable as the wild-type gene product, Suppressor-sensitive mutants are viable when a second genetic factor, a suppressor, is present, but are nonviable in the absence of the suppressor. The suppressor gene may correct or compensate for the defect in phenotype that is caused by the suppressor-sensitive mutation, or it may render the gene product, altered by the mutation, nonessential.

Most of the thousands of mutations that have been identified and studied by geneticists have been found to be deleterious and recessive. This is to be expected, considering what we know about the genetic control of metabolism and the techniques available for identifying mutations. Metabolism occurs by sequences of chemical reactions, each step of which is catalyzed by a specific enzyme coded for by one or more genes. Mutations in these genes frequently produce blocks in metabolic pathway. These blocks occur because changes in the base-pair sequences of genes often (but not always) cause changes in the amino acid sequences of polypeptides, which may, in turn, result in loss of function. This, in fact has been the most commonly observed effect of easily detected mutations. Given a wild-type allele coding for an active enzyme and mutant alleles coding for less active or totally inactive enzymes, it is apparent why most of the observed mutations might be recessive, as is observed. If the enzyme is metabolically important, such mutations will also be deleterious. If the enzyme catalyzes an essential reaction, the mutations causing total loss of activity will be recessive lethals.

But why should most mutations with phenotypically recognizable effects result in decreased gene produce activity or no gene-produce activity? This result can be predicted if one accepts the effectiveness of natural selection and if one accepts the effectiveness of natural selection and if one assumes the existence of a semiconstant environment during the recent (on the evolutionary scale) evolution of life forms on earth. A "wild-type" allele of a gene coding for a "wild-type" enzyme or structural protein will have been selected for optimal activity for many generations. Mutations resulting in amino acid changes that increased the efficiencies of enzymes in carrying out particular functions will have been preserved by natural selection, and, as the most "fit," they will have become the new "wild-types". Given a sufficient period of time in semiconstant environment, most, if not all, sequences of amino acids (at least all sequences of amino acids that differ form the "wild-type" by a single mutation) will have been tried, and natural selection will have preserved the most efficient one. It will now be the wild-type. Mutations, which produce changes in these very specific sequences of amino acids, will usually result in less activity or no activity at all. As such, they will most frequently be recessive and deleterious.

An analogy can be made with any complex, carefully engineered machine. If you randomly modify any one essential component (e.g., of a watch or an automobile), it seldom performs as well as it did prior to the random change.

Radiation-Induced Mutation

That portion of the electromagnetic spectrum containing wavelengths that are shorter and of higher energy than visible light (wavelengths below about 0.1 μm) can be subdivided into ionizing radiation (X rays, gamma rays, and cosmic rays) and nonionizing radiation (ultraviolet light). Ionizing radiations such as X rays (about 0.1 to 1 nm) are of high energy and thus are useful for medical diagnosis because they can penetrate living tissues. In the process of penetrating matter, these high-energy rays collide with atoms and cause there lease of electrons, leaving positively charged free radicals or ions. These ions, in turn, collide with other molecules, causing the release of further electrons. The net result is that a "core" of ions is formed along the track of each high-energy ray as it passes through matter of living tissues. This process of ionization (thus the name ionizing radiation) is induced by machine-produced X rays, protons, and neutrons, as well as by the alpha, beta, and gamma rays released by radioactive isotopes of the elements (e.g., ^{32}P, ^{35}S, radium, cobalt-90 etc.). Ultraviolet rays having lower energy, penetrate only the surface layer of cells in higher plants and animals and do not induce ionization. Ultraviolet rays dissipate their energy to atoms that they encounter, raising the electrons in the outer orbitals to higher energy levels, a state referred to as excitation. Molecules containing atoms in either ionic forms or excited states are chemically more reactive than those containing atoms in their normal stable states. The increased reactivity of atoms present in DNA molecules is the basis of the mutagenic effects of ultraviolet light and ionizing radiation.

Ionizing Radiation

In 1927, H. J. Muller first demonstrated that mutation could be induced by an external factor. Muller demonstrated that X-ray treatment markedly increased the frequency of sex-linked recessive lethal mutations in D. melanogaster. Muler's unambiguous demonstration of the mutagenicity of X rays became possible by his development of a technique facilitating the simple and accurate identification of lethal mutations in the X chromosome of Drosophila. This technique, called the ClB method, involves the use of females heterozygous for a normal X chromosome and X chromosome (The ClB chromosome) specifically constructed for Muller's experiment.

The ClB chromosome has three essential components. (1) The C (for crossover "suppressor") refers to the presence of a long inversion, that prevents recombination of genetic markers on the *ClB* chromosome and alleles on the normal X chromosome. The inversion does not actually prevent crossing over, but causes gametes containing X chromosomes produced by crossing over between the *ClB* chromosome and the normal X chromosome to be inviable. Chromosomes resulting from crossing over between a chromosome containing an inversion (an inverted segment of the chromosome) and a normal chromosome will contain duplication and deficiencies (repeated and missing sets of genes). The inversion is required in Muller's experiment to assure that the markers on the *ClB* chromosome stay together through meioses. (2) The *l* refers to a recessive lethal in the *ClB* chromosome. (3) The *B* refers to the presence of the partially dominant mutation that causes the bar eye phenotype, which is a narrow, slit-shaped eye. Because it is partially dominant, it allows females heterozygous for the *ClB* chromosome to be readily identified. Both the recessive lethal (*l*) and the bar eye mutation (*B*) are located within the inverted segment of the *ClB* chromosome.

Given females heterozygous for the *ClB* chromosome. Muller's experiment was operationally quite simple. Males flies were irradiated and mated with *ClB* females. The bar-eyed irradiated and mated with ClB females. The bar-eyed daughters of this mating will carry the *ClB* chromosome of the female parent and the irradiated X chromosome of the male parent and the irradiated X chromosome of the male parent. Since the entire population of reproductive cells of the males was irradiated, each bar-eyed daughter carries a potentially mutated X chromosome. That is, each male is likely to produce some sperm that contain X chromosomes carrying new lethal mutations and some sperm without X-linked lethal mutations. The bar-eyed daughters were then mated individually (in separate bottles) with wild-type males. If the irradiated X chromosomes carried by a bar-eyed daughter contains a sex-linked lethal, all of the progeny of the mating will be female. Since males are hemizygous for the X chromosome, those receiving the *ClB* chromosome will die due to the recessive lethal (*l*) that it carries. Those receiving the irradiated X chromosome will also die if a recessive lethal has been induced in it. Matings of bar-eyed daughters carrying an irradiated X chromosome, in which no lethal mutation has bee induced, with wild-type males will produce female and male progeny in a ratio of 2:1 (only the males with the *ClB* chromosome will die). Scoring for the presence of recessive sex-linked lethals is thus unambiguous and error free using the *ClB* technique—simply scoring for the presence or absence of male progeny. By using this technique. Muller was able to demonstrate an increase in mutation rate of up to 150-fold after X-ray treatment.

Another technique that facilitates the detection of mutations in Drosophila, in this case sex-linked mutations with visible effects on phenotype (often called "visible mutations"), involves the use of *attached-X-chromosomes*. Attached-X-chromosomes undergo compulsory nondisjunction (failure of homologous chromosomes or chromatids to disjoin or separate during anaphase) since the two X chromosomes are joined to single centromere. If females with two attached-X chromosomes plus a Y chromosome (XXY) are mated to normal males, any mutation that occurs on the X chromosome of the male will be expressed in the surviving male progeny. In such attached-X matings, the male progeny receive their X chromosome from their male parent, rather that from their female parent as in a normal mating. If the male parent is treated with a mutagenic agent such as X rays, the increased frequency of recessive visible mutations can be easily assessed by screening the male progeny of the attached-X mating.

X rays and most other forms of ionizing radiation are quantitated in roentgen units (r units, pronounced "runtgen"), which are measured in terms of the number of ionizations per unit volume under a standard set of conditions. More specifically, one roentgen unit is the quantity of ionizing radiation that produces one electrostatic unit of charge in a one cm^3 volume. Note that the dosage of irradiation in roentgen units does not involve a time scale. The same dosage may be obtained by a low intensity of irradiation over a long period of time or a high intensity of irradiation for a short period of time. This is very important because in most studies the frequency of induced point mutations is directly proportional to the dosage of irradiation. In Drosophila sperm, for example, there is an increase of approximately 3 percent in the mutation rate for each 1000 r in increase in irradiation dosage. This linear relationship between mutation frequency and dosage in indicative of so called "single-hit- kinetics." That is, only one event (ionization?) or one "hit" is required to cause a mutation. Or, stated differently, every ionization has some fixed (under a specific set of conditions) probability of inducing a mutation. If the cumulative effects of many ionizations were required to induce a mutation, would plot as a curve that was concave upward.

The linear relationship between mutation rate and radiation dosage is important because it speaks directly to the frequency asked question of What is a safe level of irradiation? Even very low levels of irradiation have certain low, but very real, probabilities of inducing mutations. The question is thus meaningless. There is, no such thing as a safe level. In *Drosophila* sperm, for example, very low levels of irradiation over long periods of time (chronic irradiation) are as effective in inducing mutations as the same total dosage of irradiation administered at high intensity for short periods of time (acute irradiation). This clearly has major practical significance in evaluating the effects of the increased exposure of living organisms to radiation that results from the testing and use of nuclear weapons and nuclear reactors in generators, spaceships, and so on.

In mice, chronic irradiation has been found to induce somewhat fewer mutations than the same dosage of acute irradiation. Moreover, when mice were treated with intermittene doses of irradiation, the mutation frequency was slightly lower than when they were treated with the same total amount of irradiation in a continuous dose. It should be emphasized that all of these irrdiation treatments were mutagenic, albeit, to different degrees, to both Drosophila and mice. The different responses of fruit flies and mice to chronic irradiation may result from differences in their ability to repair damaged DNA. Repair mechanisms may exist in the spermatogonia and oocytes of mice that do not exist in Drosophila sperm.

The single-hit theory implies that one ionization can produce one mutation, but it does not imply anything about the efficiency with which this happens. Several factors have been shown to affect the efficiency with which irradiation induces mutations. The receptivity of a cell at different stages of its metabolic cycle is an important factor in determining rates for induced mutations. A. H. Sparrow has shown marked variations in numbers of chromosome fragments, assumed to be directly related to mutational changes, at different stages in meiosis and cleavage in the plant genus Trillium. Chromosome aberrations were induced about 60 times more frequently at metaphase than it interphase. Nondividing cells in Trillium showed little radiation damage, whereas rapidly dividing cells were very sensitive.

Oxygen tension and temperature change, when associated with irradiation, also may significantly alter the frequency of mutations. Low-oxygen tension decreases mutations. Oxygen can magnify the effect of radiation, but only if it is present during the irradiation. Oxygen has less effect with intense conditions than with moderate conditions of ionization. Environmental agents that protect germ cells from radiation damage often do so by lowering the oxygen concentration of tissue, and those that enhance the effectiveness of radiation and oxygen.

Ionizing radiation also induces various kinds of gross changes in chromosome structure (chromosome aberrations) such as deletions, duplications, inversions, and translocations. These changes in chromosomes structure result from breaks in chromosomes caused by ionizing radiation. Since they require two breaks, the kinetics of induction are two "hit" as expected, rather than single "hit."

Ultraviolet Radiation

Ultraviolet rays do not possess sufficient energy to induce ionizations. They are, however, readily absorbed by certain substances such as purines and pyrimidines, which then enter a more reactive or excited state. Because of their lower energy, they penetrate tissues only slightly, usually only the surface layer of cells in multicullular organisms. Nevertheless, ultraviolet light (UV) is at a wavelength of 254 nm. Maximum mutagenicity also occurs at 254 nm, suggesting that the UV-induced mutation process is mediated directly by the absorption of UV by purines and pyrimidines. In vitro studies show that the pyrimidines (especially thymine) absorb strongly at 254 nm and, as a result, become very reactive. The two major products of UV absorption by pyrimidines appear to be pyrimidine hydrate and pyrimidine dimers. Several lines of evidence indicate that thymine dimerization is probably the major mutagenic effect of UV. Thymine dimers appear to cause mutations indirectly in two ways. (1) Dimers apparently perturb the DNA double helix and interfere with accurate DNA replication. (2) Occasional errors are made during the processes that cells possess for the repair of "damaged" DNA, such as DNA containing thymine dimers.

The relationship between mutation rate and UV dosage is highly variable, depending on the type of mutation, the organism, and the conditions employed. "single-hit kinetics" are only occasionally observed, in contrast to ionizing radiation.

Mutation Frequency

Mutation is necessary to provide the genetic variability required for the evolutionary adaptation of species to environmental changes. On the other hand, most are deleterious. Thus, if mutation were to become too frequent in a species, it would create a sizable "genetic load" of deleterious effects. Clearly, if this "genetic load" became too large, the species would face extinction. Human technology has already contaminated the earth with increased levels of radiation and chemicals that are known to be mutagenic. While the consequences of the present increased level of mutagenes in the environment cannot yet be accurately assessed, most scientists agree that further increases in the levels of mutagens in the environment should be avoided. Yet significant quantities of hundreds of new chemicals are introduced into the environment each year, most of them with insufficient, if any, mutagenicity tests. Whether they will cause harmful increases in mutation rate (and/or cancer incidence) is a question of utmost concern to everyone.

Each gene probably has its own characteristic mutational behaviour. Some genes mutational behaviour. Some genes undergo mutations more frequently than others in the some organism. Those with unusually high mutation rates are called unstable or mutable, but a wide range of mutation rates exists among genes that are considered stable. The mutation rate per gene in bacteria is of the order of 1 in 100,000 to 1 in 10 million (10^{-5} to 10^{-7}) per cell generation. For fruit flies, the average for mutation in a particular gene is in the order of 1 in 100,000, with a range from 1 in 200,000 to 1 in 100,000, with a range from 1 in 20,000 to 1 in 200,000 gametes. Since most of the data on mutation rates in fruit flies have been obtained from experiments with males, questions have arisen concerning a possible sex difference in overall mutation rates. B. Wallace has shown through extensive experiments that mutation rates are not significantly different in the two sexes of D. Melanogaster. However, mutation rates do differ in different strains.

Estimates of mutation rates humans indicate a somewhat greater frequency than those cited for stable gens in most other organisms. Samples collected thus far have been small, and the methods used were indirect and subject to large errors. Genes associated with such human traits as intestinal polyposis and muscular dystrophy have been estimated to mutate once in 104 to 105 people. A human generation is equal to about 50 cell generations. By expressing any mutation rate as probability of mutation per cell per generation, a mutation rate is defined independently of exact physiological conditions and stage in life cycle. This definition is based on a time unit proportional to a cell's division time. When expressed in terms of cell generations, rates for fruit and humans are generally comparable with those for bacteria.

Estimating Mutation Rates

Mutation rates are usually defined in terms of mutation events per generations or, less frequently mutations per unit time. The direct experimental determination of mutation rates is complex. Because mutation is must be sampled to get accurate estimates of mutation rates. In addition, recurrent sampling is required unless the initial population is sufficiently small that its probability of containing a mutant organism is negligible. Simply enumerating the number of mutant individuals in a population does not indicate how many mutational events have occurred since the mutants will usually undergo exponential growth like the nonmutants, although often at a slower rate than the latter.

Consider a "wild-type" allele a+ mutating to a mutant allele a with a mutation rate μ (defined as a constant a probability of a mutational event per cell duplication or per organism duplication), that is,

$$a^{+} \rightarrow a$$

clearly, the number of mutation events will depend on the number of a+ alleles in the population. For simplicity, consider a haploid organism. If one starts with population in which the number of mutant organisms equals *M* and the total population size equals *N*, then

$$dM = \left(\mu + \frac{M}{M}\right) dN$$

This *assumes* that (1) M is very small relative to N, so that the difference between N and N – M is negligible; (2) the mutant and nonmutant organisms duplicate at the same rate; (3) reversion of a → a+ does not occur or is negligible. If one starts with a population in which M is zero, and makes all the same assumptions, then the relationship simplifies to

$$dM = \mu dN$$

These equations can be integerated and used to obtain estimates of mutation rates in experimental populations. More frequently, however, populations are analyzed in terms of allele frequencies, or changes in allele frequencies due to mutation, selection, or migration. Moreover, mutation is not a unidirectional process; reverse mutations occur. A more realistic picture is thus

$$a^{+} = \Leftrightarrow a$$

in which the "wild-type" allele a+ "wild-type" gene to a mutant form (usually a nonfunctional or only slightly functional form) is investigated, what is actually measured is the summation of many different mutation events at many different sites in the gene. The "average gene" is usually considered to be a DNA sequence of about 1000 nucleotide pairs coding for polypeptide that is about 333 amino acids long. Amino acid changes at many different positions in the polypeptide (resulting from base-pair substitutions at many different positions in the structural gene) may be expected to result in an inactive gene product. Thus, when one measures the mutation rate of a "wild-type" gene to the nonfunctional mutant from, one will actually be measuring the sum of many different mutations, each occurring at its own specific rate.

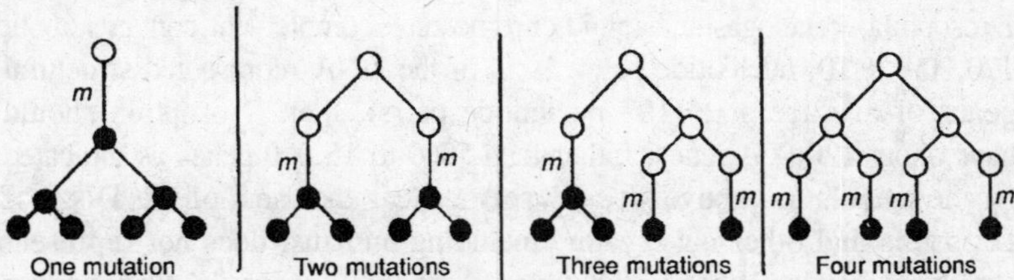

Fig. 3.6. A given number of mutant organisms in a population can result from various number of mutational events, depending on when the mutation occurs during the exponential growth of the population.

MUTATION "LOAD" VERSUS GENOME SIZE

In the preceding section, an average mutation rate of 1 per 100,000 (or 10^{-5}) per gene per generation was cited for Drosophila. Estimates of the total mutation rate—the summation of mutation rates of the entire genome – in Drosophila are of the order of 5 percent (or 5 × 10^{-2}) per generation (per haploid complement, or per gamete). These values can be used to estimate the number of genes in the Drosophila genome (haploid complement). If the mutation rate per gene in m and the mutation rate per total genome is M, then the number of genes in the genome (N), will equal M/m. Using the above estimates, N = 5 × 10–2/10–5 = 5000. This estimate agrees well with estimates of the number of genes in Drosophila obtained by other genetic criteria. On the other hand, one biochemical estimate suggests that Drosophila has about three times that many genes.

In the Drosophila genome (haploid) contains only 5000–15,000 genes, there is a major difference in the organization of the Drosophila genome and the genomes of the extensively studied bacteria and viruses. This difference, in fact, appears to be a basic difference between prokaryotes and eukaryotes. In prokaryotes, essentially all of the DNA of the genome appears to represent structural genes. Estimates of the number of genes from mutation studies (in some case, identification of all or most of the genes of the organs) agree well with estimates obtained by dividing the total DNA content in nucleotide pairs) of the genome by 1000 (103 nucleotide pairs per "average" gene). The phage lambda chromosome consists of 45 × 10^3 nucleotide pairs and about 40 known genes. The phage T4 chromosome contains about 200 × 10^3 nucleotide pairs. Over 100 genes have been mapped in phage T4, and a significant number remain to be identified. The E. coli genome contains about 4000 × 10^3 nucleotide pairs, while mutation analyses suggest that it contains about 3000 genes. In these prokaryotic organisms, then, the genomes are composed almost entirely of structural genes. The Drosophila melanogaster haploid chromosome complement contains about 120,000 × 10^3 nucleotide pairs. If all of the DNA represented structural genes of average size (103 nucleotide pairs), then Drosophila should have about 120,000 genes, rather than 5000 to 15,000 genes as indicated by the calculation above. It now seems clear the most of the DNA of Drosohila and other eukaryotes, including humans, does not represent structural genes. What is the function of this "excess" or noncoding DNA? Many geneticists believe that this noncoding DNA is regulatory, playing important roles in the regulaion of gene expression. Others believe that it has an important role in some aspect of chromosome structure. Still others believe that much of the noncoding DNA is just "junk" DNA with no important function, possibly a reservoir of nucleotide-pair sequences available for the evolution of new genes. In any case, this DNA does not code for proteins. This "noncoding" DNA is of two types: DNA that is transcribed, but for which the transcripts never leave the nuclei, and (2) nontranscribed DNA. These two types of DNA may have very different functions. The first type of noncoding DNA clearly includes many of the noncoding intervening sequences or introns of eukaryotic genes.

An estimate of the maximum number of essential genes per genome can also be made from considerations of average mutation rates and the maximum mutation "loads" that a species could be expected to survive. For example, consider an average mutation rate of 4×10^{-6} recessive lethal mutation per essential gene per generation (per gamete). J. L. King, and others, have emphasized that it is unlikely that a species could tolerate more than 0.8 new lethal mutation per zygote (or 0.4 per gamete). Dividing 0.4 new recessive lethal mutation per gamete by 4×10^{-6} new recessive lethal mutation per essential gene per gamete gives a maximum number of 10^5 essential genes per gamete. At 10^3 nucleotide pairs per gene, the 105 essential genes would represent a total for 10^8 nucleotide pairs. The haploid chromosome complement of mammals, including humans, contains about 3×10^8 nucleotide pairs. Thus, according to thee estimates, essential genes can represent a maximum of a only about 3 percent of the total DNA in the genome of mammals. The actual number of essential genes in mammals is probably closer to $1\text{–}2 \times 10^4$, or less than 1 percent of the total DNA.

Mutable Genes

Most gene are relatively stable and mutate infrequently, but in some organisms a few genes mutate spontaneously so often that individuals carrying them are mosaics of mutated and unmutated genes. The R locus, which is involved with anthocyanin pigment synthesis in maize, for example, was found by R.A. Emerson to undergo alteration much more frequently than other loci. The change from Rr to rr, for example, was found to occur, at the rate of 1 per 20,000 gametes. These "mutable" genes are either more unstable than others or they are influenced by other factors in the genetic environment. McClintock's conclusion from extensive studies on maize was that a mutable gene is not an autonomous entity, but is derived from an agent that is integrated at the site of the mutable gene to cause instability.

Examples of highly mutable genes have been found in both plants and animals, but they appear to be more common in plants. Mutations in highly mutable genes occur frequently in somatic tissue and occasionally in germ cells. Somatic mutations may show their effects as colour variegations (mosaics) in such plant part as endosperm, leaves, and petals. Many common plants—including the larkspur, snapdragon, sweet pea, four-o'clock, and morning glory—have colour variegations suggesting unstable or mutable genes.

The classical investigations of M. Demerec (1941) on a mutable gene called miniature-alpha in Drosophila virilis provided the first substantial data on the genetic properties of mutable gens in animals. These propertie are: (1) mutation occurs primarily before meiosis; (2) mutation occurs in both females and males, implying that meiotic crossing over is not involved (crossing over occurs only rearely in Drosophila males) and (3) mutation is strongly influenced by neighbouring genes. More recently, M.M. Green and others have described several mutable gene systems involving the white locus (eye colour) and other genes in D. melanogaster. White-crimson (w^c), for example, mutates to wild-type and phenotypes other than white-crimosn at a frequency of 10–3. This mutable system and several others at the w locus are associated with chromosome alterations, particularly deficiencies. This led to the hypothesis that a "*controlling element*" from the cytoplasm is integrated into the chromosome at the site of mutability, and that this agent is responsible for chromosome aberrations.

Many of these "controlling elements" have now been identified by G. Rubin, P. M. Bingham, and colleagues, and shown to be transposable elements with structures similar to the TN elements of bacteria. The unstable allele ww^c mentioned above has been shown to result from the insertion of an approximately 10,000 nucleotide-pair-long transposable element belonging to the class called FB (for "foldback") elements.

Another unstable allele, w^{a1} has been shown to have a transposable element called *copia* (because its sequence is present in RNA in *copious* amounts) inserted at the site of mutation. Copia has been isolated and sequenced. It is about 5,000 nucleotide pairs long with 276 nucleotide-pair perfect direct repeats at its ends. These 276 nucleotide-pair repeats, in turn, have 17 nucleotide-pair inverse repeats at each end. Note the similarity of *copia* to E. coli elements Tn 9 and Tn 10.

Mutator And Antimutator Genes

Genes in maize were shown by McClintock to influence the stability of other genes. These have been called mutator genes. A striking example of the action of a mutator gene with a specific effect on a basic colour gene in maize was described by M. M. Rhoades. The colour of maize leaves and other plant parts is dependent on a complex of three complementary genes, symbolized A, C and R. A colour other than green is produced only when the dominant alleles (A, C, and R) of all three genes are present. The colour may be purple if gene P is also present, or red (pp), or some other colour depending on what other genes are included along with A-C-R. Plant soft genotype aa, cc, or rr have green leaves regardless of alleles present at the other loci. Plants with the genotype aaC-R- would be expected to be green, but in the presence of a mutator gene called Dt, they are variegated. Light-coloured corn kernels have purple spots at locations where somatic mutations have occurred. The Dt gene produces its effect by influencing one or more of the a alleles of the aa genotype to mutate to A. Patches of cells scattered throughout the plant carry A alleles resulting from these mutate to A. Patches of cells scattered throughout the plant carry A alleles resulting from the mutations. On the leaves and kernels, these patches give a speckled appearance. The size of the spots depends on the stage of development at which the mutations occurred. Green cells contain unmutated genes; that is, they are of genotype aa. In this case, the allele (Dt or dt) present at one locus thus influences the mutation rate of an allele (a) present at another locus.

J. F. Speyer and others have found broad-spectrum mutator genes in bacteriophage T4. Temperature sensitive (ts) mutants of gene 43, for example, alter the mutation rates of point mutations in other genes. Some mutator genes exert their mutagenic effect during DNA replication by altering polymerase activity, producing mutagenic base analogs, or modifying DNA bases, thus influencing the mutation rates of other genes. One mutator in phage T4 gene 43 (ts L88) produces a DNA polymerase that utilizes incorrect nucleotides at a higher frequency than does the wild-type enzyme.

Several mutations in gene 43 exhibit powerful negative or antimutator activities, particularly during the formation of A : T → C : G substitutions. Experiments have shown that DNA polymerase (gene 43 products) that are isolated from E. coli that were infected with mutator, antimutator and wild-type strains for T4 bacteriophage discriminate between adenine and 2-aminopurine to different degrees during DNA synthesis in vitro. Significantly larger amounts of 2-aminopurine are incorporated into DNA by wild-type and mutator than by antimutator enzymes. This indicates that organisms have the potential to evolve mechanism that result in mutation rates that are lower than those presently existing in wild-type strains of somatic organisms.

When the mutator and antimutator DNA polyemerase of phage T4 were studied in vitro, they were found to have altered ratios of polymerase activity to 3'→5' exonuclease activity. Mutator have increased polymerase/exonuclease activity. Antimutators exhibit decreased polymerase/exonuclease activity. This suggests that the mutation rate is, at least in part, controlled by the relative rates of polymerization and proofreading rates decrease mutation rates (antimutator). Decreased proofreading efficiencies (or increased polymerization rates) increase mutation frequencies (mutator).

Several mutator genes have also been identified and characterized in E. coli.Some increase the frequency of only certain types of base-pair substitutions. Others cause an increase in all types of point mutations. R. C. von Borstell and others measured spontaneous mutation rates in yeast and isolated many mutator genes with different kinds of mutator and antimutator activity.

Decreases as well as increases in mutation rates, as compared with wild-type, can thus result from new mutations. With both mutators and antimutaors operating in the same system, particular spontaneous mutation rates may be optimized through natural selection. Mutators and antimutators thus become relative terms, because no standards are available for optimum rates. Results of studies on yeast have borne out the conclusions of those on viruses and bacteria; that spontaneous mutation rates are under the genetic control of the cell itself.

Insertion Sequence ("Is Elements") As Mutators

A significant proportion of the mutations that occur in bacteria and some bacteriophages are now known to be effects of small sequences of DNA called IS elements or insertion sequences. These DNA sequences, from about 800 to about 1400 nucleotide paris in length are present in E. coli chromosomes, for example, in several copies. The first five IS elements to be characterized were: ISI (768 nucleotide pairs long) and IS2, IS3, IS4, and IS5 (all between 1200 and 1400 nucleotide pairs in length). The IS elements are transposable; that is, they have the ability to move from one position in the chromosome or to other chromosomes in the same cell. They can move, for example, from the E. coli chromosome to bacteriophage chromosomes or to plasmids (small circular molecules of DNA, or "minichromosomes," often present in bacteria.

The chromosome of the strains of E. coli that have been studied contain about eight copies of ISI elements are physically and covalently inserted as linear sequences into the chromosomes when an IS element is inserted (or insert itself?) into a gene, it destroys the function of, mutates, that gene. While insertion of IS elements occur at many sites in the E. coli chromosomes, it is not completely at random. Preferred sites of insertion have been demonstrated in some case.

Detectable IS-induced mutations occur with a frequency of about 10^{-6} to 10^{-7} per cell generation in E. coli. IS-induced mutations are revertible. They can be distinguished from all mutations with similar effects in that their reversion frequency (usually in the range 10^{-6} to 10^{-7}) can not be enhanced with mutagens. The fact that IS-induced mutations are revertible means that IS elements can excise themselves from the chromosome with precision to the single nucleotide pair. Reversion to the functional state requires restoration of the original nuclotide-pair sequence of the gene; no base-pairs can be added or deleted during the insertion-excision process. The failure of mutagens to hence reversion is to be recombination mechanism, not a mutation process. The "*controlling elements*" and mutable loci (or unstable genes) in higher plants and animals are probably caused by sequences of DNA analogous to the IS elements in prokaryotes.

Induced Mutations

Mutations can be induced by either physical or chemical means: such mutations are called induced mutations. Irradiation is an example of a physical mutagen, with x-rays, gamma-rays, and ultraviolet light being the most common examples used. One consequence of x- or gamma-ray irradiation is the breakage of chromosomes, which may result in chromosomal rearrangements, or the events may be lethal to the cell.

5-Bromouracil

5-Bromouracil (5-BU) is a base analog; that is, its structure closely resembles one of the bases normally found in DNA. 5-BU can exist in two states. In its usual keto state it exhibits properties similar to those of thymine and thus will pair with adenine in DNA. Rarely it switches to the enol state, and in this form it will pair specifically with guanine.

Mutations can be induced by 5-BU (and in general by base-analong muta-gens) in two ways. The first involves the incorporation of the usual form of 5-BU into DNA during replication. If 5-BU shifts to

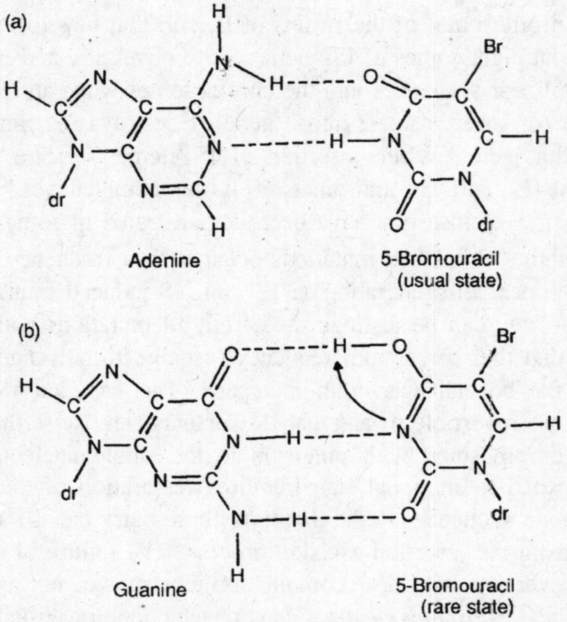

Fig. 3.7. Pairing properties of a 5-Bromouracil (5-BU): (a) In its usual keto state, 5-BU pairs with adenine; (b) In its rare enol state, 5-BU pairs with guanine. (dr = deoxyribose).

its rare enol state during the next round of replication, the result will be a transition mutation from AT to GC.

The second way that 5-BU can induce mutations is if the base analog g is incorporated in the DNA while it is the rare enol state. This dictates insertion opposite a G on the complementary strand, and subsequent replication with a shift of the 5-BU to the usual keto state will result in a transition mutation from GC to AT.

Thus 5-BU can induce either AT to GC or CG-to-AT transition mutations. (In the jargon of this area, 5-BU is said to induce two-way transition mutations.) Therefore it is possible to correct a 5-BU induced transition mutation by treating with 5-BU for a second time. This is called *reversion* of the mutation.

2-Aminopurine

2-Aminopurine (2-AP) is also a base analog and, like 5-BU, it can exist in two states. In its usual state it behaves like adenine and will form two hydrogen bonds with thymine. In its rare amino state 2-AP behaves like guanine and forms two hydrogen bonds with cytosine. Thus 2-AP can induce transition mutations both from AT-to-GC and

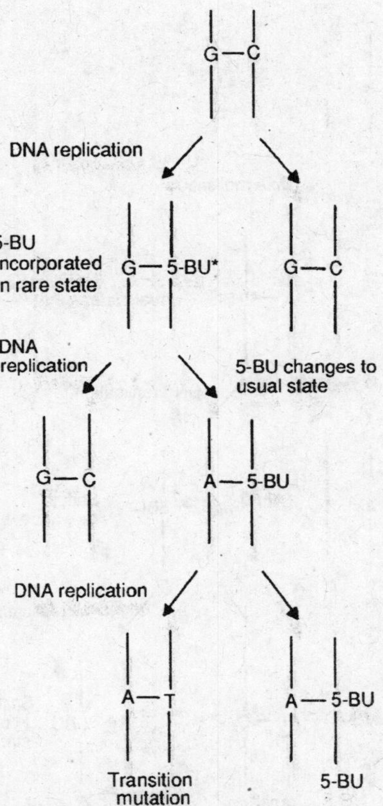

Fig. 3.8. Mutagenic action of 5-BU when it incorporates into DNA in its usual keto state and then shifts to its rare state during the next round of replication.

from GC-to-AT. 2-AP induced mutations can therefore be reverted by 2-AP treatment.

Nitrous Acid

Nitrous acid (NA : HNO_2) is a deminating, agent; it acts by removing amino groups (NH_2) from the bases. In some but not all instances this alters their base-pairing abilities and hence induces mutations. The three bases that have amino groups are adenine, guanine, and cytosine. When adenine is treated with NA, it is changed to hypoxanthine, which will pair with cytosine. This results in an AT-to-GC transition mutation.

Treatment of guanine with NA removes the amino group from the 2-carbon position and produces xanthine. However, since both guanine and xanthine pair with cytosine, no base-pair mutation results.

A—T
Add 5BU
DNA replication
A—T
A—5 BU Usual state
DNA replication
A—T
G—5BU* Shift to rare state
DNA replication
G—C
Transition mutation
A—5BU Shift back to usual state

Fig. 3.9. Mutagenic action of 5-BU when it incorporates into DNA in the rare state and then shifts to the usual keto state during the next round of replication.

Deamination of cytosine by NA produces uracil, which, or course, pairs with adenine. This results in a GC-to-AT transition mutation–the opposite of NA's effect on adenine. Thus mutations induced by nitrous

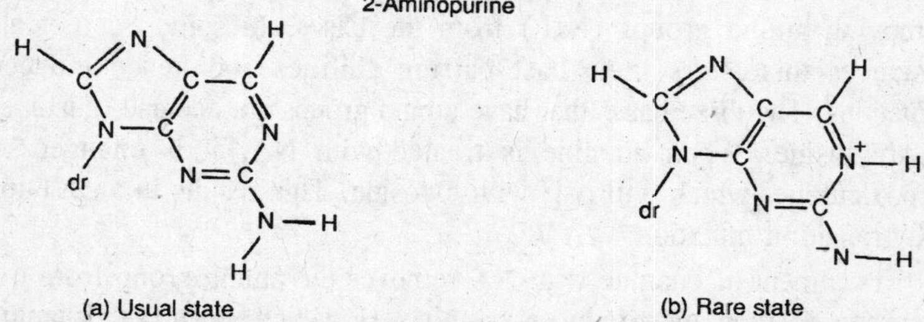

Fig. 3.10. Structure of 2-Aminopurine: (a) In its usual state (pairs with thymine) and (b) in its rare imino state (pairs with cytosine)

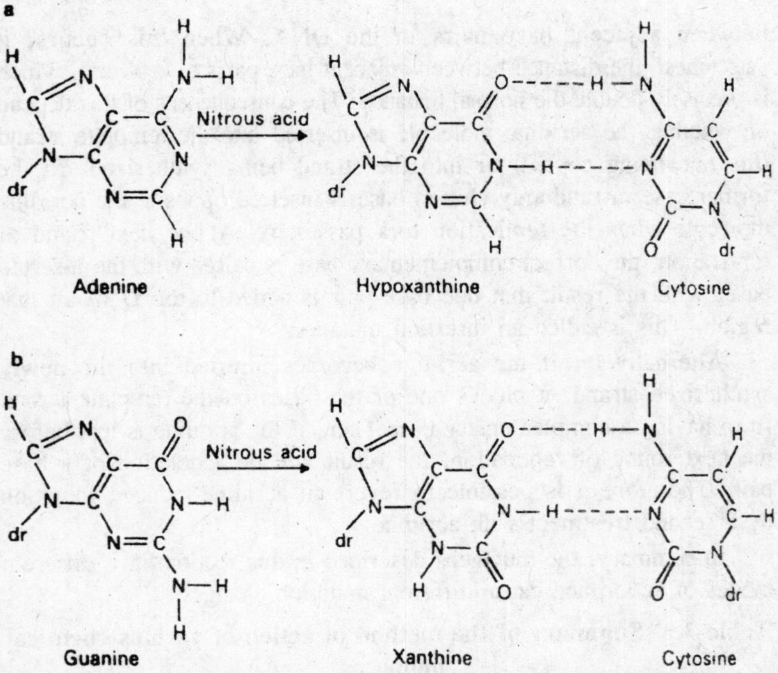

Fig. 3.11. Mutagenic action of nitrous acid. (a) Deamination of adenine by nitrous acid treatment produces hypoxanthine, which pairs with cytosine; (b) Deamination of guanine produces xanthine, which pairs with cytosine.

acid can be reverted by nitrous acid treatment: in other words, nitrous acid induces two-way transition mutations.

Hydroxylamine

Hydroxylamine (NH_2OH) reacts only with cytosine, hydroxylating it so that it can then only with adenine . Thus hydroxlamine induces one-way transition mutation from GC to AT. Because of this, mutations induced by hydroxylamine cannot be reverted to revert by 5-BU. 2-AP, or NA treatment since these mutagens can bring about a GC-to-AT transition.

Acridines

Acridine treatment results in the addition or deletion of one base pair in the DNA. This has serious consequences, since the amino acid sequence of a protein coded for by a stretch of DNA altered in this fashion will be changed drastically. This will become more apparent in later discussions of messenger RNA translation. When present at relatively low concentrations, acridine acts by becoming inserted between adjacent base pairs in the DNA. When this occurs, it "stretches" the distance between adjacent base pairs to 0.68 nm, which is precisely double the normal distance. The consequences of this depend on whether the acridine molecule is inserted into the template strand (the one being copied) or into the strand being synthesized. In the former case, a randomly chosen base is inserted opposite the acridine molecule when the replication fork passes by. At the next round of replication, the correct complementary base is paired with the inserted base, with the result that one base pair is added to the DNA in that region. This is called an insertion mutation.

Alternatively, if the acridine becomes inserted into the newly synthesized strand, it blocks one of the bases on the template strand from having a complementary base Then, if the acridine is lost before the next round of replication, the result will be a deletion of a base pair. Therefore it is possible to revert an acridine-induced mutation by a second treatment with acridine.

In summary, the mutagens described in this section have different modes of action and cause different mutation changes.

Table 3.3. Summary of the method of action of various chemical mutagens.

Mutagen	*Base-pair changes*
5-Bromouracil	AT ↔ GC two-way transitions
2-Aminopurine	AT ↔ GC two-way transitions
Nitrous acid	AT ↔ GC two-way transitions
Hydroxylamine	GC → AT one-way transitions
Acridines	+1 or −1 insertion or deletion

Some of the chemical mutagens described in this section are commonly used in the laboratory. Many other chemicals appear to cause mutations, and public awareness of this is increasing as industrial effluents, cosmetic ingredients, food additives, etc. are examined carefully for any mutagenic activity in test organisms.

Variations in Chromosome Number

Somatic cells of higher plants and animals usually have chromosomes in pairs (2n); that is, two of each kind of chromosome are present in each cell. Mature germ cells, having undergone reduction division, normally have one number of each pair (n). Many individual plants and animals, however, have local areas of somatic tissue characterized by a multiple of the basic chromosome number. A doubling process in cell division is the usual explanation for these deviations. With the exception of sex differences, somatic doubling, and minor variations that occur in natural and experimental populations, all members of a species of plants or animals have the same basic chromosome number. Chromosome number can be overemphasized as a criterion for species identification, but it represents a valid characteristic to be used along with others for distinguishing species. The range or reported chromosome numbers in animals extends from 2 pair in a rhabdocoel Gyratrix hermaphroditus and some mites, midges, and scale insects, to more than 100 in some butterflies and Crustacea. The Crustacean, *Paralithodes camtschatica*, for example, has 208 chromosomes or 104 pairs. The reported range in plants is from 2 pairs in the small composite plant Haplopappus gracilis to several hundred in some ferns. A species of fern-like plants of the genus Ophioglossum is reported to have 768 chromosomes.

Where all individuals within a species, with the exceptions noted above, have the same chromosome number, different species within a genus often have different numbers. Cytological investigations of chromosomes help to unravel problems of species formation. The evolutionary path of a certain species can be followed in some cases by comparing numerical and structural relations of its chromosomes with those of other species within the genus. The essential genetic material is a major factor in determining evolutionary patterns, but chromosome number itself represents merely the number of packages into which the genetic material is divided. Chromosome number is probably more constant, however, than any other single morphological characteristic that is available for species identification.

Changes in the number of chromosomes may be reflected in phenotypic variations, which constitute a useful tool for identifying the influence of individual chromosomes. If, for example, phenotypically distinguishable individuals with different chromosome numbers can be identified in natural populations or produced experimentally, it is sometimes possible to determine the effect of adding or removing certain chromosomes. Some plants with increased chromosome numbers have phenotypic changes in morphological or physiological characteristics which are of practical importance to man. Grape and tomato plants with chromosome numbers above 2n are larger and produce more desirable fruit than do corresponding varieties with the usual 2n number.

Classifications of chromosome changes are arbitrary and superficial because these changes are necessarily interpreted in terms of obvious

Table 3.4. Chromosome number of some common animals and plants

Species	*Number of chromosomes pair*
Plants	
Garden pea, *Pisum sativum*	7
Sorghum, *Sorghum vulgare*	10
Maize, *Zea mays*	10
Johnson Grass, *Sorghum halepense*	20
Alfalfa, *Medicago sativa*	16
Barley, *Hordeum vulgare*	7
Oats, *Avena sativa*	21
Tomato, *Lycopersicon esculentum*	12
Tobacco, *Nicotiana tabacum*	24
Trillium, *Trillium erectum*	5
Animals	
Gypsy moth, *Lymantria dispar*	31
Mouse, *Mus musculus*	20
Rabbit, *Oryctolagus cuniculus*	22
Cow, *Boss tarus*	30
Horse, *Equus caballus*	32
Donkey, (ass) *Equus asinus*	31
Dog, *Canis familaris*	39
Monkey, *Macaca rhesus*	21
Chimpanzee, *Pan troglodytes*	24

additions or eliminations of parts of chromosomes, whole chromo-somes, or whole chromosome sets. The presently accepted classification system, therefore, is merely a working tool. Two main classes are euploidy and aneuploidy ("ploid," Greek for unit; "eu," true or even; and "aneu," uneven). Euploids have chromosome complements consisting of whole sets or genomes. The chromosome number of euploid organisms is basically represented by the monoploid (n). Euploids with chromosome numbers above the monoploid level may be diploid (2n), triploid (3n), tetraploid (4n), or have some other "polyploid" number.

Aneuploidy

The first critical study of aneuploid plants was made by Blakeslee and Bellingusing the common Jimson weed Datura stramonium, which normally has 12 pairs of chromosomes in the somatic cells. In 1924, these investigators announced the discovery of a "mutant type" having

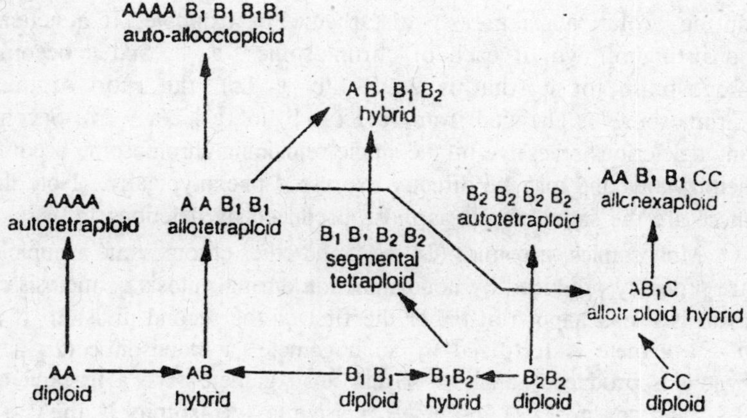

Fig. 3.12. Mode of formation of different kinds of polyploid.

25 rather than 24 chromosomes. At the meiotic metaphase, one of the 12 pairs was found to have an extra member; that is, one trisome was present along with 11 disomes. This originally discovered trisomic plant differed from wild-type plants in several specific ways. Conspicuous deviations were observed in shape and spine characteristics of seed capsules. The chromosome complement with one extra member in addition to the regular set was illustrated by the formula 2n + 1. Theoretically, because the some have, however, been divided successfully into 7 groups identified with letters A to G. Numbers 1 to 22 are associated with the autosomes in descending order by length. All autosomes can be placed satisfactorily within a group but the numbering within the groups is more or less tentative. The X chromosome is difficult to distinguish from members of the C group and the Y chromosome shows considerable variability in different preparations.

Nullisomics (2n – 2)

Although nullisomy is a lethal condition in regular diploids, an organism like wheat (which "pretends" to be diploid but is fundamentally hexaploid) can tolerate nullisomy. In fact, all of the possible 21 wheat nullisomics have been produced. Their appearances are different from normal wheat; furthermore, most of them show less vigorous growth.

Monosomics (2n – 1)

Monosomic chromosome complements are generally deleterious for two main reasons. First, the balance of chromosomes that is necessary for a finely tuned cellular homeostasis, carefully put together during evolution, is grossly disturbed. For example, if a genome consisting of two of each of chromosomes, a, b, and c becomes monosomic for c (that is 2a + 2b + 1c), the ratio of these chromosomes is changed from 1c:1 (a+b) to 1c : 2(a + b). Second, any deleterious recessive on the single remaining chromosome becomes hemizygous and may be directly expressed phenotypically. (Note that these are the same effects as those produced by deletions.)

Monosomics, trisomics (2n +1), and other chromosome aneuploids are probably produced by nondisjunction during mitosis or meiosis. In meiosis it can happen at either the first or the second division. If an n – 1 gamete is fertilized by an n gamete, a monosomic (2n – 1) zygote is produced; an n + 1 and an n gamete give a trisomic 2n +1; and an n + 1 and n + 1 give a tetrasomic if the same chromosome is involved or a double trisomic if different chromosomes are involved, and so on.

In Neurospora (a haploid), the n – 1 meiotic products abort, and do not darken like the normal ascospore; so MI and MII nondisjunctions are detected as asci with 4:4 and 6:2 ratios of normal to aborted spores. For loci on the aneuploid chromosomes, what ascus genotypes are produced?

In humans, the sex-chromosome monosomic (44 autosomes + 1X) produces a phenotype known as Turner's syndrome. Affected people have a characteristic, easily recognizable, phenotype: they are sterile females, are short in stature, and often have a web of skin extending between the neck and shoulders. Their intelligence is near-normal, although some specific cognitive functions are defective. Their frequency is about 1 in 5000 female births. Monosomics for all autosomes die in utero.

If viable, nullisomics and monosomics are useful in locating newly found recessive genes on specific chromosomes in plants. In one such method, different monosomic lines lacking a different chromosome in each line are obtained. Homozygotes for the new gene are crossed with each monosomic line, and the progeny of each cross are inspected for expression of the recessive phenotype. The cross in which the phenotype appears identifies its chromosomal location. In nullisomics and monosomics, of course, n - 1 gametes are produced. In general, these gametes tend to be more viable in a female parent than in a male. It is the union of these n – 1 gametes within n gametes, bearing the new mutation, that provides the crucial progeny types for the linkage test.

A similar approach can be used in humans. For example, two people whose vision is normal may produce a daughter who has Turner's syndrome and is also red-green colour-blind. This shows that the allele for red-green colour blindness is recessive, that it was on the X chromosome of the mother, and the nondisjunction must have occurred in the father.

Trisomics (2n + 1)

In trisomics, trivalents are regularly seen. For genes that are tightly linked to the centromere of a trisomic chromosome set, the random segregations can be represented a trisomic Aaa. All types occur equally frequently, and a gametic ratio of 1A:2Aa:2a:1aa is produced. Trisomics are sometimes recongnised by these ratios, which are also useful in locating genes on chromosomes. We have already observed a complete set of trisomic lines in Datura. Once again, note that chromosome imbalance produces highly chromosome-specific deviations from the normal appearance.

In humans there are several examples of viable trisomics. The combination XXX (1/1000 male births) results in Klinefelter's syndrome, producing males that have lanky builds, are mentally retarded, and

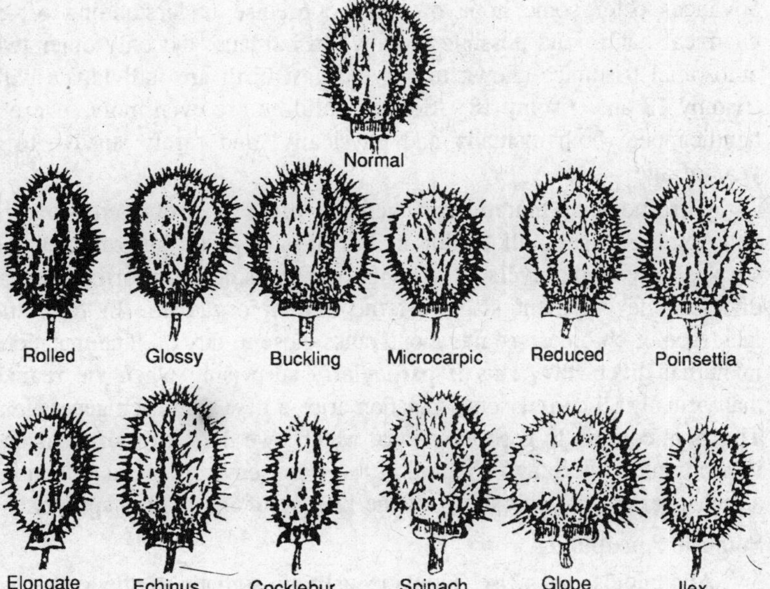

Fig. 3.13. Fruit capsules of the 12 primary trisomics of Datura stramonium, each with its particular phenotype.

sterile. Another combination, XYY, also occurs in about in 1000 male births. A lot of excitement was aroused when an attempt was made to link the XYY condition with a predisposition toward violence. This is still hotly debated, although it is now clear that an XYY condition in no way guarantees such behaviour. Nevertheless, several enterprising lawyers have attempted to use the XYY genotype as grounds for acquittal or compassion in crimes of violence. The XYY males are usually fertile. We have already looked at the generation of Down's syndrome through adjacent segregation in translocation heterozygotes. Down's syndrome also occurs much more commonly as a result of nondisjunction during meiosis, and it is then called trisomy 21. In this form of Down's syndrome, there is generally no family history of the phenotype; however, the frequency of this form is dramatically higher among children born to older mothers. The overall incidence of this abnormality is about 0.15 percent of births.

Down's syndrome is a severely incapacitating condition. Affected individuals are mentally retarded, and about one-third die by the age of 10 years. Recent advances in mapping the human genome will allow the identification of precisely those genes on the long arm of chromosome 21 that must be trisomic to produce this syndrome; these advances offer some hope of a more precise understanding of its chemical nature and possible therapy. In humans, the only other two autosomal trisomics known to survive past birth are individuals with trisomy 13 and trisomy 18. Affected children are even more severely handicapped, both mentally and physically, and rarely survive to 1 year of age.

Chromosome mutation in general plays a prominent role in determining genetic ill health in humans. Figure summarizes the surprisingly high levels of various chromosomal abnormalities at different development stages of the human organism. In fact, the incidence of chromosome mutations ranks close to that of gene mutations in human livebirths. This is particularly surprising when we realize that virtually all chromosome mutation arise a new with each generation. This is in contrast to gene mutations, which owe their level of incidence to a complex interplay of mutation rates and environmental selection, acting over many generations of the history of the human species.

Somatic Aneuploids

Aneuploids can arise spontaneously in somatic tissue or tissue culture. In such cases, the initial result is a genetic mosaic of cell types. Good examples are provided by certain conditions in humans.

Table 3.5. Relative incidence of human ill health due to gene mutation and to chromosome mutation

Type of mutation	*Percentage of live birth*
Gene mutation	
Autosomal dominant	0.90
Autosomal recessive	0.25
X-linked	0.05
Total gene mutation	1.20
Chromosome mutation	
Autosomal trisomies (mainly Down's syndrome)	0.14
Other unbalanced autosomal aberrations	0.06
Balanced autosomal aberrations	0.19
Sex chromosomes	
XYY, XXY, and other ♂♂	0.17
XO, XXX, and other ♀♀	0.05
Total chromosome mutation	0.61

Sexual mosaics provide the first example. These are people whose bodies are a mixture of male and female tissue. One type of sexual mosaic is XO/XYY. This mosaic can be explained by postulating an XY zygote in which an early mitotic division involved a nondisjunction of the Y chromosomes, so that both went to one pole:

The phenotypic sex of such individuals depends upon where in the body the male and female sectors end up. In this case, if nondisjunction occurred at a later mitotic division, there would be a three-way XY/XO/XYY.

Aneuploidy in Man

More recent studies on individuals have related chromosome numbers below and above 46 with intersex conditions and other irregularities manifesting physical, reproductive, and mental abnormalities. Participants in the Chicago Conference agreed on a system of nomenclature for identifying numerical and structural chromosome alterations. In a description of a karyotype, the first item to be recorded is the total number of chromosomes, including the sex chromosomes, followed by the sex chromosome constitution and any autosomal aberrations. A complement of 44 autosomes and one X, for example, is symbolized 45, X. This monosomic chromosome complement has been associated with an abnormal female condition known for many years as Turner's syndrome and which occurs in one of about 5000 people in the general population.

The Turner Syndrome (45,X)

This monosomic has a chromosome complement of 44 autosomes and one X chromosome. The chromosome anomaly is associated with an abnormal female phenotype described in 1938 by H. H. Turner and associates and known as the Turner syndrome. It occurs in about 1 per 2500 live female births. More than 90 percent abort spontaneously. A rough estimate for 45,X adults in the general population is in 1 in 5000. These adults have virtually no ovaries, have limited secondary sexual characteristics, and are sterile. Microscopic sections of the ovaries show fibrous streaks of tissue representing remnants of ovaries. Affected females have short stature, low-set ears, webbed neck, and shieldlike chest. Mental deficiency is not usually associated with this syndrome. Epithelial cells of 45,X patients are X chromatin negative, as expected when only X chromosome is present.

X monosomic probably originate from exceptional eggs or sperm with no sex chromosome or from the loss of a sex chromosome in mitosis during early cleavage stages, after an XX or XY zygote has been formed. This latter probability is supported by the high frequency of mosaics that result from postzygotic events in patients with the Turner syndrome. Mosaics with X/XX sex chromosomes show symptoms of the Turner syndrome but are usually taller than X and have fewer anomalies that nonmosaic 45,X females. They show more feminization, more normal menstruation, and may be fertile. Many cases of the somatic Turner phenotype without the typical 45,X chromosome constitution are now known. Most of these have one normal X chromosome and a fragment of a second X chromosome. Both arms of the second X chromosome are apparently necessary for normal ovarian differentiation. Individuals with only the long arm of the second X are short in stature and show other somatic symptoms of the Turner syndrome, whereas those with only the short arm of the second X have normal stature and do not show as many signs of the Turner syndrome. This indicates that the Turner phenotype is mostly controlled by genes on the short arm of the X chromosome.

Patients with partial deletion of one X chromosome are X chromatin positive and therefore may be misdiagnosed if a buccal smear is the only test used. The deficient X chromosome always forms the X chromatin body. A Y chromosome also occurs in some individuals with the Turner phenotype. These patients are usually mosaic for 45,X/

46,XY, with a normal Y. People with one X and a Y fragment, not including the Y short arm, have only streak ovaries but are normal in phenotype. This suggests that male-determining genes are in the short arm of the Y chromosome, and those that prevent Turner phenotype are in the Y long arm as well as the X short arm. Major features of the Turner phenotype occur in some males as well as in females. The male Turner syndrome is characterized by defective development of the testes, sterility, and limited male secondary sexual characteristics, along with somatic features of the Turner phenotype. These people have normal male karyotypes.

The Klinefelter Syndrome (47,XXY)

An extra X chromosome in addition to the usual male (XY) chromosome complement (47,XXY) has been associated with the abnormal male syndrome described (in 1942) by H.F. Klinefelter and known as the *Klinefelter syndrome*. It is estimated to occur in 1 per 500 live male births. Individuals with this syndrome are phenotypically males but with some tendency toward femaleness, particularly in secondary sex characteristics. Such features as enlarged breasts, underdeveloped body hair, small testes, and small prostate glands are a part of the syndrome. Presumably, the XXY constitution originates either by fertilization of an exceptional orginates either by fertilization of an exceptional XX egg by a Y sperm or of an X egg by an exceptional XY sperm. Studies of Klinefelter syndrome and Turner syndrome indicate that the Y chromosome in human beings, unlike that in *Drosophila*, determines male sex.

The most common karyotype (about three-quarters of the cases) for the Klinefelter syndrome is 47,XXY, but the symptoms of the syndrome will usually occur whenever more than one X chromosome is present along with a Y chromosome. More complex karyotypes associated with the Klinefelter syndrome include: XXYY, XXXY, XXXYY, XXXXY, XXXXYY, and XXXXXY. All patients with the Klinefelter syndrome have one or more X chromatin bodies in the their cells. Mental retardation is usually found when there are more than two X chromosomes. The XY/XXY mosaicism in patients with Klinefelter syndrome is associated with less severe physical and reproductive anomalies.

Aneuploidy of X Chromosomes and Mental Deficiency

Other irregular combination of X chromosomes have also been recognized among females with X chromosome aberrations. About 1 percent of all mentally defective women in institutions have been shown to have one or more extra X chromosomes. This chromosome abnormality occurs in about 1 in 700 live births in the general population. Individuals with the "triple X syndrome" are comparable in some ways with Drosophila metafemales (XXX). In Drosophila, however, such individuals are usually lethal, and those that survive are strikingly abnormal and sterile. Human XXX individuals are sometimes visibly undistinguished from normal XX females, but there is considerable range in phenotypic expression. They may be mentally abnormal.

The best-known symptoms in this syndrome are abnormalities associated with functional processes such as menstruation. One patient cited by P. A. Jacobs was a 37-year-old female who reported that the first suggestion of an abnormality was highly irregular menstruation. When the abdominal wall was opened, the ovaries appeared as if they were postmensopausal. Microscopically, they showed deficient ovarian follicle formation. Of 63 cells observed, 51 had 47 chromosomes; the extra chromosome was an X. Nondisjunction in the production of the egg from which this woman developed was postulated as the mechanism for the occurrence of extra chromosome. Buccal smears showed two sex chromatin bodies in the epithelial cells as expected when three X chromosomes are present. Individuals with tetrasomic X chromosomes (48,XXXX) are all mentally defective. The degree of mental deficiency increases with the number of X chromosomes present.

47,XYY and Behaviour

P. A. Jacobs and her associates reported in 1965 that seven XYY males were detected in a population of 197 male, mentally subnormal inmates of a penal institution in Scotland. The XYY men were unusually tall, with an average height of 73.1 inches, compared with 64 inches for XY men in the same prison. Numerous other studies, mostly in institutionalized populations, have since confirmed that a high proportion of XYY individuals are tall, subnormal in intelligence (with IQs individuals are tall, subnormal in intelligence (with IQs ranging from 80 to 95), and antisocial. The aggressive behaviour that brought them into conflict with the law was usually against property rather than people.

XYY trisomy occurs about once in 1000 live male births in the general European population. Only a few of these can be accounted for in the criminal population. Furthermore, most XYY men have been described as perfectly normal in behaviour. Hook has shown that only 3.6 percent of all XYY men are institutionalized for any reason.

Environmental factors are presumed to be involved in the development of aggressiveness. Since some XYY men are subnormal in intelligence and excessively tall in stature, particular environmental situations in childhood or adulthoood may lead to withdrawal from society or aggressive behaviour. Unfavourable social conditions such as frustration in personal accomplishment and taunting from associates may encourage physical aggression as a means of adaptation. Males with this sex trisomy have not been found to transmit the extra Y chromosome to their sons. This extra chromosome seems to be weeded out in gametogenesis. A wide range of physical and mental abnormalities has been detected in institutionalized XYY men, but most of these are irregular in occurrence and do not form a syndrome. Tallness of stature and mental dullness, however, are fairly constant characteristics among institutionalized XYY men.

Chromosomal Mosaics

Individuals who have at least two cell lines, with different karyotypes derived from one zygote, originate from nondisjunction in a cleavage division after fertilization. One daughter cell would thus receive one too many and the other would be one deficient. Each cell would give rise to cell line with its irregular chromosome number. Proportions of cells representing the different cell lines would vary in different tissues, making the extent of the mosaicism and the effect on the organism difficult to predict.

Many sex chromosome mosaics have been detected in human beings. The main phenotypic characteristic is extreme variability. Some sex chromosome mosaics have been reported —X/XX, X/XY, XX/XY, XXY/XX, XX/XXX, XXX/X XXX/XXXXY—and several other combinations reflecting two or three cell lines. Mid to severe phenotypic symptoms have been associated with these sex chromosome mosaics.

Abnormal Euploidy

Monoploids

In this section we shall consider monoploidy as an unusual condition. Monoploid individuals can arise spontaneously in natural populations as rare aberrations, but in several forms (such as bees, wasps, and ants) the males are normally monoploid, having derived from unfertilized eggs. In the germ cells of a monoploid, meiosis cannot occur normally because the chromosomes having no pairing partners. Thus monoploids are characteristically sterile. (However, meiosis can be bypassed in some monoploid animals, such as male honeybees, which produce gametes essentially by mitotic division). If meiosis occurs and the single chromosomes segregate randomly, then the probability of their all going to one pole is ($1/2)^{x-1}$, where x is the number of chromosomes. This will determine the frequency of viable (whole-set) gametes, obviously a vanishingly small number if x is large.

Monoploids have a major role in modern approaches to plant breeding. Diploidy is an inherent nuisance in the induction and selection of new favourable plant mutations and of new selection of new favourable plant mutations and of new combinations of genes already present. Monoploids provide a way around some of these problems. In some plants, monoploids may be artificially derived from the products of meiosis in the plant's anthers. A cell destined to become a pollen grain may be induced by cold treatment to grow instead into an embryoid, a small dividing mass of cells. The embryoid may be grown on agar to form a monoploid planter, which can then be potted in soil to mature.

Monoploids may be exploited in several ways. In one method, they are first examined for favourable traits or gene combinations. These may arise from heterozygosity already present in the parent or induced in the parent by mutagens. The monoploid can then be subjected to chromosome doubling to achieve a completely homozygous diploid with a normal meiosis, capable of providing seed. How is this achieved? Quite simply, by the application of a compound called colchicine to meristematic tissue. Colchicine, an alkaloid drug extracted from the autumn crocus, inhibits the mitotic spindle, so that cells with two chromosomes sets are produced. These may proliferate to form a sector of diploid tissue that can be identified cytologically.

Another way the monoploid may be used is to treat its cells, basically like a population of haploid organisms, in a mutagenesis-and-selection procedure. The cells are isolated, their walls are removed by enzyme treatment, and they are treated with mutagen. They are then plated on selective medium— perhaps a toxic compound normally produced by one of the plant's parasites, or an insecticide— to select resistant cells. Resistant plantlets grow eventually into haploid plants, which can then be doubled (using colchicine) into a pure-breeding resistant type. These are potentially powerful techniques that can circumvent the normally slow process of what is basically meiotic plant breeding. The techniques have been successfully applied in several important crop plants, such as soybeans and tobacco. This is, of course, another aspect of somatic-cell genetics in higher organisms.

The another technique of or producing monoploids does not work in all organism or in all genotypes of an organism. Another useful technique has been developed in barley, an important crop plant. When diploid barley, Hordeum vulgare, is pollinated using a diploid wild relative called Hordeum bulbosum, fertilization occurs, but during the ensuing somatic cell divisions, the chromosomes of H. Bulbosum are preferentially eliminated from the zygote, resulting in a haploid embryo. (The haploidization process appears to be caused by a genetic incompatibility between the chromosomes of the different species.) The resulting haploids can be doubled with colchicine. This approach has led to the rapid production and widespread planting of several new barley varieties. It is being used successfully in other species too.

Polyploids

Once into the realm of polyploids, we must distinguish between autopolyploids and allopolyploids. *Autopolyploids* are composed of multiple sets from within one species, whereas *allopolyploids* are composed of sets from different species. Allopolyploids form only between closely related species; however, the different chromosome sets are homeologous (only partially homologous), not fully homologous as they are in autopolyploids.

Triploids

Triploids are usually autopolyploids. They are constructed from the cross of a 4x (tetraploid) and a 2x (diploid). the 2x and the x gametes unite to form a 3x triploid.

Triploids also are characteristically sterile. The problem again involves pairing at meiosis. Although pairing can take place in several ways, it usually occurs between only two chromosomes at a time. The

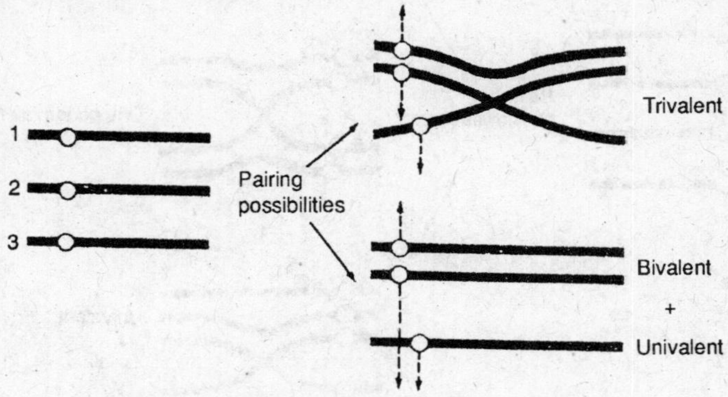

Fig. 3.14. Meiotic pairing possibilities in a triploid.

net result is always the same, an unbalanced segregation of one of the following types:

$$\frac{1+2}{3} \text{ or } \frac{1+3}{2} \text{ or } \frac{2+3}{1}$$

This happens for every chromosome threesome, and the probability of obtaining either a 2 x or x gamete is $(\frac{1}{2})^{x-1}$, where x is the number of chromosomes in a set. The other will be unbalanced gametes, having two of one chromosome type, one of another, two of another, and so on, and most will be nonfunctional. Even if the gametes are functional, the resulting zygotes will be unbalanced. A practical application of the sterility associated with triploidy lies in the production of seedless varieties of watermelons and bananas.

Autotetraploids

Autotetraploids occur either naturally, by the spontaneous accidental doubling of a 2x genome to 4x, or artificially, through the use of colchicine. Autotetraploids are evident in many commercially important crop plants because, as with other polyploids, the larger number of chromosome sets is often associated with increased size of the plant. This is manifested in increased cell size, fruit size, stomata size, and so on. Because 4 is an even number, autotetraploids can have a regular meiosis, although this is by no means always the case. The crucial factor is how the four chromosomes of one type pair and segregate. The two bivalent and the quadrivalent pairing modes tend to be most

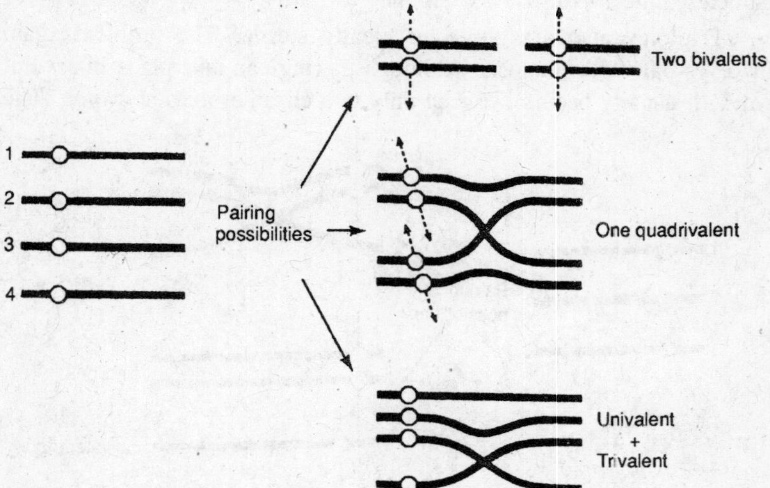

Fig. 3.15. Meiotic pairing possibilities in tetraploids.

regular in segregation, but even here there is no guarantee of a 2 → 2 segregation. If a regular 2 → 2 segregation is achieved at each chromosome type, as is the case in some species, than a formal genetic analysis can be developed for autotetraploids.

Let's hypothesize an experiment in which colchicine is used to double the chromosomes of an *Aa* plant into an *AAaa* autotetraploid, which we will assume shows 2 → 2 segregation. We now have a further worry because autotetraploids give different genetic results in their progeny, depending on whether or not the locus concerned is tightly linked to the centromere. First we consider a centromeric gene. The three possible pairing and segregation patterns are presented in Figures, these occur by chance and with equal frequency. As the figure shows, the 2x gametes will be *Aa, AA, or aa,* and these will be produced in a ratio of 8:2:2, or 4:1:1. If such a plant is offspring is obviously 1/6 × 1/6 = 1/36. In other words, a 35:1 phenotypic ratio will be observed if *A* is fully dominant over three *a* alleles.

If, in the same kind of plant, a genetic locus *B/b* is very far removed from the centromere, crossing-over must be considered. This forces us to think in terms of chromatids instead of chromosomes, and we have for *B* chromatids and for *b* chromatids. Because the number of crossovers in a such a long region will be large, the genes will become effectively unlinked from their original centromeres, and the packaging of genes two at a time into gametes is very much like grabbing two balls at random from a bag of eight balls, four of one kind and four of another. The probability of picking two *b* genes is then

4/8 (the first one) × 3/7 (the second one) = 12/56
= 3/14

So, in a selfing, the probability of a *bbbb* phenotype will be equal 3/14 × 3/14 = 9/196 = 1/22. Hence there will be a 21:1 phenotype ratio of *B – – –:bbbb.* For genetic loci of intermediate position, intermediate ratios will, of course, result.

Allopolyploids

The "classical" allopolyploid was synthesized by G. Karpechenko in 1928. He wanted to make a fertile hybrid between the cabbage (*Brassica*) and the radish (*Raphanus*) that would have the leaves of the former and roots of the latter. Each of these species has 18 chromosomes, and they are related closely enough to allow intercrossing. A variable hybrid progeny individual was produced from seed. However, this hybrid was functionally sterile because the nine chromosomes from the cabbage parent were different enough from the radish chromosomes that homology was insufficient for normal synapsis and disjunction.

However, one day a few seeds were in fact produced by this (almost) sterile hybrid. On planting, these seeds produced fertile individuals with 36 chromosomes. These individuals were allopolyploids. They had apparently been derived from spontaneous accidental chromosome doubling in the sterile hybrid, presumably in tissue that eventually became germinal and underwent meiosis. Thus, in $2n_1 + 2n_2$ tissue, there is a pairing partner for each chromosome, and balanced gametes of the type $n_1 + n_2$ are produced. These fuse to given $2n_1 + 2n_2$ allopolyploid progeny, which are in turn fertile also. This kind of allopolyploid is sometimes called an amphidiploid. (Unfortunately for Karpechenko, his amphidiploid had the roots of a cabbage and the leaves of a radish.)

If the allopolyploid is crossed to either parent species, sterile offspring result. In the case of the cross to radish, these offspring would be $2n_1 + n_2$, constituted from an $n_1 + n_2$ gamete from the allopolyploid, and an n_1 gamete from the radish. Obviously, the n_2 chromosomes will have no pairing partners, so sterility will result. Consequently, Karpechenko had effectively created a new species, with no possibility of gene exchange with its parents. He called his new species *Raphanobrassica*.

Nowadays, allopolyploids are routinely synthesized as a major tool in plant breeding. The goal obviously is to combine some of the worthwhile features of both parental species into one type. This kind of endeavor is very uncertain, as Karpechenko found out. In fact, only one amphidiploid has ever been intentionally produced that is of potentially widespread use. This is *Triticale*, an amphidiploid between wheat (*Triticum, 2n = 6x = 42*) and rye (*Secale,* 2n = 2x = 14). *Tricale* combines the high yields of wheat with the ruggedness of rye. A massive international *Triticale* testing program is now under way, and many breeders have great hopes for the future of this artificial amphidiploid. In mature, allopolyploidy seems to have been a major force in speciation of plants. There are many different examples. One particularly satisfying one is shown by the genus *Brassica*. Here three different parent species have been hybridized in all possible pair combinations to form new amphidiploid species. This has all taken place in nature, but *Brassica* amphidiploids also have been artificially synthesized.

A particularly interesting natural allopolyploid is bread wheat, *Triticum aestivum* (2n = 6x = 42). By a study of various wild relatives, it has been possible to reconstruct a probable evolutionary history of breat wheat. In a wheat meiosis, there are always 21 pairs of chromosomes. Furthermore, it has been possible to establish that any given chromosome has only one specific pairing partner (homologous pairing)—not five other potential ones (homologous pairing). The suppression of such homeologous pairing (which would lead to much reduced stability of the species) is maintained by a gene *Ph* ensures a diploid-like genetics for this basically hexaploid species. Without *Ph*, bread wheat could probably never have arisen. It is interesting to speculate on whether Western civilization could have arisen or progressed without this species—in other words, without *Ph*.

Somatic Allopolyploids from Cell Hybridization

Another innovative approach to plant breeding is to try to make allopolyploid-like hybrids by asexual methods. Theoretically, such a technique would permit combination of widely differing parental species. The technique does indeed work, but so far the only allopolyploids that have been produced are those that can also be made by the sexual methods we have considered already. The procedure is as follows. Cell suspensions of the two parental species are prepared and stripped of their cell walls by special enzyme treatments. The stripped cells are called *protoplasts*. The two suspensions (protoplast suspensions) are combined with polyethylene glycol, which enhances protoplast fusion. The parental cells and the fused cells will proliferate to form colonies (in much the same way as microbes) on agar medium. If these colonies, or calluses, are examined, a fair percentage of them are found to be allopolyploid-like hybrids with chromosome number equal to the sum of the parental types. Thus, not only do the protoplast cell membranes fuse to form a kind of heterokaryon, but the nuclei fuse too.

A good example of an allopolyploid-like hybrid is commercial tobacco, *Nicotiana tabacum*, which has 48 chromosomes. This species of tobacco was originally found in nature as a spontaneously occurring amphidiploid. The two probable parents are N. Sylves and N. Tomentosiformis, each of which has 24 chromosomes. A sexual cross between N. Tabacum and either of the other two gives a 36-chromosome hybrid n which there are 12 chromosome pairs plus 12 unpaired chromosomes. A cross between N. Sylvestris and N. Tomentosiformis gives a 24-chromosome hybrid n which there is no pairing at all. Hence, it appears that part of the N. Tabacum genome is from N. Sylvestris and part from N. Tomentosiformis. This amphidiploid can be re-created either sexually, by processing involving colchicine as described previously, or somatically by cell fusion. When cells or the prospective parental species are fused, a 48-chromosome hybrid cell line is produced from which may be grown plants whose behaviour is identical to that of N. Tabacum. (Note that in the latter method, colchicine is not required, since the fusion product is already amphidiploid.)

The recovery of somatic hybrids may be enhanced if a selective system is available. For example, two different monoploid lines of *N. Tabacum* had light-sensitive yellowish and light-resistant, as a result of complementation between the parental genotypes. The calluses can be grown into plantlets, which then either are grafted onto a mature plant to develop or are themselves potted.

Application of Polyploidy

Among the cultivated varieties of wheat, three different chromosome numbers are represented: 14, 28, and 42 (x = 7). For example, the primitive small-grained einkorn type of Europe and Asia, Triticum monococcum, has 14 chromosomes in its vegetative cells. Its yield is low and it is of comparatively little value. An emmer wheat (durum), T. dicoccum, grown chiefly in southern Europe but also in the United States, has 28 chromosomes. It has thick heads with large hard kernels and issued mainly for macaroni, spaghetti, and stock feed. The bread wheats, T. aestivum, with 42 chromosomes, were postulated by J. Percival in England to have come from a cross between emmer wheat and goat grass (Aegilops), both of which are native to the Babylonian region where bread wheat originated.

When techniques for artificial chromosome doubling became established, investigations of the origin of bread wheat confirmed Percival's theory. Experimental evidence obtained by E. S. McFadden and E. R. Sears and separately by H. Kihara traced the pathway for the origin of one type of bread wheat, T. Spelta.

Aegilops squarrosa (*n* = 7) was found to carry a group of major characteristics that distinguish the hexaploid (n=21) T. Spelta from the tetraploids (n = 1) T. dicoccum and T. dicoccoides. Hybrids between these tetraploid species of wheat and A. squarrosa proved to have all of the major taxonomic characters of T. spelta but the hybrids were completely or nearly sterile. When the F_1 hybrids of T. dicoccoides × A. squarrosa were treated with colchicine, highly fertile allopolyploids with 42 chromosomes were obtained. These synthetic hexaploids closely resembled the cultivated. T. spelta, and they produced highly fertile hybrids with that species and with T. vulgare, known to be in the ancestry of the bread wheats. This demonstrated that the genome of the hexaploid wheats corresponded to one chromosome set of A. squarrosa. It was postulated that T. spelta is the ancestral hexaploid wheat of Europe, having arisen, possibly in fairly recent times, in southeastern Europe or southwestern Asia following chromosome doubling of natural hybrids of T. dicoccoides (or its cultivated close relative, T. dicoccum) × A. squarrosa. T. spelta is believed to have been carried over the northerly route into central and western Europe. Experiments of McFadden, Sears, and Kihara reconstructed the pathway through which a moderately useful wheat and a goat grass hybridized in nature and produced forerunners of a most valuable crop, bread wheat.

New World Cotton

Crosses can be made between distinct species of cotton, members of the benes Gossypium. The hybrids show a wide range of vigor and fertility, making the material favourable for studies of origins. Three cytological groups have been found to correspond with the major world distributional areas. Old World cotton had 13 pairs of large chromosomes. American cotton, which originated in Central or South America, has 13 pairs of small chromosomes. New world cotton (the cultivated long-staple type) has 26 pairs, 13 large and 13 small. Evidently, hybridization and chromosome duplication occurred somewhere in the ancestry of the New World Cotton.

J. O. Beasley used the colchicine technique and succeeding in doubling the chromosomes of a hybrid between the Old World and American cotton. The resulting hybrids, with four set of chromosomes (amphidiploids), crossed readily among themselves and produced fertile plants resembling New World cotton. The process by which the valuable polyploid cotton may have originated in nature was thus duplicated in the laboratory.

Primrose Hybridization

The primrose, Primula kewensis, is an allotetraploid with 36 (2n) chromosomes. It was derived from a cross between two diploids, P. floribunda (x= 9) and P. verticillata (x= 9). Plants from these two species crossed readily, producing hybrids with 18 chromosomes in their vegetative cells. 9 from P. floribunda and 9 from P. verticillata, but the hybrids were sterile. Eventually, however, a branch on a hybrid plant developed from a cell in which the chromosome number was doubled (36), so that each chromosome had a homologous partner. This branch was propagated and gave rise to a fertile primrose plant with cells containing 36 chromosomes of the two diploid parents, the sterile diploid hybrid, and the fertile allotetraploid are shown.

Tobacco Resistance

Induced polyploidy has been exploited to a great extent. Practical applications may become more common as additional data are accumulated. By artificially induced polyploidy, disease resistance and other desirable qualities have been incorporated into some commercial crop plants. Tobacco, Nicotiana tabacum, for example, is susceptible to the tobacco mosaic virus (TMV), whereas N. glutinosa appeared at first observation to be resistant. Further investigation, however, showed that in N. glutinosa the virus killed the cells that were invaded and the virus particles became isolated in the dead cell. The apparent resistance thus was attributable to hypersensitivity. When the two tobacco species were crossed, the hybrid was found to be "resistant" to the virus, but totally sterile. When the chromosomes were doubled, it was possible to secure a fertile polyploid "resistant" to the virus.

Polyploid Fruits, Flowers, and Wheat

Some varieties of plants that serve human needs more effectively than others have now been identified as polyploids. Many polyploids were selected and cultivated because of their large size, vigor, and ornamental values, before their chromosome numbers were known. Giant "sports" from twings of McIntosh apple trees that were found to be tetraploid (4n) were propagated into whole trees, which produce extra-large fruit. The texture of the giant apples is as fine as that of diploids, but the yield is inferior. Mass selection of seedlings may overcome this difficulty. Bartlett pears, several varieties of grapes, and cranberries have also produced sports with giant fruits. Some of these show promise of practical usefulness. With colchicine treatment, a number of polyploids have been developed artificially. This technique has provided a way to explore the mechanism involved in polyploid formation and to make use of the good qualities of polyploids. Tetraploid (4n) maize is more vigorous than the ordinary diploid and produces some 20 percent more vitamin A. Its fertility is somewhat reduced, but this drawback responds to selection. Polyploid watermelons have been developed from colchicine treatment by Kihara and others.

The tetraploid with 44 chromosomes is large and has practical value. Triploid watermelons with 33 chromosomes are especially desirable because they are sterile and have no seeds. Among the flower garden varieties, 4n marigolds and snapdragons are widely cultivated. Polyploid plants respond to artificial selection and hybridization, as do diploid species. The recent history of plant breeding has been characterized by a marked improvement in many polyploid plant crops. The yield of wheat, for example, has increased appreciably. This has been accomplished by developing disease-resistant strains and breeding for increased hardiness and greater efficiency so that crops may survive under the various environmental conditions found in wheat-growing areas.

A constant threat to the wheat crop is rust—a fungus that attacks the stems and leaves of the growing plants and destroys the ripening grain. Spores are borne by wind and, when conditions are right, they spread like fire through wheat fields. The disease can be combated by developing rust-resistant strains and by eradicating barberry bushes, which are hosts to the spores during the spring months. But new varieties of rust that destroy previously resistant grain keep evolving, thus perpetuating the job of plant breeders. The larger kernels at the left are from a new strain of rust-resistant spring wheat. At the right are shown kernels of wheat, similar in other respects but not resistant, that are dwarfed from infection with stem rust. The number of kernels of grain per plant as well as the size of the kernels is decreased by rust infection. Investigators in agricultural experiment stations are constantly alert for new rusts. When a new one is found, the standard wheat varieties are tested against it. If they are not resistant, breeding programs are initiated immediately to develop new strains resistant to that particular rust.

Chromosome Anomalies in Spontaneous Abortions in Humans

A wide variety of chromosome numbers and chromosome structural aberrations is found in spontaneoulsy aborted human fetuses. The types of aberrations found vary according to differences in the age of the fetus at the time of abortion. For example, 40 percent of spontaneously aborted fetuses under 90 days of gestational age (i.e., length of time since the last menstrual period of the mother) exhibit chromosome anomalies. For 91-to 120-day-old fetuses, 25 percent show chromosomal anomalies, and only 5 percent of fetuses over 120 days old exhibit chromosome anomalies. Thus, chromosomal anomalies cause most fetuses to die and be aborted in early developmental stages.

Before the percentage of spontaneous abortions resulting from chromosomal anomalies can be calculated, one must first define what constitutes an aborted fetus. Apparently a large number of conceptions occur in humans, and the rechronic myelogenous leukemia possess two cell lines; one cell line has a normal chromosome complement, whereas the other appears to be missing the long arm of chromosome 2. This condition was originally thought to be a monosomy; however, using band staining techniques to identify the long arm, it was learned that the long arm was translocated to one of the larger chromosomes, usually chromosome 9 (referred to as the Philadelphia chromosome). The role of this chromosomal aberration in the induction, development, and progression of cancer is unknown.

Inherited autosomal recessive disorders, such as Bloom's syndrome, Fanconi's anemia, ataxia-telangiectasia, and xeroderma pigmentosum, have been associated with chromosomal instability and or deficiency in mutation repair mechanisms that result in chromosomal aberrations. These individuals have a high incidence of cancer.

Mutation Analysis of Large Genomic Regions in Tumor DNA using Single-strand Conformation Polymorphism

Detection of Point Mutations in Tumor DNA

In recent years, we have seen a dramatic improvement in our ability to detect nucleotide changes in tumor DNA using a number of techniques for mutation detection that have become routine instruments in many laboratories. The choice of a suitable method or methods of mutation analysis is governed by many factors, including the costs, experimental sensitivity, expected mutation pattern in the target sequence and its functional consequences, as well as staff expertise, personal experience, and preference. The primary selection criterion for such a method is the ability of a technique to search for the presence of unknown mutations in the analyzed regions (scanning methods) as opposed to looking for known mutations already characterized at the nucleotide level. Scanning procedures represent a cost-effective alternative to nucleotide sequencing, but usually at a price of an inferior detection rate. The former group of techniques includes procedures based on conformation polymorphism changes, denaturing gradient gel electrophoresis, constant denaturant capillary electrophoresis, and mismatch repair and RNase cleavage methods. The latter group, exemplified by techniques using sequence-specific oligonucleotides, oligonucleotide liagation assay, and ligase chain reaction, is less frequently used for analyzing molecular changes in tumor samples. A wise choice of most appropriate procedures is a crucial step for the identification of molecular changes underlying cancer development and for the correct interpretation of mutation screening.

Single-Strand Conformation Polymorphism Analysis

Single-strand conformation analysis (SSCP) is one of the simplest scanning techniques for detecting unknown mutations. Sequence variants usually exhibit differences in mobility of single-stranded fragments under nondenaturing electrophoretic conditions. Mobility shifts of DNA fragments result from mutation-induced changes of the tertiary structure of DNA. The term *polymerase chain reaction* (PCR)-SSCP refers to a PCR-amplified product analyzed by SSCP.

SSCP is particularly useful when searching for small deletions or insertions and single-base mutations and polymorphisms. Note that large insertions or deletions on the order of kilobases encompassing the amplified region are likely to go undetected.

MATERIALS

Polymerase Chain Reaction

1. Template: high-molecular DNA or cDNA extracted from tumor/normal cells.
2. *Taq* polymerase.
3. PCR buffer.
4. dNTPs.
5. Tested oligonucleotide primers.
6. Double-distilled H_2O.
7. α-^{32}P-dCTP or α-^{33}P-dCTP for isotopic detection.
8. Suitable restriction endonucleases, if the fragment size is too large for sensitive detection.
9. Formamide buffer: 95% formamide, 0.05% bromophenol blue, 0.05% xylene cyanol, 50 m*M* NaOH.
10. Thermal cycler.

Gel Electrophoresis

1. Gel electrophoresis apparatus.
2. Power pack.
3. Gel plates.
4. Combs.
5. Plastic film.
6. Filter papers.
7. Optional: temperature control of gel plates (water jacket, fans).

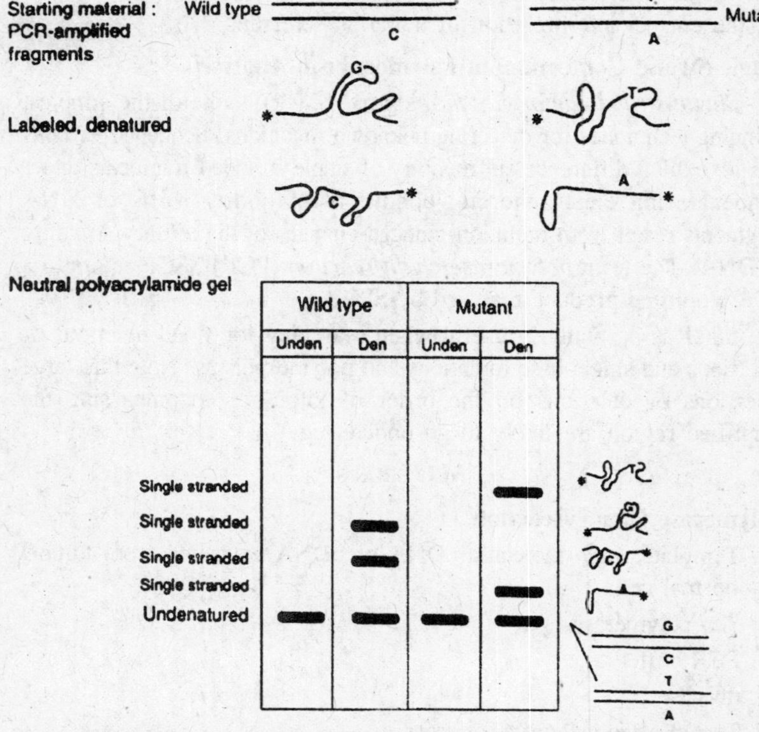

Fig. 3.16. The principle of single strand conformation polymorphism analysis.

8. Acrylamide/bisacrylamide
9. Ammonium sulfate.
10. TEMED.
11. Glycerol.
12. 10X Tris-borate EDTA (TBE) buffer: 0.9 *M* Tris-borate, 20 m*M* EDTA.
13. For isotopic detection of labeled fragments: Kodak X-OMAT films, X-ray cassettes, developer.

Methods

Polymerase Chain Reaction

PCR usually involves the incorporation of a label, either directly into the product or via an isotopically or nonisotopically labeled oligonucleotide primer. Alternatively, DNA fragments can be labeled after electrophoresis (e.g., by silver staining). The PCR should be tested using an agarose gel before running SSCP gels to determine whether the product is clean. PCR products with spurious bands should be avoided. A meticulous computer-assisted oligonucleotide primer design will pay off here.

A typical 100-μL PCR setup for direct isotopic labeling includes 10 μL of 10X PCR buffer (containing 1.5 m*M* $MgCl_2$), 5 μL of dNTP (2.5 m*M* stock solution), 5 μL of primer mix (final concentration 0.1–1 μ*M*), 5 × 5 μL of DNA (10–100 mg/μL), 0.5 μL of *Taq* polymerase (5 U/μL), approx 0.1–0.5 μL of α-^{32}P or α-^{33}P-dCTP (10 mCi/mL, 3000 Ci/mmol), and ddH_2O up to 100 μL. This amount is for at least five separate PCR reactions. A 20-μL reaction contains 5 μL of the template, which is convenient for dispensing multiple samples. The concentration of the labeled dNTPs depends on the sequence composition of the amplicon. After adding the enzyme-containing mixture to the template, thermal cycling should commence as soon as possible.

When using multiple samples, the amount of each template in the reaction tube should be the same. The usual amount of DNA per reaction is 50–100 ng. If the efficiency of PCR is markedly different from sample to sample (e.g., owing to the presence of enzyme inhibitors following DNA extraction from paraffin-embedded tissue), the template concentration should be further adjusted. However, loading different amounts of differentially labeled PCR products may result in altered mobilities of DNA fragments, and this may lead to difficulties in the interpretation of SSCP patterns. Different signal intensities from different samples are generally associated with a suboptimal detection rate, and every effort should be made to normalize the signal to allow the accurate evaluation of fragment mobility.

After completing the PCR, a restriction endonuclease digestion may help achieve a suitable fragment size for SSCP if the initial amplicon is too large. However, this extra step may be costly when analyzing multiple samples, and a subsequent complex SSCP pattern may be difficult to interpret.

Before running the electrophoresis, a formamide buffer is added in excess. No mixing is necessary before denaturing samples on a PCR cycler and loading onto an SSCP gel.

Gel Electrophoresis

1. Assemble glass plates for the gel.
2. In a beaker, mix the following components for a 100-mL gel solution: 5 mL of 10X TBE, 12 mL of 40% acrylamide/bisacrylamide (crosslinking 2.5%), 5 mL of glycerol, 1 mL of 10% ammonium persulfate, and ddH2O up to 100 mL.

3. Add 50 μL of TEMED and immediately pour into the gel plate assembly. Insert the comb and leave for at least 1.5 h to polymerize.
4. Remove the comb, clean the plates, assemble the gel, and fill the tank reservoir with 0.5X TBE. Check that there are no air bubbles in the gel, that the wells are undamaged, and that there is no leakage between the wells. Loading bromophenol dye to suspected wells is helpful for identifying leakages.
5. Denature the PCR products at 95°C for 5 min and load the wells. If the gel is run at room temperature, the applied power should not lead to an increased temperature of the plates. A thermometer attached to the plate is useful for monitoring the electrophoresis.
6. After completing the electrophoresis, transfer the gel to a sheet of filter paper, cover with Saran Wrap, and dry using a gel dryer. Expose the dried gel to an X-ray film for a few hours to overnight. Several exposures may be required for the correct reading of the autoradiogram.

Sensitivity of PCR-SSCP

The sensitivity of the PCR-SSCP method has been subject to controversy. Although the technique is generally believed to be efficient with the detection rate of >85% in a single run for fragments shorter than 300 bp, some previous estimates were lower. The sensitivity of PCR-SSCP depends on several factors, including the mutation pattern in the target sequence.

Since the higher-order structure of nucleic acids is dependent on the entire sequence of the amplified fragment, the sensitivity of SSCP in detecting a given variation will vary from one fragment to another. Unlike, e.g., denaturing gradient gel electrophoresis, there is no adequate theoretical model for predicting the three-dimensional structure of single-stranded DNA under a given set of conditions. Can we still say how sensitive our SSCP analysis is for a sequence of interest?

Because the tertiary structure of single-stranded fragments depends on physical conditions such as pH, ionic strength, and temperature, these factors are likely to influence SSCP patterns and need to be controlled. Although not previously endorsed, adding glycerol to SSCP gels was found to improve detection rate by reducing the pH of the Tris-borate buffer by the reaction of glycerol and borate ion. Temperature is a particularly important variable. If not controlled, an excessive running power may generate heat, resulting in the disappearance of mobility shifts. Optimized crosslinking and polyacrylamide gel concentrations are generally recommended.

The analysis of globin, *p53,* and rhodopsin mutations suggested that the type of mutation (transition vs transversion) did not play a major role in determining whether a mutation was detected by SSCP analysis. Although the position of the base substitutions was found to be more important than the type of base substitution, it appears that the sequence flanking mutated residues plays an even more significant role. Although the sensitivity was found to vary dramatically with the size of the DNA fragments analyzed, with the optimal size fragments for the detection of sensitive base substitution at about 150 bp, subsequent studies did not support such a steep decline in sensitivity. The blind quality control study of fragments larger than 450 bp reported a detection rate of 84%, an and even higher rate was found by running fragments between 300 and 800 bp in low-pH buffer systems. Since a single base change contributes to the tertiary structure in a larger fragment less than in small one, the probability of detecting a base change in fragments larger than 300 bp is generally considered to be lower than for optimally sized fragments.

The fact that a shift of a mutated fragment is detected under certain physical conditions led the authors to suggest the use of varying running conditions. This approach is warranted together with the use of complementary methods for mutation detection of single nucleotide changes, if a high or 100% detection rate is desired. The most commonly changed variables are polyacrylamide and buffer concentrations, use of an alternative gel matrix such as the MDE gel, and changing glycerol concentration in the gel.

In practice, however, the use of too thick gels, excessive amounts of loaded DNA (sometimes owing to insufficient labeling of fragments), inappropriate pH of the gel, a high voltage leading to gel overheating, and analyzing PCR products with spurious fragments are among the most common mistakes of inexperienced users. Each of these factors drastically affects the sensitivity of detection of conformational changes in single-strand fragments. These may have been reasons behind a controversy in the estimates of sensitivity. The sensitivity is generally considered to be very high if SSCP is performed using optimal conditions.

Mutation Analysis of ATM Using PCR-SSCP

The ability of PCR-SSCP to detect mutations also reflects the size of analyzed region. The analysis of multiple PCR-amplified fragments from large genes or genomic regions may decrease the sensitivity to an unacceptably low level.

We have partially addressed this concern in the PCR-SSCP analysis of the human *ATM* gene. *ATM* is deficient in patients with ataxia telangiectasia (A-T), a multisystem recessive condition with a high risk of developing lymphoreticular malignancies. The gene contains 66 small coding exons of the average size of 253 bp spanning about 184 kb of genomic sequence. Since the size of exons is suitable for SSCP analysis, all coding exons were individually amplified using oligonucleotides primed to the flanking intronic sequence.

By analyzing cDNA prepared from A-T patients, the mutation pattern in patients' germlines was previously found to be dominated by small insertions, deletions, and point mutations, whereas most mutations were private. Assuming that A-T patients had two mutated copies of *ATM* and all mutations were in the regions covered by the oligonucleotide primers, we could estimate the detection rate of our SSCP mutation assay at 70%. This figure may be an underestimate, if the assumptions are not met. Such an estimate, however, applies to the whole gene represented by 65 amplicons. The probability of detecting a mutation in an average PCR segment (approx 1√65 of ≅ the screened region) would be 65 0.7 0.995. Such a high detection rate is likely to reflect the mutation pattern found in the germline of A-T patients, dominated by small deletions, insertions, and point mutations, changes readily identified by SSCP. The detection rate is likely to be different when analyzing genes with a distinct mutation pattern.

As the majority of SSCP changes in the germline of A-T patients result in a premature termination of the ATM translation product, the protein truncation test, is an obvious method of choice for the identification of unknown A-T alleles in the germline. However, this test may not be the most appropriate for analyzing the same gene in tumor cells. By using the SSCP analysis of tumor DNA extracted from presentation samples of patients with sporadic T-cell prolymphocytic leukemia (T-PLL), a malignancy exhibiting phenotypic similarities to a leukemia seen in A-T, *ATM* was found to be mutated in about one-half of T-PLL cases.

A variety of techniques for mutation detection have now indicated that the gene is likely to be inactivated or mutated in most, if not all, T-PLL patients. The presence of loss-offunction mutations, frequent loss of the wild-type allele in tumor cells, and clustering of missense mutation in the highly conserved 3' part of the gene suggest that *ATM* functions as a tumor suppressor gene in the develoment of T-PLL. Although mutations have not been found in all cases, the detection rate using a single pass of SSCP was found similar to that in the germline of A-T patients, suggesting that the inactivation or mutation of *ATM* is probably an essential step among genetic alterations leading to T-PLL. Although the possibility of a predisposing heterozygote change could not be excluded in T-PLL samples with mutations identical to those previously reported in the germline (normal cells were not available), the vast majority of T-PLL cases contained mutations not previously found in A-T, suggesting somatic changes. The *ATM* mutation pattern in T-PLL was found to be markedly distinct from that found in the germline of A-T patients. While the frame-shift mutations predominate in the germline, most mutations in T-PLL tumor samples were missense mutations, a characteristic type of mutation in tumor cells.

Thus, although the *protein truncation test* (PTT) appears to be a method of choice for analyzing the germline changes with reported sensitivity similar to that of SSCP, PTT alone would be unlikely to detect missense mutations that characterize the somatic mutation pattern in the same gene in tumor cells. The PTT might even miss T-PLL alterations altogether. This case illustrates the need for employing a combination of wisely selected, preferably complementing techniques, particularly in the absence of our knowledge about the mutation pattern of the analyzed gene or genomic segment.

Negative results of PCR-SSCP mutation screening need a cautious interpretation. The absence of *ATM* mutations in a large number of breast cancer samples analyzed does not exclude the presence of mutations in this malignancy. However, it is unlikely that the gene would be frequently altered in breast cancer, certainly not to an extent similar to that found in T-PLL. No somatic *ATM* mutations have been identified so far in tumor DNA isolated from breast cancer, but, given a high population prevalence of breast tumors as compared to T-PLL, it is possible that this may be the case in a small proportion of breast tumors. To address this area of question, large sets of samples will need to analyzed.

SSCP is also sensitive in detecting mutations in mixed populations of cells containing normal and mutated alleles. A study of the *p53* gene detected mutations against the background of 85–95% of the wild-type allele, a figure sufficient to identify clonal changes in tumors containing a substantial proportion of normal cells.

In conclusion, PCR-SSCP is a rapid, simple, and cost-effective scanning method for mutation detection. It is particularly useful for the initial screening of optimally sized PCR-amplified fragments for point mutations, small deletions, and insertions. It serves well as an inexpensive method of choice for screening candidate cancer susceptibility genes and in situations in which the detection rate of mutation screening is not required to be absolute. If the expected mutation pattern is not known, a combination of suitable techniques discussed in this book should provide a more sensitive and specific tool for analyzing a growing number of cancer susceptibility genes and also more accurate estimates of cancer risk conferred by genetic alterations.

4

Chromosome in Cancer

Cancer is a genetic disease. Gene mutations are not only responsible for rare hereditary forms of human cancer, but for the sporadic forms of human malignancies as well. Many of these specific genetic defects in cancer cells can be visualized as chromosomal aberrations. Conventional cytogenetic analysis of metaphase chromosomes from human malignancies is a first screening step to identify chromosomal aberrations. Since the introduction of chromosome banding techniques in 1970 by Caspersson et al., significant knowledge of chromosomal aberrations especially in hematologic malignancies as well as sarcomas has been gained. In these malignancies, specific balanced translocations were identified and have led to the cloning of the genes involved at many breakpoints. These aberrations have proven to be of significant etiologic, diagnostic, prognostic, as well as therapeutic relevance, especially in leukemias. While cytogenetic analyses have been exceedingly valuable for the description of chromosomal abnormalities in hematologic malignancies and in sarcomas, epithelial cancers were more difficult to study. This is owing, in part, not only to the accessibility of malignant cells and subsequently metaphases for cytogenetic analysis in leukemias, but also to the nature of reciprocal translocations, which provided more immediate entry points for positional cloning efforts.

Although cytogenetic methodologies for the analysis of solid tumor specimens have improved, the difficulty in obtaining good-quality metaphase chromosomes remains. The interpretation of cytogenetic abnormalities in epithelial cancers is further confounded by the often vast number and complex nature of chromosomal aberrations in these tumors. Still, recurrent aberrations and recurrent chromosomal imbalances have been identified, but their clinical relevance is less firmly established.

Some of the limitations of chromosome banding techniques were overcome by the introduction of molecular cytogenetic techniques such as *fluorescence in situ hybridization* (FISH) with chromosome-painting probes and *comparative genomic hybridization* (CGH). For example, in hematologic malignancies, the t(12;21)(p13;q22) was detected by chromosome painting, because the telomeric regions involved in this translocation are indistinguishable by banding techniques. The 12;21 translocation was ascertained to be the most common chromosomal aberration in pediatric B-ALL and has been associated with a favorable prognosis. In solid tumors, the application of CGH has led to the identification of recurring patterns of genomic imbalances, both for different tumors and for distinct tumor stages.

Herein we focus on recently introduced molecular cytogenetic screening techniques that allow one to visualize all human metaphase chromosomes in specific colors.

Methodology of SKY

Two alternative techniques were developed for color karyotyping: combinatorial multifluor FISH (M-FISH) and spectral karyotyping (SKY). Whereas M-FISH employs a conventional imaging approach requiring multiple exposures through a series of single bandpass filters, SKY utilizes a novel approach by combining Fourier spectroscopy with epifluorescence microscopy and *charge-coupled device* (CCD)-imaging, thereby measuring the entire spectrum at all points in a single exposure.

For SKY, 24 differentially labeled chromosome libraries are produced by amplifying flow-sorted chromosomes utilizing a degenerate oligonucleotide primed polymerase chain reaction (DOP-PCR). Subsequently, the probes are labeled through the incorporation of either haptenized (*biotin* and *digoxigenin*) or directly labeled nucleotides, again via PCR. The use of five fluorochromes, either alone or in combination, allows one to discern up to 31 targets simultaneously. The generated chromosome-specific probes are pooled, precipitated with an excess of Cot-1 DNA to suppress repetitive sequences (suppression hybridization), and hybridized onto metaphase chromosomes. The use of an epi-fluorescence microscope equipped with a single, custom-designed triple bandpass filter allows for the simultaneous excitation of all fluorochromes as well as measurement of the entire emission spectrum of one metaphase in a single exposure. The emitted light from each point of the metaphase is passed through the collection optics and subsequently the Sagnac interferometer, where an optical path difference is created. The resulting interferogram is measured for every pixel of the CCD camera and, using Fourier transformation, is converted to spectral information. The spectral image can be displayed first in RGB colors (obtained by assigning red, green, and blue to specific sections of the emission spectrum) to evaluate the quality of the hybridization (i.e., homogeneity). Every pixel with the same spectral information is subsequently assigned a pseudo-color allowing the spectral classification of all chromosomes.

Advantages and Limitations

SKY, which is a screening tool, combines the respective advantages of chromosome banding techniques with the advantages of FISH. SKY is especially useful for the detection of interchromosomal structural aberrations that lead to color changes of the aberrant chromosome, such as translocations and insertions. It therefore facilitates the identification of cryptic translocations as well as the clarification of complex aberrations. In addition, SKY assists in the identification of material not recognizable by banding techniques such as marker and ring chromosomes. Other aberrations important in tumor cytogenetics such as double minute chromosomes as well as homogeneously staining regions, which are aberrations that harbor amplified DNA sequences, can be better resolved and contribute to the identification of critical oncogenes. Since its introduction, the value of SKY for use in cancer cytogenetics has been amply demonstrated.

Limitations of the technique pertain to intrachromosomal changes, such as para- or pericentric inversions as well as small deletions or duplications that do not lead to a color change or change in size of the respective aberrant chromosome, which then can be identified more readily in conjunction with the inverted DAPI image or other banding techniques. However, very small marker chromosomes or double minute chromosomes cannot in all instances be classified unambiguously, perhaps owing to the fact that their euchromatin content is low. Therefore, for a comprehensive analysis of tumor metaphases, a combination of molecular cytogenetic methods and banding techniques is advocated.

Applications of SKY

The usefulness of SKY for cancer cytogenetics, of hematologic malignancies as well as solid tumors, has been shown. Although the difficulty in obtaining good metaphase chromosomes from primary solid tumors remains, SKY analysis of the often complex karyotypes contributes to a more comprehensive cytogenetic analysis and might assist in the identification of stage-specific aberrations.

In contrast to the common assumption that cytogenetic changes in cell lines are frequently the result of culture artifacts, the molecular cytogenetic analysis of tumor cell lines showed that the karyotype is surprisingly stable after years of culturing. Furthermore, results of the SKY analysis of pancreatic cell lines correlated well with those of the CGH analysis of primary tumors. In contrast to CGH, SKY can detect the specific type of aberrations that result in chromosomal gains, the amplification of putative oncogenes (e.g., duplications, double minute chromosomes, homogeneously staining regions, jumping translocations), as well as loss of chromosomal material that may harbor tumor suppressor genes [e.g., deletions, isochromosomes such as i(17)(q10)]. Therefore, SKY analysis might not only contribute to the comprehensive analysis of complex aberrations, but also to our understanding of the mechanisms leading to these changes.

Mouse models of human disease become more and more important for our understanding of malignancies. As they often can be studied at earlier stages of carcinogenesis, they hold the promise for identification of tumor-initiating events as well as the dissection of genetic events responsible for tumor progression. Nevertheless, the analysis of mouse chromosomes is challenging because mouse chromosomes are all acrocentric and of similar size. The adaptation of SKY to the mouse karyotype by Liyanage et al. has proven to be a very valuable tool in the analysis of several mouse models. Comprehensive SKY analyses have shown that chromosomal aberrations in the aforementioned mouse tumors are similar to the changes in the respective human tumors, thereby validating these models.

Further Tools and Future Goals

To collect the increasing amount of emerging SKY data and to expedite the identification of new recurrent tumor or tumor stage-specific aberrations, a database has been developed.

This database is linked to the *Cancer Chromosome Aberration Project* (CCAP), which integrates the physical and sequence maps with the cytogenetic map of the human genome. This project provides STS-tagged and sequenced BAC clones for the entire human genome, whose cytogenetic location has been determined by high-resolution FISH mapping with a resolution of 1 to 2 Mb. CCAP facilitates the high-resolution mapping of chromosomal breakpoints and the subsequent cloning of the genes located at the breakpoints, and potentially will provide new diagnostic tools for interphase cytogenetics.

Furthermore, the combination of a comprehensive cytogenetic analysis with gene and protein expression profiling will provide in the near future a wealth of information on the consequences of chromosomal aberrations in cancer, and it is hoped that this will identify entry points for the identification of new therapeutic targets and strategies.

MATERIALS

Preparation of SKY Kits

1. PCR cycler.
2. Gel electrophoresis setup.
3. Speedvac.
4. Temperature-controlled microcentrifuge.
5. Primer: Telenius 6 MW(5'-CCGACTCGAGNNNNNNATGTGG-3') (100 μ*M*).
6. Nucleotides for DNA amplification: 100 m*M* dNTPs, 2 m*M* stock solution.
7. Nucleotides for labeling:
   (a) Spectrum Orange dUTP; dilute 1:5 to 0.2 m*M*.
   (b) Texas Red dUTP; dilute 1:5 to 0.2 m*M*.
   (c) 0.1 m*M* Rhodamine 110-dUTP.
   (d) 1 m*M* Biotin-16-dUTP.
   (e) 1 m*M* Digoxigenin-11-dUTP.
   (f) For the labeling PCR, prepare a stock solution of dNTPs with a final concentration of dATP, dCTP, and dGTP of 2 m*M*, but only 1.5 m*M* of dTTP.
8. Polymerase: native *Taq* (5 U/μL).
9. Buffer: 10X PCR Buffer.
10. Human Cot-1 DNA (1 mg/mL).
11. Salmon sperm DNA (9.7 mg/mL).
12. 3 *M* Na-acetate.
13. Deionized formamide (pH 7.0).
14. Master mix: 20% dextran sulfate in 2X *saline sodium citrate* (SSC), pH 7.0; autoclave and store aliquots at –20°C.

Pretreatment, Denaturation, and Hybridization of Slides for SKY

1. Thermomixer or water bath.
2. Hot plate.

3. Shaker.
4. Hybridization chamber at 37°C.
5. 2X SSC.
6. RNase A (stock solution: 20 mg/mL).
7. Pepsin (stock solution: 100 mg/mL).
8. 0.01 *N* HCl.
9. 1X Phosphate-buffered saline (PBS).
10. 1X PBS/$MgCl_2$ (50 m*M*).
11. 1% Formaldehyde in 1X PBS/$MgCl_2$ (50 m*M*).
12. Ethanol (70, 90, 100%).
13. 70% Formamide/2X SSC (pH 7.0).

Detection

1. 50% Formamide/2X SSC (adjust to pH 7.0).
2. 1X SSC.
3. 4X SSC/Tween-20 (0.1%).
4. Blocking Solution: 3% *bovine serum albumine* (BSA) in 4X SSC/ Tween-20; store at 4°C.
5. 1% BSA in 4X SSC/Tween-20.
6. DAPI: 80 ng/mL in 2X SCC (stock solution: 2 mg of DAPI/10 mL of sterile water).
7. Antifade: Dissolve 100 mg of 1,4-phenylenediamine in 2 mL of 1X PBS. Adjust pH with carbonate-biocarbanate buffer (pH 9.0) to 8.0, add 1X PBS to 10 mL, mix with 90 mL of 86% glycerol, aliquot and store at –20°C, and protect from light during use.
8. Mouse antidigoxin.
9. Fluorolink-Cy5-avidin.
10. Fluorolink-Cy5.5-sheep-antimouse-IgG.

Image Acquisition and Analysis

1. Epifluorescence microscope equipped with a DAPI filter and SKY filter V 3.0.
2. 150-W Xenon lamp.
3. SpectraCube SD200, Spectral Imaging Acquisition Software, and SkyView software.

Methods

The protocols in this chapter are for SKY analysis of human chromosomes. Nevertheless, the procedure is quite similar for the mouse genome.

Preparation of SKY Kits

Primary DOP-PCR

Flow-sorted chromosomes are amplified by PCR using a DOP as described by Telenius et al. The DNA amplification with DOPs is sequence unspecific. Therefore, employment of sterile techniques is extremely important in order to avoid contamination with genomic DNA.

Each chromosome-specific primary PCR product is labeled with a single fluorescent dye in a second DOP-PCR step for quality control purposes. Individual hybridization of all painting probes onto normal control slides should result only in specific hybridization signals for the respective pair of homologous chromosomes with low overall background. Otherwise, the primary PCR product cannot be used for the secondary and labeling DOP-PCR.

Secondary DOP-PCR

The primary PCR products are further amplified in a second DOP-PCR. Great precautions should be taken to avoid contamination also during this step.

1. Mix the following components for the PCR reaction: 2 μL of DNA (150–200 ng), 10 μL of PCR buffer (10X), 8 μL of $MgCl_2$ (25 m*M*), 10 μL of dNTP (2 m*M*), 65 μL of dH_2O, 4 μL of primer (100 m*M*), 1 μL of *Taq* polymerase (5 U/μL) for a total volume of 100 μL.
2. Run the following DOP-PCR program:
   (a) Step 1: 94°C for 1 min.
   (b) Step 2: 56°C for 1 min.
   (c) Step 3: 72°C for 3 min with addition of 1 s/cycle.
   (d) Step 4: Repeat steps 1–3, 29 times.
   (e) Step 5: 72°C for 10 min.
   (f) Step 6: 4°C for ∞.
3. Of the PCR product, run 2 μL on a 1% agarose gel as a quality control (intense smear between 500 bp and 2 kb).
4. Freeze DNA at –20°C.

DOP-PCR for labeling

Five different fluorochromes (either directly labeled or haptenized nucleotides) are used to accomplish the differential labeling of 24 painting probes. Table 4.1 was devised in order to achieve good color differences among chromosomes.

Table 4.1. Labeling scheme

Chromosome	*Rhodamine 110*	*Spectrum Orange*	*Texas Red*	*Cy 5 (biotin)*	*Cy 5.5 (digoxigenin)*
1		x			x
2					x
3	x			x	x
4			x	x	
5	x	x	x		x
6			x		x
7	x			x	
8	x				
9	x	x			x
10				x	x
11		x			
12	x		x	x	x
13	x	x			
14			x		
15		x	x	x	
16	x		x	x	
17				x	
18	x	x	x		
19		x		x	
20	x	x		x	
21	x				x
22		x	x	x	x
X	x		x		
Y	x	x		x	x

1. The setup in Table 4.1 leads to 57 reactions. Label 57 autoclaved PCR tubes accordingly.
2. Mix the following components for the PCR reaction: 4 μL of DNA (400–600 ng), 10 μL of PCR buffer (10X), 8 μL of $MgCl_2$ (25 m*M*), 5 μL of dNTP (2 m*M*), dTTP (1.5 m*M*), 65 μL (for direct)/67 μL (for indirect) of dH_2O, 2 μL of primer (100 m*M*), 1 μL of *Taq* polymerase (5 U/mL); x-dUTP: 5 μL of Rhodamine 110 (0.1 m*M*), 5 μL of Spectrum Orange (0.1 m*M*), 5 μL of Texas Red (0.2 m*M*), 3 μL of biotin (1 m*M*), 3 μL of digoxigenin (1 m*M*) for a total volume of 100 μL.

3. Run the following PCR program:
   (a) Step 1: 94°C for 1 min.
   (b) Step 2: 56°C for 1 min.
   (c) Step 3: 72°C for 3 min with addition of 1 s/cycle.
   (d) Step 4: Repeat steps 1–3, 29 times.
   (e) Step 5: 72°C for 10 min.
   (f) Step 6: 4°C for ∞.
4. Run 2 μL of each DNA on a 1% agarose gel as a quality control (intense smear between 500 bp and 2 kb).
5. One SKY Kit should be precipitated according to the protocol and hybridized onto normal chromosomes to assess the quality. If the SKY Kit is of good quality, the automated classification of a normal metaphase using the SkyView software should be correct. The following points should be evaluated for quality assessment:
   (a) The overall painting homogeneity as well as the suppression of heterochromatin.
   (b) The signal-to-noise ratio: Using the software for image acquisition, the highest and lowest values for the fluorescence intensity within the image are displayed. A difference of at least 100 counts between the intensity along chromosomes and background must be achieved.
   (c) The color separation between chromosomes displayed in red, green or blue in the RGB image.
   (d) The spectra of the single dyes: The spectra of this test hybridization should be compared with and should match the reference spectra stored in the combinatorial table (ctb)-file.
6. If the quality of the test hybridization was good, all SKY Kits can be precipitated and stored at –20°C until further use.

Precipitation of SKY kits

1. Combine 4 μL of each chromosome-painting probe (400–600 ng), 20 μL of human Cot-1 DNA and 1 μL of salmon sperm DNA in an Eppendorf tube for every SKY Kit.
2. Add 1/10 vol of 3 *M* Na-acetate and 2.5 to 3.0 times the total volume of cold 100% ethanol.
3. Vortex and precipitate at –20°C overnight or at –80°C for 30 min.
4. Centrifuge the precipitated DNA at 4°C and 11,700*g* for 30 min.
5. Remove the supernatant and dry the DNA pellet in a Speedvac for 5–10 min.

6. Add 6 μL of deionized formamide (pH 7.0), and shake in a thermomixer at 37°C until the pellet is completely dissolved (at least 1 h).
7. Add 6 μL of Master Mix, vortex, and spin briefly.
8. Store SKY Kits at –20°C until used for hybridization.

Preparation of Metaphase Chromosomes

Metaphase chromosome preparation for SKY follows standard cytogenetic protocols. Best hybridization results are generally obtained with slides aged for 1 wk either at room temperature or in a drying oven at 37°C, if they are exposed to humidity at room temperature. Prepared slides can be stored for several years in an airtight container with desiccant at –20 or –80°C after dehydration through an ethanol series.

Pretreatment, Denaturation, and Hybridization of Slides for SKY

Pretreatment of slides

1. Equilibrate slides in 2X SSC (room temperature).
2. Dilute the RNase stock 1:200 in 2X SSC, apply 120 μL per slide, and cover with a 24 × 60 mm coverslip.
3. Incubate at 37°C for 60 min.
4. Prepare 100 mL of 0.01 *N* HCl, adjust to pH 2.0, and pre-warm at 37°C.
5. Remove the coverslips and wash three times for 5 min each in 2X SSC on a shaker at room temperature.
6. Pepsin treatment: Add 5–30 μL of pepsin to a Coplin jar, and then add 100 mL of prewarmed HCl, and incubate the slides at 37°C for 2 min.
7. Wash twice for 5 min each in 1X PBS at room temperature, shaking.
8. Wash once for 5 min in 1X PBS/$MgCl_2$.
9. Incubate the slides for 10 min at room temperature in 1% formaldehyde in 1X PBS/$MgCl_2$ for postfixation.
10. Wash again one time for 5 min in 1X PBS at room temperature, shaking.
11. Dehydrate the slides in 70, 90, and 100% ethanol for 3 min each.
12. Let the slides air-dry.

Denaturation of SKY kit

1. Prewarm SKY Kits at 37°C for 30 min.

2. Denature SKY Kits at 80°C for 5 min in a thermomixer or water bath,
3. Before applying to the slide, allow the SKY Kit to preanneal at 37°C for 1 to 2 h.

Slide denaturation

1. Apply 120 μL of 70% formamide/2X SSC to a 24 × 60 mm coverslip and touch slide to coverslip.
2. Denature the slides at 75°C on a slide warmer for 1 min, 30 s. Denaturation of slides can also be performed by preheating 70% formamide/2X SSC in a Coplin jar in a water bath to 72°C. This is especially applicable for G-banded slides, for which denaturation times are shorter (10–30 s).
3. Shake off the coverslips and immediately place the slides in freshly prepared 70% ethanol (precooled to 0°C) for 3 min, followed by 3 min in 90% and 100% ethanol each.
4. Let the slides air-dry.

Hybridization

1. After preannealing, add the SKY Kit to the preselected hybridization area on the denaturated slides and cover with an 18-mm^2 coverslip.
2. Seal the coverslips with rubber cement and incubate in a hybridization chamber at 37°C for 48 h. Drying out of the SKY Kit during the hybridization time should be avoided.

Detection

1. Prepare solutions (formamide/SSC, 1X SSC, 4X SSC/Tween-20) and prewarm at 45°C for 30 min before starting the detection.
2. After the hybridization time, carefully remove the rubber cement and dip the slides in formamide/SSC until the coverslips slide off.
3. Wash the slides three times for 5 min each in formamide/SSC, shaking.
4. Wash the slides three times for 5 min each in 1X SSC, shaking.
5. Dip the slides in 4X SSC/Tween-20.
6. Incubate the slides with blocking solution (120 μL/slide, covered with a 24 × 60 mm coverslip) in a hybridization chamber at 37°C for 30 min.
7. Spin all the fluorescent dyes for 3 min at 13,000 rpm.
8. Dip the slides in 4X SSC/Tween-20.
9. Add 120 μL of antibody solution containing mouse antidigoxin (1:200 dilution in 1% BSA) per 24 × 60 mm coverslip, touch the slide

to the coverslip, and incubate in a hybridization chamber for 1 h at 37°C.

10. Wash the slides three times for 5 min each in 4X SSC/Tween-20, shaking.
11. Add 120 μL of antibody solution containing avidin-Cy5 and Cy5.5 antimouse (1:200 dilution in 1% BSA each) per coverslip (24 × 60 mm), touch the slide to the coverslip, and incubate in a hybridization chamber for 1 h at 37°C.
12. Wash the slides three times for 5 min each in 4X SSC/Tween-20, shaking.
13. Stain with DAPI for 5 min in a light-protected Coplin jar.
14. Wash for 5 min in 2X SSC, shaking.
15. Dehydrate the slides in an ethanol series (70, 90, 100%) for 3 min each.
16. Let the slides air-dry in the dark.
17. When the slides are completely dry, apply 30 μL of antifade, cover with 24 × 60 mm coverslips, and store in the dark at 4°C until image acquisition.

Image Acquisition and Analysis

For each metaphase, a spectral image and the corresponding DAPI image is acquired using an epifluorescence microscope connected to the SpectraCube (Applied Spectral Imaging; a combination of a Sagnac-Interferometer and a CCD-camera). For the spectral image, a custom-designed SKY filter is employed; the DAPI image is acquired using the TR1-filter. The subsequently inverted DAPI-image gives a chromosomal banding pattern comparable with the one obtained by G-banding. During image acquisition, heat protection filters should normally be placed into the light pass but can be removed if the intensity of the fluorescent dyes with emission in the far red range (Cy5 and Cy5.5) is weak.

For image analysis, the spectral image is first displayed in RGB (red-green-blue) colors. This allows for the evaluation of hybridization quality. Using the SkyView software, both the spectral and the DAPI image are then analyzed simultaneously. Through correlation of the spectral information with the labeling scheme and the reference spectra of the five fluorescent dyes (stored in a ctb–file) a specific pseudocolor is assigned to each image point. Thus, all material belonging to the same chromosome will be displayed in the same pseudocolor, and chromosomal aberrations will be easily visible.

Notes

1. Pretreatment with pepsin to remove residual cytoplasm is a crucial step because overtreatment with pepsin leads to reduced signal intensity and impaired chromosome morphology and therefore compromises SKY results. Pepsin concentration and time must therefore be adjusted according to the amount of cytoplasm; that is, use low concentrations of pepsin (5–10 μL; 2 min) if there is little cytoplasm, and 20–30 μL, 5 min, for cells with high amounts of cytoplasm. Cytoplasm is visible as opaque material around the metaphase chromosomes. If no cytoplasm is present, pepsin treatment may not be necessary at all.
2. During the detection avoid exposure to light as much as possible and avoid air-drying of the slides between the different steps. Slides should be handled carefully in order to avoid scratching the surfaces.

Detection of Chromosome Abnormalities in Leukemia Using Fluorescence In Situ Hybridization

Cytogenetic analysis plays a pivotal role in the diagnosis and management of patients with hematologic malignancies. In research, the identification of specific chromosomal rearrangements associated with defined clinical groups has led to an explosion in the knowledge of basic mechanisms contributing to leukemogenesis. The strength of cytogenetic analysis is as a direct method for screening the whole genome. However, the interpretation of the banding pattern of highly rearranged chromosomes is often unreliable. Since the advent of molecular cytogenetic technologies based around *fluorescence in situ hybridization* (FISH), the accuracy of cytogenetic diagnosis has been considerably enhanced.

Specific problems hampering the accurate analysis of leukemic karyotypes such as the low mitotic index, heterogeneity of the sample, and often poor morphology of chromosomes are also largely overcome by FISH. One of the most significant advances is the use of interphase FISH, which permits the use of nondividing cells as DNA targets and enables a large number of cells to be evaluated. This has advantages for monitoring disease progression, response to treatment, and success of bone marrow transplantation. The simultaneous identification of cell type (by morphology or immunophenotype) and chromosome abnormality (by FISH) is also possible, allowing the identification of cell lineages involved in the neoplastic clone.

The application of FISH to metaphase chromosomes provides unequivocal evidence of chromosome rearrangements. Whole-chromosome painting probes, derived from chromosome-specific libraries, or *polymerase chain reaction* (PCR) amplification of flow-sorted or microdissected chromosomes can be used to identify accurately the components of complex rearrangements and marker chromosomes. Chromosome-specific centromeric probes, targeting the tandemly repeated alpha (or beta) satellite sequences present in the hetero-chromatin of chromosome centromeres, are invaluable for the rapid visualization of numerical chromosome abnormalities. Specific gene probes for the detection of leukemia-associated translocations and inversions allow accurate detection of these rearrangements, especially in complex or masked versions of the translocation, and are particularly useful for interphase analysis. A significant advance in the resolution of FISH for the visualization of translocations is provided by hybridization to extended DNA fibers, so-called fiber-FISH. This is particularly valuable for the analysis of chromosome rearrangements with highly variable breakpoints, provided there is a well-characterized contig of the region.

One of the most appealing aspects of FISH is the ability to identify several targets simultaneously using different colors (so-called multicolor FISH). The most recent developments in this area are those that enable "*color karyotyping*," using whole-chromosome painting probes that delineate each of the 22 pairs of autosomes and the sex chromosomes in a different color. The related techniques of multiplex-FISH (M-FISH) and spectral karyotyping (SKY) provide the prospect of a molecular analysis of karyotype. Herein we outline the basic FISH methodologies, as well as some of the more advanced techniques, with particular reference to specific applications in hematologic malignancy.

MATERIALS

Preparation of Bone Marrow Metaphase Chromosomes

1. Bone marrow aspirate collected into sterile bottles containing transport medium (RPMI 1640 plus 50 U/mL of penicillin, 50 μg/mL of streptomycin, and 10 U/mL of preservative-free lithium heparin).
2. Thymidine, crystalline: 100 μM stock.
3. 5-Fluorodeoxyuridine: 100 μM stock.
4. Uridine: 400 μM stock.
5. Colcemid (10 μg/mL).

6. Culture medium: RPMI 1640, 50 U/mL of penicillin, 50 μg/mL of streptomycin, 2 m*M* L-glutamine, 20% *fetal calf serum* (FCS).
7. Hypotonic solution: 0.075 *M* KCl.
8. Fixative: 3:1 AnalaR methanol:glacial acetic acid, at 4°C.
9. Precleaned microscope slides (Superfrost, BDH).

Pretreatment of Chromosomes and Nuclei

1. Pepsin (100 mg/mL).
2. Phosphate-buffered saline (PBS)/50 m*M* $MgCl_2$: 50 mL of 1 *M* $MgCl_2$ + 950 mL of 1X PBS.
3. PBS/50 m*M*$MgCl_2$/1% formaldehyde (make up fresh each time): 2.7 mL of formaldehyde in 100 mL of PBS/$MgCl_2$.
4. PBS (1X): 8 g of NaCl, 0.2 g of KCl, 1.44 g of Na_2HPO_4, 0.2 g of KH_2PO_4 in 800 mL of H_2O, pH to 7.4 with HCl. Add H_2O to 1 L.
5. RNase A (10 mg/mL).
6. Formaldehyde (40% [w/v]).

Preparation of Probe DNA

Cosmids, P1 artificial chromosomes (PACs)

1. 2X TY medium (1 L): 16 g of Bacto tryptone, 10 g of yeast extract, 5 g of NaCl.
2. Glucose/EDTA/Tris (GET): 0.9% glucose, 10 m*M* EDTA, 25 m*M*Tris-HCl, pH 7.0.
3. NaOH/sodium dodecyl sulfate (SDS): 0.2 *M* NaOH, 1% SDS.
4. 3 *M* KOAc, pH 5.5.
5. RNase A (DNase free) (10 mg/mL) (Sigma).

Yeast artificial chromosomes (YACs)

1. YEPD medium (1L): 10 g of Bacto yeast extract, 20 g of Bactopeptone, 20 g of dextrose, 10 mL of adenine sulfate (0.5% in 0.5 *M* of HCl).
2. GDIS: 2% Triton X-100, 1% SDS, 100 m*M* NaCl, 10 m*M* Tris-HCl, pH 7.4, 1 m*M* EDTA.
3. Phenol:chloroform:isoamyl alcohol (25:24:1).
4. RNase A (DNase free) (10 mg/mL).
5. Glass beads, 710–1180 μm, acid washed.

Nick Translation Labeling

1. Purified probe DNA (1 μg).
2. 10X Nick translation buffer: 0.5 *M* Tris-HCl, pH 7.5, 50 m*M* $MgCl_2$, 0.5 mg/mL of nuclease-free *bovine serum albumin* (BSA).

3. 1 m*M* Biotin-16-dUTP (bio-16-dUTP), 1 m*M* digoxigenin-11-dUTP (dig-11-dUTP).
4. 100 m*M* Dithiothreitol (DTT).
5. dNTP mix: 0.5 m*M* each dATP, dCTP, dGTP, and 0.1 m*M* dTTP.
6. DNase 1 (200,000 U).
7. DNase 1 dilution buffer: 50% glycerol, 0.15 *M* NaCl, 20 m*M* sodium acetate, pH 5.0.
8. DNA polymerase 1 (10 U/μL).
9. MicroSpin G50 columns.
10. *Escherichia coli* tRNA (10 mg/mL).
11. Salmon sperm DNA (5 mg/mL, sonicated to 200–500 bp).
12. TE: 10 m*M* Tris-HCl, pH 7.5, 1 m*M* EDTA.
13. Gel-loading buffer (5X bromophenol blue): 10% (w/v) Ficoll, 0.1 *M* Na_2 EDTA, 0.5% (w/v) SDS, 0.1% (w/v) bromophenol blue.
14. Electrophoresis buffer (10X TBE): 108 g of Tris base (89 m*M*), 55 g of boric acid (89 m*M*), 40 mL of 0.5 *M* EDTA, pH 8.0 (2 m*M*) per liter.
15. *Phi*X174 *Hae*III size marker.

Competitive In Situ Suppression Hybridization

1. Human Cot-1 DNA.
2. 3 *M* Sodium acetate.
3. Denaturing solution: 70% (v/v) formamide, 2X saline sodium citrate (SSC), 0.1 m*M* EDTA, pH 7.0.
4. Hybridization buffer: 50% (v/v) formamide, 10% (w/v) dextran sulfate, 1% (v/v) Triton X-100, 2X SSC, pH 7.0.
5. Formamide (purified).
6. 50% Dextran sulfate.
7. 20X SSC: 1X SSC = 150 m*M* sodium chloride, 15 m*M* sodium citrate, pH 7.0.
8. Blocking solution: 3% (w/v) BSA in 4X SSC, 0.05% (v/v) Triton X-100 (make up fresh).
9. Wash solution: 4X SSC, 0.05% (v/v) Triton X-100.

Detection of Bound, Labeled Probe

1. Fluorescence microscope (epifluorescence illumination), with suitable fluorescence objectives and filter sets (usually need separate filter sets for fluorescein isothiocyanate [FITC], Texas red/rhodamine and 4,6-diamidino-2-phenylindole [DAPI]/AMCA, as well as a double or triple filter block).

2. Avidin-DCS-FITC (1 mg/mL).
3. Biotinylated anti-avidin D (0.5 mg/mL).
4. Propidium iodide.
5. Vectashield mountant.
6. Avidin DCS-Texas red (2.5 mg/mL stock).
7. Diluent for antibodies: blocking solution, filtered through a 0.45-μm syringe filter. Stock antibody solutions are stored at –20°C.
8. Monoclonal antidigoxigenin.
9. Rabbit antimouse Ig-FITC.
10. Monoclonal antirabbit-FITC.

Degenerate Oligonucleotide Primer-PCR Amplification of Flow-Sorted Chromosomes

1. Flow-sorted chromosomes (approximate concentration: 500/μL).
2. 2X PCR buffer: 10 m*M* $MgCl_2$, 100 m*M* KCl, 20 m*M* Tris-HCl, pH 8.4, 0.2 mg/mL of gelatin.
3. dNTP mix: 2 m*M* each dATP, dCTP, dGTP, dTTP.
4. 6-MW primer: 5' CCGACTCGAGNNNNNNATGTGG 3' (30 μ*M*).
5. *Taq* 1 (2.5 U/μL) polymerase.
6. 1 m*M* Biotin-16-dUTP or 1 m*M* dig-11-dUTP.

Alkaline Phosphatase Antialkaline Phosphatase Staining

1. Thin bone marrow smears (store unfixed wrapped in foil at –20°C).
2. Tris-buffered saline (TBS): 1 *M* Tris, 0.5 *M* NaCl.
3. Appropriate primary monoclonal antibody.
4. Rabbit antimouse antibody diluted 1:500 in TBS.
5. Monoclonal alkaline phosphatase antialkaline phosphatase (APAAP) complex (1:500 dilution).
6. Alkaline phosphatase substrate: Dissolve 2 mg of naphthol AS mix into 10 mL of 0.1 *M* Tris buffer (pH 8.2). To this add 10 mg of Fast Red TR mix and dissolve. Then add levamisole (0.1 *M*) to block endogenous alkaline phosphatase. Filter before use.

Methods

Preparation of Target Material

Culture and harvesting of mitotic chromosomes from leukemic bone marrow

1. Set up between one and four cultures, depending on the white cell count. Each culture should contain approx 1×10^6 cells/mL. In most cases, the following will suffice:

(a) Direct harvesting after 1 h exposed to colcemid (0.1 μg/mL).

(b) A 24-h incubation with the addition of colcemid for the last hour.

(c) Twenty-four hour synchronized cultures. For these, add fluorodeoxyuridine (0.1 *μM*) and uridine (4 *μM*) after 24 h and reincubate the cultures overnight (16–18 h). Finally, add thymidine (10 *μM*), and reincubate for 5 to 6 h before adding of colcemid for 10 min before harvesting.

2. Centrifuge at 100*g* for 5 min. Discard the supernatant and resuspend the pellet in hypotonic solution (prewarmed to 37°C). Incubate at 37°C for 20 min.
3. Centrifuge, discard the supernatant, and mix the pellet in the small volume of hypotonic solution remaining. Add freshly made fixative dropwise, with mixing. Add the first milliliter of fixative slowly, and then make up to 10 mL.
4. Leave in fixative for 30 min at 4°C. Centrifuge at 100*g* for 5 min, then wash in three to five changes of fixative before making slides.
5. Wipe Superfrost slides clean with absolute ethanol just before use.
6. Place a drop of cell suspension on each slide and air-dry. Monitor the quality of chromosome spreading under phase contrast. Chromosomes should be well spread without visible cytoplasm and should appear dark gray under phase contrast (not black and refractile or light gray and almost invisible).

The "direct" culture can be replaced by overnight incubation with colcemid (0.5 μg/mL). For cell lines, culture according to their specified growth requirements, then harvest when growing logarithmically, usually 24–48 h after a change of medium. Add colcemid for the final 1 h before harvesting.

Preparation of interphase nuclei

Interphase nuclei are present in large numbers on slides from leukemic bone marrow or blood prepared. Interphase nuclei can also be prepared from fresh bone marrow after Ficoll separation of mononuclear cells. After washing pellets in culture medium (RPMI, without FCS), fix the cell pellet in several changes of methanol:acetic acid (3:1). Drop onto clean slides. Nuclei from a variety of tissues and culture types can be prepared by cytospin, then fixed in methanol (10–20 min). Bone marrow smears are prepared in the usual way and stored unfixed, wrapped in foil at –20°C until required.

Pretreatment of Chromosomes and Nuclei

The methanol/acetic acid fixation of metaphase chromosomes removes some basic proteins that might interfere with hybridization. However, there is still a variable amount of other protein and cytoplasmic contaminants on metaphase chromosome preparations that may block hybridization, or cause nonspecific background. We routinely use an RNase treatment and postfixation with formaldehyde. For interphase FISH, it may be necessary to add a proteolytic digestion (e.g., pepsin) treatment to this, to aid access of the probe and detection reagents. However, overdigestion can cause loss of cells from slides, so use only when absolutely necessary.

1. Place 100 μL of RNase A (100 μg/mL) on slides under a 24 × 50 mm coverslip and incubate at 37°C for 30 min to 1 h.
2. Wash three times (3 min each) in 2X SSC (with agitation).
3. Pepsin treatment (optional): 50 μg/mL in 0.01 *M* HCl. Incubate for 10 min at RT.
4. Wash (two times for 5 min each) in 1X PBS.
5. Wash (once for 5 min) in 1X PBS/50 m*M* $MgCl_2$.
6. Fix in PBS/50 m*M* $MgCl_2$/1% formaldehyde (2.7 mL of formaldehyde in 100 mL of 1X PBS/50 m*M* $MgCl_2$ [fresh solution]) for 10 min.
7. Wash in 1X PBS for 5 min (with agitation).
8. Dehydrate slides through an alcohol series (70%, 95%, absolute) and allow to airdry. Slides can be stored desiccated at 4°C for up to 1 mo before use.

Preparation of Probe DNA

Cosmid, P1, and PAC DNA

Any DNA purification method that produces DNA suitable for sequencing will generally also work for FISH. The following medium-scale alkaline lysis method gives a high yield of cosmid, PAC, or P1 DNA. However, this is relatively impure and may require additional purification steps. As a guide, if the DNA fails to cut with DNase I, purify with phenol/chloroform or CsCl gradient centrifugation.

1. Inoculate 250 mL of 2X YT medium plus antibiotic (final concentration: 30 μg/mL of kanamycin, 50 μg/mL of ampicillin) in a 500-mL sterile plugged flask with a single well-separated colony.
2. Grow at 37°C with shaking (300 rpm) until approaching saturation (approx 18 h)

3. Transfer to a 250-mL bottle. Centrifuge at 4000*g* for 10 min.
4. Discard the supernatant medium and drain briefly. Add 50 mL of cold glucose/EDTA/Tris (GET). Resuspend by drawing up in a 10-mL pipet.
5. Add 50 mL of NaOH/SDS at room temperature. Mix by very gentle, minimal inversions. Leave for 5 min (room temperature).
6. Add 50 mL of cold 3 *M* KoAc. Mix by very gentle, minimal inversions. Place on ice for 20 min.
7. Centrifuge at 9000*g* for 20 min (4°C).
8. Carefully transfer the supernatant to a fresh 250-mL bottle through a mesh.
9. Add 90 mL of isopropanol (0.7X vol) and mix. Leave at room temperature for 5 min.
10. Centrifuge at 5000*g* for 15 min at room temperature. Discard supernatant.
11. Add 25 mL of 70% ethanol, and rotate the bottle to rinse the inner surface. Transfer pellet to 50-mL Falcon tubes.
12. Centrifuge at 5000*g* for 5 min (4°C). Discard the supernatant.
13. Allow to stand for 1 min, and then remove final traces of 70% ethanol with a Gilson.
14. Air-dry. Resuspend in approx 200 μL of H_2O (or TE).
15. Incubate with RNase A (final concentration: 30 μg/mL) at 37°C for 30 min.

Yeast artificial chromosome DNA

The following method yields high quantities of total yeast DNA suitable for FISH. The average yield from a 10-mL culture is 10–20 μg.

1. Culture cells at 30°C for up to 2 d in 10 mL of YEPD medium (grow to saturation).
2. Centrifuge (1500*g*, 10 min) to pellet the cells, and discard the supernatant. Transfer to an Eppendorf tube, and wash the cells with 500 μL of distilled water.
3. Centrifuge and then resuspend in 200 μL of GDIS. Add 0.35 g of glass beads and 200 μL of phenol. Vortex continuously for 5 min.
4. Add 200 μL of distilled water to the suspension, mix well, and spin for 4 min in a microcentrifuge.
5. Extract once more with phenol, then once with phenol:chloroform: isoamyl alcohol.

6. Precipitate the DNA as usual (0.1X sodium acetate, 2X absolute ethanol) followed by a 70% ethanol rinse.
7. Remove the aqueous layer and treat this with 50 μg/mL of RNase A for 20 min at 37°C.
8. Dry the pellet and resuspend in 20 μL of distilled water.
9. Measure the DNA concentration accurately, preferably in a fluorometer.

Nick Translation Labeling of Probes

Nick translation is the most widely used method for labeling probes for *in situ* hybridization, because the fragment size can be controlled by the amount of DNase I in the reaction mixture. As nick translation is highly efficient for labeling double-stranded circular DNA molecules, there is no need to isolate the insert from the vector sequences. The size of labeled probe fragments is a critical factor in *in situ* hybridization protocols, with an average size of 300 bp being optimal (range 100–500 bp). Larger probe fragments will result in bright background fluorescence all over the slide, obscuring any specific signal. If the labeled probe fragments are too small (<50 bp), the site of hybridization may not be visible owing to the resulting weak fluorescent signal.

To ensure the correct size of labeled fragments, it is necessary to run a small aliquot of labeled probe on a 2% agarose gel. Other labeling methods (e.g., random primer labeling, PCR) can be used to produce labeled probes for FISH. However, in all cases the size of the labeled fragments must be checked, and recut with DNase I, if necessary. Probes for localization by FISH are usually labeled with either biotin or digoxigenin, available conjugated to dUTPs by a spacer arm of variable length (e.g., bio-16-dUTP, dig-11-dUTP). Various fluorochromes including FITC, and the cyanine dyes Cy3, and Cy5 are now available directly conjugated to dUTP, enabling direct labeling of DNA.

1. Add the following (in order) to a 1.5-mL Eppendorf tube on ice:
   (a) 1 μg of probe DNA.
   (b) 1.2 μL of 1 m*M* bio-16-dUTP, dig-11-dUTP, or fluorochrome-dUTP.
   (c) 5 μL of dNTP mix.
   (d) 5 μL of 10X nick translation buffer.
   (e) 5 μL of 100 m*M* DTT.

   (f) Sterile-distilled water to make up to a final volume of 50 μL.
   (g) 3–5 μL of 100 U/mL DNase I (need to establish amount for each new batch).
   (h) 1 μL of 10 U/μL DNA Polymerase I.
2. Mix well.
3. Incubate at 15°C for 90 min.
4. Stop reaction by placing tubes on ice.
5. Check the size of the labeled products by running an aliquot on a 2% agarose gel (in TBE and containing 5 μL of 5 mg/mL ethidium bromide/100 mL) as follows:
   (a) 5 μL of labeled probe (approx 100 ng).
   (b) 4 μL of gel-loading buffer (5X bromophenol blue).
   (c) 11 μL of sterile distilled water.
6. Run at 50 V for 1–1.5 h with *Phi*X174 *Hae*III (20 μL = 250 ng) as a size marker.
7. View on a transilluminator and photograph. The optimal size range for *in situ* hybridization is 50–500 bp. A smear of products from 100 to 300 (corresponding to the six smallest bands of *Phi*X174) is suitable. If the size range is larger than this, add a further 5 μL of DNase I, place at 15°C for an additional 30–60 min, and run another aliquot on a gel to test the size.
8. Purify to remove unincorporated nucleotides by passing the labeled probe through a MicroSpin G50 column (designed for biotinylated probes) according to the manufacturer's instructions.
9. Measure the volume of eluate and then ethanol precipitate the purified, labeled probe by adding the following:
   (a) 50 μg of *E. coli* tRNA.
   (b) 50 μg of salmon sperm DNA.
   (c) 0.1 vol of 3 *M* sodium acetate, pH 5.6.
   (d) 2–2.25 vol of ice-cold ethanol.

   Mix well and place at –70°C for 1–2 h or –20°C overnight.
10. Centrifuge in a microcentrifuge for 15–25 min at 4°C. Pour off the supernatant and dry the pellet (either air-dry or dry in a vacuum desiccator). Resuspend the pellet in 20 μL TE pH 8.0 to give a final concentration of 50 ng/μL. Allow the DNA to dissolve at room temperature for 1 to 2 h or at 4°C overnight with occasional mixing. Purified, labeled probes are stable for several years when stored at –20°C.

Competitive In Situ Suppression Hybridization

Clones containing large DNA fragments (i.e., phage, cosmid, YAC, P1) and whole-chromosome paints require an additional step before hybridization to remove ubiquitous repetitive sequences. This is achieved by a short incubation prior to hybridization, with unlabeled human competitor DNA, in the form of either total human DNA (placental DNA, sheared and sonicated to 50–300 bp) or human Cot-1 DNA (Gibco-BRL). When all of the probe sequences contribute to the hybridization signal (e.g., repetitive DNA probes, unique cDNA probes), there is no need to add competitor DNA. Hybridization is carried out in a moist chamber. This can be achieved by using a plastic microscope slide box containing moist tissue paper (wring out excess water), placed in an incubator or floated in a water bath. Alternatively, we use metal trays for both hybridization and detection steps.

Table 4.2 Suggested amount of probe and competitor (10 μL hybridization volume)

Type of probe	*Amount*	*Cot-1 DNA (μg)*
Single fragment cloned in plasmid	200 ng	
Single fragment cloned in phage	200 ng	2.5
Single fragment cloned in cosmid	50–100 ng	2.5
YAC, total yeast DNA	400 ng–1 μg	5–7.5
PAC, P1	200–400 ng	3–5
Alphoid DNA repeat (centromere)	10 ng	
Whole-chromosome paint, libraries	100–400 ng	5–7.5
Whole-chromosome paint, PCR amplified flow-sorted chromosomes	100 ng	6.25

1. Dry down the appropriate concentration of probe and competitor either in a vacuum desiccator (Speedivac) or by ethanol precipitation; e.g., for cosmids:
   (a) 100 ng of labeled probe.
   (b) 2.5 μg (2.5 μL) of Cot-1 DNA.
   (c) 0.1 vol of 3 *M* sodium acetate.
   (d) 2 vol of ice-cold ethanol.
   Allow to precipitate for 1 to 2 h at –70°C.
2. Centrifuge and dry down the pellet as for labeled probes. Resuspend the pellet in 11 μL of hybridization buffer (warmed to room temperature).

3. Denature the probe mixture at 95°C in a hotblock for 10 min. Plunge the tubes on ice for a few minutes, and then centrifuge briefly in a microcentrifuge.
4. Place the probe mixture at 37°C for 15 min to 2 h.
5. Just prior to hybridization, denature the chromosomal DNA as follows:
   (a) Incubate the slides in denaturing solution (in a water bath in a fume hood) at 70°C for 5 min.
   (b) Wash the slides in cold 2X SSC, followed by two changes of 2X SSC.
   (c) Dehydrate through a cold alcohol series (70%, 90%, absolute).
6. Air-dry the slides and place on a hot plate at approx 42°C.
7. Centrifuge the probe mixture quickly to get the liquid to the bottom of the tube. Place this mixture on the previously treated slide containing chromosomes and cover with a 22 × 32 mm coverslip (do not let drop dry). Seal the coverslip with rubber solution, and place the slides in a moist chamber at 37°C for overnight to 4 d.
8. Remove the rubber solution. The coverslips can then be removed either by soaking in 2X SSC or by gently tipping them off into the glass disposal bin (never pull them off).
9. Carry out the following washes:
   (a) Three washes (3 min each) in 2X SSC at room temperature (with agitation).
   (b) Two washes (20 min each) in 0.1X SSC at 65°C.
   (c) One 5-min wash in 0.1X SSC at room temperature (with agitation).
10. Wash the slides in wash solution for 3 min.
11. Incubate the slides in blocking solution for 10–20 min (room temperature).
12. Wash in wash solution for 3 min before carrying out the appropriate detection steps.

Detection of Bound, Labeled Probe

For directly fluorochrome labeled probes, no immunologic detection steps are required. For repetitive centromeric probes and whole-chromosome paints, usually only one layer of detection reagent is required (i.e., fluorochrome-conjugated avidin or antibody). For single-copy probes, we use the following protocols, using three detection layers. The signal can be amplified further by adding several layers of detection reagents. However, increasing the number of layers to more than three will result in high background and reduced signal:noise ratio.

Biotin-labeled probes

1. Dilute 2.5 μL of stock avidin DCS-FITC in 1 mL of blocking solution (final concentration: 5 μg/mL). Add 100 μL of this under a 24 × 50 mm coverslip. Incubate in a moist chamber at 37°C for 30 min.
2. Flick off the coverslips and wash the slides three times (for 3 min each) in wash solution.
3. Dilute 10 μL of stock biotin anti-avidin D in 1 mL of blocking solution (final concentration: 5 μg/mL). Add 100 μL of this under a 24 × 50 mm coverslip. Incubate in a moist chamber at 37°C for 30 min.
4. Flick off the coverslips and wash the slides three times (for 3 min each) in wash solution.
5. Add 100 μL of avidin-FITC (same as the first layer). Incubate for 30 min as before.
6. Carry out the following final washes:
   (a) Wash once for 3 min in wash solution.
   (b) Wash twice (5 min each) in PBS.
   (c) Dehydrate the slides through an ethanol series. Air-dry.
7. Mount the slides in 40 μL of Vectashield containing 1.5 μg/mL of DAPI and 0.75 μg/mL of propidium iodide under a 24 × 50 mm coverslip. Seal the edges of the coverslip with rubber solution or nail varnish. The signal keeps well for several weeks when slides are stored at 4°C.

Digoxigenin-labeled probes

1. Prepare all antibody dilutions in blocking solution, filtered before use. Make up the following antibody dilutions in 1 mL of blocking solution:
   (a) First layer: 1.5 μL of mouse monoclonal antidigoxigenin.
   (b) Second layer: 1 μL of rabbit antimouse-FITC.
   (c) Third layer: 10 μL of monoclonal antirabbit-FITC.
2. Incubate in each antibody layer (100 μL under a 24 × 50 mm coverslip) for 30 min at 37°C in a moist chamber.
3. After each antibody layer, wash three times (3 min each) in wash solution.

4. Carry out the final washes as for biotin detection
5. Mount in Vectashield containing 1.5 μg/mL of DAPI and 0.75 μg/mL of propidium iodide.

Dual-color detection of biotin- and digoxigenin-labeled probes

1. Prepare all antibody dilutions in blocking solution, filtered before use. Make up the following antibody dilutions in 1 mL of blocking solution:
   (a) First layer: 1 μL of avidin-Texas red + 1.5 μL of mouse monoclonal antidigoxigenin.
   (b) Second layer: 10 μL of biotin antiavidin + 1 μL of rabbit antimouse-FITC.
   (c) Third layer: 1 μL of avidin-Texas red + 10 μL of monoclonal antirabbit-FITC.
2. Incubate in each antibody layer for 30 min at 37°C in a moist chamber.
3. After each antibody layer, wash three times (3 min each) in wash solution.
4. Carry out the final washes as for biotin detection.
5. Mount in Vectashield containing only 1.5 μg/mL of DAPI.

Microscopy

For the majority of FISH signals, the only equipment required is an epifluorescence microscope equipped with the appropriate filter sets. Both metaphase and interphase FISH analysis can be performed directly at the microscope, with photographic recording of representative images. However, photomicroscopy of multicolor FISH images may be difficult, owing to the long exposure times and loss of registration of images when changing filters. Digital imaging fluorescence systems such as confocal laser scanning microscopes and *charge-coupled device* (CCD) cameras provide significant advantages in terms of both image storage and the ability for image processing. Confocal laser scanning microscopes provide complete and accurate registration of fluorescent signals on chromosomes by the simultaneous scanning of each fluorochrome through separate filter blocks. These systems are also highly suitable for three-dimensional FISH applications. However, confocal systems are limited for multicolor imaging because most standard lasers only allow excitation of up to three fluorochromes.

High-performance, highly cooled (–30°C) CCD cameras are extremely sensitive to photons over a wide range of wavelengths and are now the instrument of choice for FISH, particularly for multicolor

Table 4.3. Fluorescent dyes commonly used for FISH

Fluorochrome	*Color*	*Absorbance (nm)*	*Emission (nm)*
DAPI	Blue	350	456
SpectrumAqua	Blue	433	480
FITC	Yellow/green	490	520
SpectrumGreen	Green	497	524
Rhodamine	Red	550	575
Cy3	Red	554	568
SpectrumOrange	Orange	559	588
Cy3.5	Red	581	588
SpectrumRed	Red	587	612
Texas red	Deep red	595	615
Cy5	Far red	652	672
Cy5.5	Near infrared	682	703
Cy7	Near infrared	755	778

applications. Problems with image registration owing to the movement of microscope filter blocks can be overcome by the use of a filter wheel containing the excitation filters and situated between the lamp and the microscope. For most FISH applications ambient temperature (+15°C), video-rated CCD cameras are probably sufficient, and for whole-chromosome painting, relatively inexpensive video cameras will suffice. When purchasing a FISH imaging system, it is important to consider requirements for hardware (i.e., compatibility and storage) and software (i.e., sophisticated packages for multicolor FISH and comparative genomic hybridization in addition to standard image capture and enhancement facilities).

Interpretation of Results

Metaphase FISH

For mapping purposes and also for the assessment of *yeast artificial chromosome* (YAC) chimerism, FISH is carried out to normal male metaphase spreads. To determine the number of metaphases that need to be evaluated for these applications, it is important to consider the hybridization efficiency, which decreases proportionately with probe size. For whole-chromosome painting probes and centromeric alphoid repeats, only a few metaphases need to be evaluated. Single-copy probes cloned in cosmids, YACs, *bacterial artificial chromosomes* (BACs), P1, and PACs also hybridize very efficiently (>80% of cells with signal on all four chromatids), so that usually only a few cells (5–10) need to be scored. Small single-copy sequences (<3 kb) hybridize less efficiently (30% of cells with signal on all four chromatids), and, thus, many more metaphases need to be evaluated.

In addition to these considerations, it should be borne in mind that all leukemic cell preparations (with the possible exception of cell lines) are heterogeneous mixtures, with variable numbers of normal and clonal cells. Therefore, for assessing the presence of numerical or structural rearrangements in leukemic bone marrow, it is important to screen as many metaphases as possible. The percentage of abnormal cells from G-banding can be used as a guide. For the presence of deletions, the normal chromosome homolog serves as an internal control. For mapping the extent of chromosome deletions, it is necessary to include a probe to tag the appropriate chromosome, so that only metaphases with the abnormal chromosome are scored.

Interphase FISH

Probes used for interphase analysis should be chosen to hybridize with high efficiency (>90%). Also note that in dual- or triple-color FISH experiments, three probes with 90% efficiency will hybridize simultaneously to only 73% of nuclei. Centromeric probes are most suitable for detecting numerical abnormalities in interphase, because these exhibit compact, unambiguous signals. Choosing suitable probes is particularly important for the assessment of deletions. In this case, co-hybridization with a control probe in a second color will increase the sensitivity. The control probe should be of similar complexity, localized to a region not likely to be affected by a chromosome rearragement in the particular type of leukemia being studied. However, because of the established occurrence of false monosomy (owing to inefficient hybridization or the overlap of signals viewed in two dimensions), diagnostic cutoff levels need to be established for each probe. DNA probes are now available commercially for the majority of specific translocations in leukemia. Differential labeling and dual-color detection of these allow the direct visualization of the fusion gene. However, it is important to establish "*in-house*" cutoff levels for false positivity for such probes. This can be quite high for some translocations, owing to the variability of breakpoints.

Advanced Methods and Applications

Whole-chromosome painting probes by degenerate oligonucleotide primer-PCR amplification of flow-sorted chromosomes

One of the most significant advances in probe generation has been the ability to selectively amplify genomic regions by PCR. Whole-chromosome paints can be produced by interspersed repetitive sequence element-PCR (e.g., Alu-PCR) by selectively amplifying the human DNA content of somatic cell hybrids. However, because of the distribution of these sequences across the genome, the resultant chromosome paints produce an R-banded pattern, which may not be optimal for the detection of some rearrangements. The technique of *degenerate oligonucleotide primer* (DOP)-PCR can be used to obtain more evenly distributed whole-chromosome or region-specific chromosome paints. This technique is also the basis for the production of 24 color paint sets for SKY and M-FISH.

First-round DOP-PCR amplification

All reagents except chromosomal DNA and *Taq* 1 polymerase can be sterilized by exposure to short-wave ultraviolet irradiation (5 min on a transilluminator). All solutions, microcentrifuge tubes, and tips should be autoclaved and kept for only PCR. Use aerosol-resistant tips and add all reagents in a laminar flow hood to minimize contamination. Prepare positive (2.5 pg of genomic DNA) and negative (all of the reagents except chromosomes) controls in the same way.

1. Combine in a sterile 0.5-mL microcentrifuge tube: x μL (= 500 flow-sorted chromosomes), 50 μL of 2X PCR buffer, 10 μL of dNTP mix, 6.6 μL of 30 m*M*6-MW primer, 0.5 μL of (1.25 U) *Taq* 1 polymerase, and distilled water to a final volume 100 μL.
2. Overlay with 100 μL of mineral oil and run the following program in a DNA thermal cycler: Denature for 10 min at 93°C. 5 cycles of: 1 min at 94°C, 1.5 min at 30°C, 3 min at 30–72°C transition, and 3 min at 72°C; 35 cycles of 1 min at 94°C, 1 min at 62°C, and 3 min at 72°C, with an additional 1 s/cycle and final extension time of 10 min.
3. Run a 10-μL aliquot of the amplified products on a 1.2% agarose gel with *Phi*X174 to check the success of the amplification. There should be no amplification in the negative control.

Second-round DOP-PCR and probe labeling

1. Add the following to a new sterile 0.5-mL microcentrifuge tube: 5 μL of amplified products from first round, 25 μL of 2X PCR buffer, 5 μL of nucleotide mix, 3.3 μL of 6-MW primer, 2.5 μL *Taq* 1 polymerase, and 12 μL of 1 m*M* biotin-16-dUTP.
2. Mix well, overlay with 50 μL of mineral oil, and run the following PCR program: Denature for 10 min at 93°C. 25 cycles of 1 min at 94°C, 1 min at 62°C, and 3 min at 72°C, with a final extension time of 10 min.

3. Remove the mineral oil. Run 10 μL of labeled products on a 1.2% agarose gel to check the size range. If the labeled fragments are too large, recut with 5 μL of DNase I for 30–60 min.
4. Purify the labeled DNA through a MicroSpin G50 (or Sephadex G50) column. Measure the DNA concentration of the purified, labeled DNA in a fluorimeter (usually 20–50 ng/mL). Ethanol precipitate the labeled DNA with tRNA and single-stranded DNA as usual, and dry and resuspend in distilled water or TE to a suitable concentration; this is now ready for use as a chromosome paint. Use 100 ng of probe + 6 μg of Cot-1 DNA per slide.

Combined immunophenotyping and FISH

The following technique relies on the ability of the reaction product of the APAAP immunophenotyping method to remain throughout subsequent harsh FISH procedures. Staining with Fast red produces autofluorescence visible through all filter sets and can be viewed at the same time as the FISH signal. We have used this to identify the cell lineages carrying the del(5q) clonal chromosome abnormality in myelodysplastic syndrome patients. After immunostaining, FISH is carried out essentially using a pepsin pretreatment to aid probe penetration.

1. Allow bone marrow smears to reach room temperature and then unwrap.
2. Fix in either acetone:methanol (1:1) for 90 s or acetone alone for 10 min. Then transfer immediately to TBS for 5 min at room temperature.
3. Add the appropriate primary mouse monoclonal antibody and incubate the slides in a moist chamber at room temperature for 30 min. Also incubate a negative control slide (no antibody added) in PBS for 30 min.
4. Add the second layer, rabbit antimouse antibody, and incubate for 30 min in a humid chamber.
5. Add the third antibody, mouse monoclonal APAAP complex, and incubate for 30 min in a moist chamber at room temperature.
6. Wash for 5 min in TBS between each antibody layer.
7. To enhance staining, repeat the antimouse antibody and APAAP steps (steps 4 and 5) with reduced incubation times of 10 min.
8. Finally, add alkaline phosphatase substrate to the slides and incubate for 10–20 min.
9. Wash the slides in TBS, then distilled water, and allow to air-dry.

Multicolor FISH

The simplest approach to multicolor FISH uses two probes labeled with different haptens or fluorochromes, and the third probe labeled separately with both, mixed in a 1:1 ratio. An extension of this approach can be used to detect up to seven different targets using three fluorochromes. Increasing the number of fluorochromes to five allows the identification of all 24 pairs of human chromosomes. Both M-FISH and SKY use a set of whole-chromosome paints combinatorially labeled with five fluorochromes, but differ in their method for the discrimination of the fluorochrome combinations. The second detection method, M-FISH, uses a filter-based detection system, capturing the separate fluorochrome images for each of five fluorochromes using specifically selected narrow bandpass filter sets. We have used M-FISH and a set of combinatorially labeled whole-chromosome paints to analyze the complex karyotype in the myeloid leukemia-derived cell line GF-D8.

Notes

1. Proper storage of slides is important to maintain good-quality chromosomal DNA. Slides can be used for hybridization the day after they are made, or kept for up to 1 mo at room temperature. For long-term storage, keep slides in a sealed container with desiccant at –20°C.
2. Alu-PCR amplification of total yeast DNA can be used to increase the yield of YAC DNA. However, Alu-poor YACs may not amplify, and the sensitivity for determining YAC chimerism is not known. Isolation of the YAC from the yeast background by pulsed-field gel electrophoresis can be used, but this has a low yield and may be difficult if the YAC is not visible by ethidium bromide staining.
3. It is important to have an accurate measurement of DNA concentration for nick translation labeling. Spectrophotometric measurements are often inaccurate, owing to RNA and other contaminants. We measure probe DNA concentration using a fluorometer, which measures the fluorescence of a DNA-binding dye, compared to a known standard.
4. These are frequently encountered problems:
   (a) *No hybridization signal.* This may be owing to insufficient probe DNA in the hybridization mix. The DNA concentration of any new probe should be measured accurately. This may also be owing to inadequate denaturation of probe and/or chromosomes.

(b) *Probe fragment size too small.* Always check the labeled fragment size on a 2% (1.2% for PCR products) gel with *Phi*X174 *Hae*III size marker. The optimum fragment size is 100–500 bp.

(c) *High background.* High background with strong specific signal may be owing to low stringency of hybridization or posthybridization washes or incomplete competition. The stringency of hybridization can be increased by either increasing the hybridization temperature, increasing the formamide concentration of the hybridization mix and/or posthybridization washes to 60%, or decreasing the SSC concentration to 0.1% in the posthybridization washes. Alternatively, increase the Cot-1 DNA concentration: This is already present in large excess so that any increase should be substantial (up to 10-fold).

(d) *Brightly fluorescent signal all over the slide.* This occurs when the labeled probe fragments are too large: If labeled probe is >500 bp, it should be recut with DNase I. High background of this type also may be caused by insufficient blocking with BSA.

(e) *Cells lost from slide.* Handle slides with care at all stages especially during removal of cover slips (never pull them off). Agitation during posthybridization washes should be carried out on a rocking platform set at minimum speed.

(f) *Poor chromosome morphology/banding.* If chromosomes look "blown," they may have been overdenatured: Always check the temperature of the denaturing solution inside the coplin jar. Overdenatured chromosomes give a C-banding pattern with DAPI staining.

5. These are important hybridization parameters:

(a) *Temperature.* The temperature at which two DNA strands separate (T_m) is in the range of 85–95°C. The optimal DNA-DNA reassociation temperature (T_r) is approx 25°C below the T_m of the native duplex. However, fixed chromosome preparations on microscope slides will not tolerate temperatures >65°C for long periods. The presence of formamide in the hybridization buffer lowers the T_r, allowing hybridization to take place at 37–42°C, and preserving chromosome morphology.

(b) *Time of hybridization.* This depends on the size and copy number of the target sequence, as well as the complexity of the probe. Repetitive sequence probes such as alphoid centromeric probes require only 1 h for hybridization. Unique sequence probes cloned in plasmid, cosmid, or phage vector require hybridization overnight (16–18 h). Larger insert probes (large YACs) may benefit from longer times to (1–2 d), and very complex probes such as multicolor painting sets and whole genomes in comparative genomic hybridization require 2 to 3 d.

(c) *Denaturation of chromosomal DNA*. The optimal time for denaturation needs to be determined for each batch of slides. Overdenaturation results in loss of chromosome morphology and very poor DAPI banding after hybridization. Underdenaturation results in little or no signal. The pH of the denaturation solution is also important: This should be checked when the solution is up to temperature and adjusted if necessary. It is preferable to prepare the denaturing solution and use it as soon as it has reached the desired temperature to prevent pH fluctuations. Alternatively, use EDTA (final concentration of 0.1 m*M*) to stabilize the denaturing solution against pH changes.

(d) *Stringency of hybridization conditions*. Renaturation depends on specific base pairing between two complementary DNA strands and can be controlled by the stringency of the hybridization conditions. Increasing the hybridization temperature or decreasing the salt concentration increases the stringency, which has a direct effect on the accuracy of base pairing.

6. The low salt washes are comparable to the following formamide washes: 50% formamide in 2X SSC (three times for 5 min each), followed by 2X SSC (three times for 5 min each) at 45°C.

5

X Chromosome in Cancer

The understanding that human neoplasms are clonal cell proliferations ultimately derived from a single transformed somatic cell represents a major advance in cancer biology. A cell population is designated as clonal if it can be demonstrated to have arisen from a single parent or progenitor cell. The clonality of select human neoplastic cell populations can be determined in several ways. One way is by detection of stable, unique somatic chromosome abnormalities; somatic gene mutations (*H-ras*); or immunoglobulin heavy/light chain rearrangements. The drawbacks of these are that they either are rare, are fortuitous, or require labor-intensive techniques. Another way to assess clonality in human cell populations is to exploit the unique position of the X chromosome in human female development.

Histology

X-Chromosome Inactivation Phenomena

The chromosomes in eukaryotic organisms are derived from two parental organisms, male and female or paternal and maternal. One half of the chromosomes are maternally derived, the other half are paternally derived. All of the chromosomes are transcriptionally active except one of the two X chromosomes of cells found in mature females. Early in development, one of the two X chromosomes (most but not all of its genes) in the cells constituting a human female embryo becomes transcriptionally inactivated. This appears to be a random process in that some of the cells of the early human female embryo express only paternal X chromosome genes whereas other cells from the same embryo express only maternal X chromosome genes. This phenomenon of X chromosome maternal/paternal molecular mosaicism persists throughout the life of the human female and represents a gene dosage compensation mechanism whereby comparable X chromosome gene expression in males and females is ensured.

One protein whose gene is X chromosome linked is glucose-6-phosphate dehydrogenase (*G6PD*). G6PD is a rate-controlling enzyme for the hexose monophosphate shunt, which produces NADPH and pentose sugars. Deficiency of G6PD is the most common and most polymorphic red cell enzymopathy in the world known so far. The typical clinical manifestation of the common deficient variants is an acute, short-lasting nonspherocytic hemolysis in affected males and in affected heterozygous females. The study of the biology of *G6PD* mosaicism in females by Beutler et al. in the late 1950s to early 1960s inspired some of the initial research on tumor clonality. They demonstrated biphenotypic erythrocytes in females known to be heterozygous for G6PD deficiency. Erythrocyte mosaicism was first demonstrated by showing that erythrocytes from heterozygous females exhibited a glutathione consumption curve identical to that of a 50:50 mixture of cells from an affected and unaffected male, respectively. In later work, erythrocytes from two adult females heterozygous for sickle cell trait and G6PD deficiency, separated based on oxidant-induced generation of sickle cells, were either G6PD deficient or had normal G6PD activity. Davidson et al. further showed that skin cells obtained from G6PD heterozygous females, when cultured and later subjected to single-cell platings, produced clonal populations with either normal or absent G6PD activity. These results, in addition to Lyon's animal experiments and Ohno and Hauschka's observations, provided some early experimental confirmation of the Lyon hypothesis of X chromosome inactivation.

Not all *G6PD* mutations produce a hemolytic phenotype. Some exhibit differences in qualitative electrophoretic mobility relative to the wildtype molecule (designated "B" by convention). For example, G6PD A is a mutation characterized by rapid mobility on electrophoresis relative to G6PD B. G6PD A hemizygosity is associated with almost normal in vitro enzyme activity and no hemolytic phenotype. By contrast, while the G6PD A-isoenzyme has the same rapid mobility on electrophoresis as G6PD A, it has reduced red cell enzymatic activity as a result of intrinsic protein instability. This instability results in shortened red cell survival time (hemolysis) on oxidant exposure of the older erythrocytes that have very low G6PD activity since erythrocytes do not possess protein synthesis machinery.

Review of Methods Used to Study X-Chromosome Inactivation

Protein-based methods

In 1965, Linder and Gartler exploited the electrophoretic mobility differences of these three isoenzymes. They studied leimyomas obtained from females who were known G6PD A/B heterozygotes undergoing hysterectomies for multiple uterine leimyomas. Electrophoresis was performed on crude extracts of individual leimyomas. Individual leimyomas were either exclusively A or exclusively B. Electrophoresis was also performed on the surrounding uninvolved myometria; both A and B bands were observed. Finally, Beutler et al. subjected cell extracts of antemortem and postmortem neoplastic and nonneoplastic tissue obtained from two known G6PD A/B heterozygotes. One had *chronic lymphocytic leukemia* (CLL), and the other had metastatic colon cancer. The individual with CLL demonstrated exclusively A clonal lymph node tissue; the individual with colon cancer showed some neoplastic tissue specimens with exclusively A bands, others with exclusively B bands, and still others with both A and B bands. These studies emphasized the potential problem of contaminating supporting/stromal tissue cells (monocytes, fibroblasts, and so on) when evaluating fresh, unprocessed neoplastic tissue. In addition, the finding of both clonal A and B neoplastic tissue in the colon cancer patient was suggestive of more than one initial transformed cell. In summary, the first studies of tumor cell clonality exploiting the hypothesis of random X chromosome inactivation derived initially from pioneering work by Beutler et al. and his studies of G6PD mosaicism. More widespread applicability was restricted primarily by the limited ethnic distribution of the of the qualitative G6PD mutation in question.

DNA-RNA-based methods

The next phase in the study of tumor cell clonality harnessed technologic advances drawn from the detailed study of DNA and the discovery of bacterial enzymes (*restriction endonucleases*) that cleave DNA at specific (restricted) sites determined by DNA nucleotide sequence. The frequency of genomic DNA polymorphisms vastly exceeds the frequency of protein polymorphisms. Interindividual DNA sequence differences that may be exploited for clonality studies may occur between X chromosome-linked genes and also occur in exons or introns of the X chromosome-linked genes themselves. By convention, these differences in DNA sequence are referred to as polymorphisms rather than mutations if they are not associated with a disease state and if they are observed in sufficiently high frequencies. A particular gene displays a characteristic pattern on Southern blot gel electrophoresis when genomic DNA is digested with a given restriction endonuclease. If a polymorphism occurs at the restriction site of that enzyme, that pattern will be altered and this particular polymorphism would be conveniently detectable by Southern blot; this phenomenon is referred to as a restriction fragment length polymorphism. Studies of the transcriptional activity of genomic DNA also demonstrated that differential cytosine residue methylation marks some genes (X and non-X chromosome linked) as transcriptionally inactive. Not all cytosine residues in all genes are methylated when transcriptionally inactivated. However, cytosine residue methylation (typically but not always indicating transcriptional inactivation) occurs consistently at some sites in some genes. These methylated and unmethylated nucleotide sequences can be distinguished by methylation-sensitive restriction endonucleases. Thus, an ubiquitously expressed X-linked gene with a common restriction site polymorphism and differentially methylated cytosine residues (reflecting transcriptional activation/inactivation status), which constitute a separate, methylation-sensitive restriction endonuclease site, could potentially serve as a clonality marker in a very large population of females.

In the mid 1980s, Vogelstein et al. pioneered a novel clonality assay based on detection of X-linked gene restriction site polymorphisms and differential methylation as a marker for X chromosome transcriptional activation/ inactivation. The *hypoxanthine phosphoribosyltransferase* (*HPRT*) gene is an X chromosome gene encoding an essential enzyme for the purine/pyrimidine salvage pathway. The *HPRT* gene has a readily identifiable *Bam*HI restriction site polymorphism for which approximately one-third of females are heterozygous. In addition, the *HPRT* gene is hypermethylated at cytosine residues distant from the *Bam*HI site when transcriptionally active. Some of the methylation-prone cytosine residues also make up a methylation-sensitive restriction endonuclease site. DNA isolated from solid tumors obtained from females known to be heterozygous for the *HPRT Bam*HI restriction site polymorphism subjected to *Bam*HI digestion followed by methylation-sensitive endonuclease digestion, Southern blotting, and autoradiography shows only one of the two polymorphic loci. By contrast, DNA obtained from nontumor tissue close to the excised tumors showed an autoradiographic pattern consistent with hypermethylation of both polymorphic loci, indicating that this population of cells is polyclonal (i.e., composed of a mixture of cells using either the maternally derived or the paternally derived X chromosome). Other X-linked loci with restriction endonuclease site polymorphisms and cytosine residues located in methylation-sensitive restriction endonuclease sites whose methylation status coincided with transcriptional activation were found (monoamine oxidase and phosphoglycerate kinase). Another, the human androgen receptor (*HUMARA*) locus, was unique in four ways: The restriction site polymorphism consisted of a variable number of tandem repeats of a CAG trinucleotide sequence, the restriction site polymorphism was located in the coding region (exon 1), the restriction site polymorphism was very closely linked to a methylation-sensitive restriction site, and more than 90% of human females were potentially heterozygous for the restriction site polymorphism. Exploiting these properties, Busque et al. confirmed the correlation between methylation and transcriptional activation at the *HUMARA* locus.

In summary, the development of differential methylation-based clonality assays represented a significant technologic step forward. Their development expanded the potential number of females available for clonality studies. The restriction site polymorphisms discovered to date are not limited to a specific demographic grouping, as is the G6PD isoenzyme assay. However, reliance on differential DNA methylation as a marker for transcriptional activation has some limitations. The functional significance and mechanisms of regulation of DNA methylation are poorly understood. The relationship of DNA methylation to transcriptional activation is far from well understood. Some genes have methylated cytosine residues when transcriptionally inactivated; other genes have methylated cytosine residues when transcriptionally active. Furthermore, the DNA extracted from tumor cells is somewhat hypomethylated relative to nontumor DNA; this may impact interpretation of tumor clonality data derived from differential methylation assays. Finally, the differential methylation clonality assays are only applicable to nucleated cells and require large numbers of such cells for sufficient DNA. Nonnucleated cells such as erythrocytes and platelets are not suitable for differential methylation clonality assays. Reliance on differential DNA methylation as a marker for transcriptional activation may not represent an optimal method for studying clonality. As X chromosome-based clonality assays have evolved, the following has become clear. First, the assay must be applicable to large numbers of females. Second, the assay must be based on a biologically sound method of discriminating between the transcriptionally active and inactive X chromosome. Third, the X chromosome gene transcription product must be ubiquitously expressed and not tumor or tissue specific. Finally, it would be desirable for the assay to be applicable to nucleated and nonnucleated cells.

Recent sequencing of a number of X chromosome-linked genes has resulted in the discovery of polymorphisms in the coding regions of a number of ubiquitously expressed house-keeping genes. In three of these X chromosome-linked gene exonic polymorphic sequences, the polymorphism is conservative (i.e., the nucleotide substitutions in the polymorphic codon codes for the same amino acid as the wild-type sequence). These exonic X chromosome polymorphisms are present in the *G6PD*, palmitoylated erythrocyte membrane antigen (*p55*), and the iduronate-2-sulfatase (*IDS*) genes. These polymorphisms do not appear to affect mRNA stability, posttranscriptional processing, or translation. Expression-based clonality assays have been developed that can detect and quantitate the expression of coding region polymorphisms in both nucleated and nonnucleated cells and use this as a marker for clonality.

The first clonality assay based on the discrimination of the active X chromosome by its transcript was developed independently by two groups. Their work was based on observations by Vulliamy et al., who found that some individuals possessed a C-to-T transposition at nucleotide (nt) 1311 (exon 11) of the *G6PD* gene. Beutler et al. demonstrated that this transposition actually represented a very common polymorphism. One of these groups utilized this polymorphism in a study of a woman with X-linked chronic granulomatous disease. Family studies revealed that the propositus was heterozygous for the C1311T G6PD polymorphism; her mother was homozygous for the C allele and her father was hemizygous for the T allele. These investigators extracted total RNA from the propositus's granulocytes and *polymerase chain reaction* (PCR) amplified the resulting cDNA with primers complementary to the region flanking G6PD nt 1311. The products were then separated on a denaturing polyacrylamide gel, dot-blotted, and probed with radiolabeled allele-specific oligomers. The oligomers were allele specific in that they were 19–20-mers complementary to the nucleotide sequences flanking the C1311T site, differing only at the site complementary to nt 1311. A single mismatched base pair between such duplexes results in significant duplex instability; only perfect complementarity between the probe and its binding partner results in a high degree of target molecule/oligomer hybridization stability. The granulocytes of the propositus were found to express only the paternal X chromosome, demonstrating a spontaneous chronic granulomatous disease mutation in the patient's paternal X chromosome.

Prchal et al., working simultaneously to exploit the G6PD C1311T polymorphism for a transcription-based clonality assay, built on the foundation and the work of Barany and Landegren et al., who developed a method of detecting nucleotide differences using thermostable DNA ligase. DNA ligase is a nuclear enzyme that ligates juxtaposed oligonucleotides complementary to a denatured DNA target strand. The DNA ligase-based assays can distinguish single nucleotide substitutions in otherwise identical DNA target sequences with high fidelity. These thermostable ligase properties were utilized for a clonality assay that detects the *G6PD* C1311T polymorphism by a *ligase detection reaction* (LDR) assay. Since this particular polymorphism is not recognizable by any known restriction enzymes, LDR detects both alleles at this locus. In this procedure, a thermostable DNA ligase covalently binds two adjacent DNA oligonucleotides provided they are perfectly complementary to the target DNA region of interest. Thus, allele-specific oligonucleotides (of different size) can be constructed to detect the presence of either, or both, allelic transcripts. Experimental conditions were developed that allow detection of both alleles in the same tube using either PCR-amplified genomic DNA or cDNA as templates. In addition, since the ligase utilized was also thermostable, the reaction could be subjected to multiple thermal cycles to linearly amplify product.

This particular quantitative transcription technique was used for the study of clonality in a female with long-standing polycythemia vera who was heterozygous for the *G6PD* C1311T exonic polymorphism. Using 5–10 cc of peripheral blood, RNA was extracted from separated reticulocytes, granulocytes, platelets, and mononuclear cells. Total RNA from each separated cell population was reverse transcribed to cDNA and amplified using *G6PD* C1311T flanking region-specific primers. These reverse transcriptase (RT)-PCR products were then utilized in an LDR assay using variant oligomers with 3' termini specific for either the C or T allele at the *G6PD* nt 1311 polymorphism. Although heterozygous at the *G6PD* C1311T polymorphism, this individual's reticulocytes, platelets, and granulocytes displayed only one band on autoradiography. This suggested to the investigators that these cells all derived from a single stem cell (i.e., were clonal). The mononuclear cells (mostly T-lymphocytes) exhibited two bands on autoradiography, suggesting cells derived from more than one stem cell (i.e., were polyclonal), as were the cells from her nonhematopoietic tissues (oral mucosal epithelial cells, urinary epithelial cells, and hair follicle cells). In normal females heterozygous for the G6PD C1311T polymorphism, all peripheral blood cells, as well as the cells from nonhematopoietic tissues, were found to be polyclonal. These two original studies demonstrated that a common, single nucleotide polymorphism in the coding region of an X-linked housekeeping gene could be exploited in a clonality assay based on differentiation of the active X chromosome by its transcript.

The differentiation of the active from the inactive X chromosome by their transcripts was also exploited for the studies of normal hematopoiesis. In these studies using RT-PCR/LDR, the conditions for RT-PCR/LDR were developed that allowed quantitation of the X chromosome allelic transcript ratio. This methodology was shown to be reproducible with <5% interassay variability, sensitive for analysis of as few as 100 cells, and permitting studies of rare populations of cells isolated by *fluorescence activated cell sorting* (FACS) sorting. Among normal *G6PD* C1311T heterozygous females, the relative autoradiographic intensities of the two bands, in the single individual, was noted to vary from one tissue to the other, while this ratio was constant in all hematopoietic cells (platelets; reticulocytes; granulocytes; monocytes; B-, T-, and NK-lymphocytes).

By contrast, the X chromosome allelic transcript ratio of hematopoietic cells varies from one individual to another individual. This inter-individual variation in X chromosome allelic transcript ratio was subjected to computer analyses and, assuming that no preferential selection occurred, suggested that eight progenitor cells for all of the blood cells were present in the embryo at the time of X chromosome inactivation. Thus, "*skewing*" of the X chromosome allelic transcript ratio is a normal phenomenon. Longitudinal evaluation by this method of peripheral blood cells from these same normal *G6PD* C131T heterozygous females over time showed that this pattern of individual variation remained constant in all lineages for a period of 3 yr of observation. This observation provided no support for "clonal succession theory of hematopoiesis," although it could not formally exclude it.

The clonality assay based on a transcriptional polymorphism of the X chromosome using the *G6PD* C1311T polymorphism is limited by its applicability to less than one-fourth of females. A similar RT-PCR/LDR assay was developed to detect expression from a common single-nucleotide exonic polymorphism found on the X-linked gene p55

(T358G). About 60% of females are heterozygous for either the G6PD or p55 exonic polymorphisms. Of note, while the G6PD and p55 genes are adjacent to each other on the X chromosome (< 100 kb), frequent crossovers between these loci were encountered, suggesting an ancient origin of these polymorphisms in evolution.

A third exonic conservative polymorphism of the single-nucleotide X chromosome gene has been reported in the *IDS* gene (C146T). El-Kassar et al. have utilized the *IDS* exonic polymorphism for clonality study of nonnucleated platelets in essential thrombocythemia and found discrepancies between the clonality results from the methylation-based *HUMARA* assay and the transcription-based *IDS* assay when granulocytes from these subjects were used for analysis. This work suggested the superiority of the transcription-based clonality assays. When large numbers of normal females were genotyped for polymorphisms in the X-linked G6PD p55 and IDS genes, 60–70% of Caucasian and African American females were heterozygous for at least one of these three polymorphisms.

Unfortunately, while the IDS polymorphism was most informative in Caucasian and African American females, it was not informative among Asian females. A fourth X chromosome-linked gene exonic polymorphism exists at the *HUMARA* locus and has been used for a transcription-based clonality assay. We had difficulty standardizing this assay, perhaps because of different efficacy of PCR when HUMARA cDNA templates of different lengths, owing to a variable number of tandem CAG trinucleotide repeats, are used. This suggests that large numbers of women are potentially informative for expression-based clonality studies utilizing one or more of these genes.

These assays have several potential advantages over the *G6PD* isoenzyme detection or differential DNA methylation assays. They are not limited by racial specificity and are applicable to nucleated and nonnucleated cells. In addition, they can be quantitative and only a small amount of tissue is needed for analysis. In the presence of appropriate controls, these assays can also quantify the relative percentages of clonal and nonclonal cells in a particular tissue sample.

The RT-PCR/LDR assay is already providing insight and improving our understanding of a number of clinical syndromes and diseases. To date, these have been almost exclusively hematologic/immunologic diseases primarily because of the ease of accessibility of the affected tissue (blood and marrow) and the availability of established methods to separate nearly pure populations of affected cells uncontaminated by stromal/supportive cells. These have included studies of *myeloproliferative disorders* (MPD), juvenile chronic myelogenous leukemia, X-linked hyper IgM syndrome, and common variable immunodeficiency.

These assays still entail potential exposure to radioactivity and are somewhat labor-intensive. More rapid, less hazardous assays have been developed that are broadly based on principles similar to those of the RT-PCR/LDR assays. *Allele-specific PCR* (ASPCR) refers to a PCR-based technique that can accurately identify single-nucleotide base differences between two otherwise identical genomic DNA or cDNA strands. The technique requires two PCR rounds. The first round utilizes primers specific for sequences flanking the polymorphic nucleotide of interest and generates a high concentration of "*template*" products containing the polymorphic nucleotide of interest.

In the second PCR round, an aliquot of first-round products is added to two PCR reaction tubes each containing buffer, nucleotides, $MgCl_2$, and a common 3' primer. The 5' primer in each second-round reaction tube is allele specific; its 3' terminus is designed to be complementary to the polymorphic nucleotide or the wild-type allele. The second PCR round is very brief, usually only four to six cycles. If there is a lack of complementarity between the polymorphic locus on the template strand and the 3'-terminal nucleotide of the second-round 5' primer, *Taq* polymerase-mediated amplification cannot proceed efficiently, and a sufficient amount of visible product of agarose gel does not accumulate. Thus, only the template-round products are visible on agarose gel electrophoresis.

A modification of these assays was introduced by El-Kassar et al. and Harrison et al. whereby they utilized a PCR mismatch system instead of ASPCR. In their respective techniques, the target molecule (DNA or cDNA) is subjected to a single round of PCR using primers that hybridize to sequences flanking the X-linked exonic polymorphic site in question. The primers do not hybridize to the polymorphic site itself, as in ASPCR. One of the primers contains a nucleotide mismatch two or four nucleotides upstream from the primer 3' terminus (four or five nucleotides from the polymorphic site on the target molecule). PCR products generated under such conditions will substitute a new, complementary nucleotide at the site of primer/target molecule mismatch.

In the presence of one polymorphism (but not the other), this reconstitutes a cryptic restriction endonuclease site. When a target

DNA or cDNA molecule containing the other polymorphism is amplified under these conditions, no such cryptic restriction site is generated. The PCR reaction products are then subjected to restriction endonuclease digestion and gel electrophoresis; the relative expression of each allele in the cell population under study can then be determined by the band pattern generated. Since the primers do not hybridize directly to the polymorphic site in question, equal amplification of both polymorphisms is ensured. In addition, many rounds of PCR are eliminated. Both Harrison et al. and El-Kassar et al. also demonstrated a high degree of correlation between the DNA-based differential methylation *HUMARA* assay and their primer mismatch RT-PCR assays (utilizing the aforementioned *G6PD*, *p55*, and *IDS* exonic polymorphisms) in their studies of clonality in essential thrombocythemia.

Interpreting Data from DNA–RNA-Based Clonality Methods

X chromosome inactivation occurs early in development and has been hypothesized to be a gene dosage equalizing mechanism in the XX eukaryotic female. X inactivation appears to be regulated by an X inactivation–specific transcript (Xist), an RNA transcript originating from the X inactivating center (Xic) of the X chromosome. Deletion of Xist or the Xic abolishes random X inactivation. By mechanisms yet to be elucidated, the Xist transcript induces apparently random transcriptional inactivation in one of the two X chromosomes at a specific developmental stage in the female embryo. In addition, studies in murine embryos show that X inactivation is tissue specific; different embryonic tissues sequentially undergo X inactivation. The number of adult tissue progenitor cells present at the time of X inactivation in a particular embryonic tissue would thus be expected to influence the relative proportion of mature cells ultimately expressing either the maternally derived or paternally derived X chromosome. For example, if only two progenitor cells are present in the embryo at the time of tissue-specific X inactivation, it is highly likely that those two progenitor will express only the paternal or only the paternal X chromosome. If all the organism's blood cells derive from these two progenitors, then that organism would appear to have clonal hematopoiesis on X chromosome-based clonality analysis. However, if 8, 16, or 32 progenitors are present at the time of random X chromosome inactivation, it is highly likely that close to one half of the progenitor cells will express only the maternal and the other half only the paternal X chromosome, and the tissue would appear to be nonclonal on X chromosome-based clonality analysis.

The tissue specificity of embryonic X chromosome inactivation and the possibility of X chromosome allelic skewing resulting from a relatively small number of adult tissue progenitor cells present at the time of X inactivation dictates that X chromosome-based clonality data may exhibit significant interindividual variation. Such data should therefore be interpreted with caution and in the presence of appropriate tissue-specific positive controls. Clonality studies performed on peripheral blood cells from normal women show that approx 20–35% exhibit allelic skewing.

Skewing of the X chromosome allelic usage ratio in peripheral blood cells becomes more pronounced as individuals age; whether this is owing to exhaustion of the hematopoietic stem cell pool or a progressive effect of cell selection owing to expression of X chromosome alleles that are detrimental to proliferation/survival ("*pseudoclonality*") has not yet been established. It is also possible that this phenomenon may reflect the methylation differences of DNA among the cells rather than true clonal selection; since it has been observed only when methylation-based clonality assay was used and not in X-chromosome inactivation-based transcription clonality assay.

Conclusions

Overall, advances made in the understanding of the regulation of gene transcription and the biology of the X chromosome have contributed substantially to the development of widely applicable X chromosome-based clonality assays. Those assays, which rely on detection of exonic polymorphisms, require very pure study cell populations. Contaminating lymphocytes, fibroblasts, and monocytes may inadvertently contribute nonclonal RNA, and substantially alter results in small tissue specimens, thereby possibly limiting their applicability to solid tumors. Even in very uniform cell populations, the possibility of differential DNA methylation (as seen in malignant tissue when methylation-based clonality assays are used), potential interindividual variability in the number of progenitor cells present at the time of X chromosome inactivation, age-related allelic skewing, and "*pseudoclonality*" observed in females heterozygous for X-linked inherited diseases all necessitate thoughtful use of appropriate controls and, possibly, use of more than one clonality assay for proper conclusions to be reached.

There are clearly many clonality assays available to the researcher. Here we describe a rapid, reproducible, and non-radioactive clonality assay based on detection of exonic polymorphisms of the X chromosome genes p55 and G6PD using ASPCR.

MATERIALS

Isolation of Blood Cells: Preparation of Granulocyte and T-Lymphocyte Fractions from Peripheral Blood

Separation of granulocytes and mononuclear cells by density gradient centrifugation

1. Density gradient: Histopaque-1077.
2. Phosphate-buffered saline (PBS).

Separation of T-lymphocytes by rosetting with sheep red blood cells

1. Neuraminidase-treated sheep *red blood cells* (RBCs).
2. Fetal calf serum.
3. 1% Stock solution of polybrene.

Preparation of RNA

1. TRIzol reagent.
2. Chloroform.
3. Isopropanol.
4. 75% Ethanol in RNase-free water.
5. RNase-free water: Add 0.01% diethylpyrocarbonate to distilled water in glass bottles, allow to stand overnight, and autoclave).

First-strand cDNA Synthesis

1. SuperScript II RNase H-Reverse Transcriptase (200 U/mL).
2. 5X First-strand buffer: 250 m*M* Tris-HCl, pH 8.3, 375 m*M* KCl, 15 m*M* $MgCl_2$, supplied with enzyme.
3. 0.1 *M* Dithiothreitol (DTT) (supplied with enzyme).
4. 25 m*M* dNTPs (25 m*M* each of dATP, dCTP, dGTP, and dTTP).
5. RNasin (40 U/mL).
6. Random hexamer $pd(N)_6$ (1 mg/mL).
7. Single-strand DNA-binding protein.
8. RNase-free water.

Analysis of Genomic DNA for Genotype Determination by ASPCR

Polymerase chain reaction

1. 10X PCR buffer II.
2. 25 m*M* $MgCl_2$ (supplied with buffer).
3. 10 m*M* dNTPs (10 m*M* each of dATP, dCTP, dGTP, and dTTP).
4. AmpliTaq DNA polymerase (5 U/mL).
5. Single-strand DNA-binding protein.

6. Oligonucleotide primers.
7. Mineral oil.
8. Sterile distilled water.
9. Perkin-Elmer 9600 thermocycling machine.

Agarose gel electrophoresis

1. 1X TAE buffer: 50X TAE buffer contains 242 g of Tris base, 57.1 mL of glacial acetic acid, and 100 mL of 0.5 *M* EDTA, pH 8.0, adjusted to 1 L total volume with distilled water.
2. Ethidium bromide (10 mg/mL stock solution).
3. DNA-grade agarose.
4. 10X Gel-loading dye: 0.25% bromophenol blue, 0.25% xylene cyanol, 15% Ficoll-400.
5. λ*Hin*dIII DNA molecular marker.
6. Distilled water.

Methods

Isolation of Blood Cells: Preparation of Granulocyte and T-Lymphocyte Fractions from Peripheral Blood

Peripheral blood samples anticoagulated with EDTA can be used for genotyping and for determination of clonality in females known to have a clonal hematopoietic disorder. The method described here is for the separation of granulocytes and T-lymphocytes from 20 mL of peripheral blood. Further separation of the myeliod lineage may be required for some clonality studies.

Separation of granulocytes and mononuclear cells by density gradient centrifugation

1. Collect 20 mL of peripheral blood into trisodium EDTA tubes.
2. Gently layer the blood onto 25 mL of Histopaque-1077 in a 50-mL polypropylene conical tube and centrifuge at 400*g* (Sorvall RT6000B benchtop centrifuge) for 30 min at room temperature.
3. Transfer the interface (the mononuclear cell layer) to a sterile 50-mL conical tube, using a Pasteur pipet.
4. Aspirate the layers using a Pasteur pipet and discard to leave the RBC/granulocyte layer.
5. Add PBS to the RBC/granulocyte layer to give a total volume of 50 mL and mix by gentle inversion.
6. Centrifuge at 400*g* at room temperature for 10 min.
7. Remove the supernatant using a Pasteur pipet and discard.
8. Repeat steps 5–7.

9. To lyse the red cells, distribute the packed RBC/granulocyte layer into conical tubes containing freshly prepared red cell lysis buffer (approx 1 mL of RBCs/50 mL of red cell lysis buffer), and leave at room temperature for 15 min, with occasional mixing.
10. Centrifuge at 400*g* for 10 min at room temperature and pour off the supernatant.
11. Pool each granulocyte pellet into two conical tubes.
12. Fill the tubes to 50 mL with PBS and centrifuge at 400*g* for 10 min at room temperature. Pour off the supernatant.
13. Repeat step 12.
14. Pool the pellets into one conical tube and resuspend in PBS to a total volume of 10 mL.
15. Take an aliquot and obtain a cell count using an automated counter.

Separation of T-lymphocytes by rosetting with sheep RBCs

This protocol is based on the erythrocyte rosetting method of Kaplan and Clark.

1. Dilute the mononuclear cell fraction from step 3 to obtain a concentration of 2–6 $\times$ 10^6/mL white blood cells.
2. Add 1–2 vol of neuraminidase-treated sheep RBCs (TCS Biologicals), 0.5–1 vol of FCS, and 100–300 μL of a fresh 1:30 dilution of a 1% stock solution of polybrene to the cell suspension.
3. Centrifuge the suspension at 750 rpm for 5 min at 4°C, and then incubate at 4°C for a minimum of 5 h or maximum overnight.
4. Remove the supernatant from the packed cell pellet (sheep RBCs and rosetted T-lymphocytes) and add 1 vol of PBS.
5. Resuspend the cells by rotating the meniscus through the cell pellet.
6. Layer the cell suspension onto an equal volume of Histopaque and centrifuge at 400*g* for 30 min at room temperature.
7. Aspirate and discard the upper layer, interface (non-T-cell), and Histopaque layer leaving the sheep RBC/T-lymphocyte layer.
8. Add PBS to 50 mL and centrifuge at 400*g* for 10 min at room temperature.
9. Remove the supernatant using a Pasteur pipet and discard.
10. Repeat steps 8 and 9.
11. To lyse the sheep RBCs, distribute the cell pellet into conical tubes containing freshly prepared red cell lysis buffer (approx 1 mL of cells/50 mL of lysis buffer), and incubate at room temperature for 15 min with occasional mixing.

12. Centrifuge at 400*g* for 10 min and pour off the supernatant.
13. Treat the T-cell pellets exactly as the granulocyte pellets.

Preparation of RNA

RNA preparation is perfomed using TRIzol reagent according to the manufacturer's instructions, with minor modifications.

1. After counting, pellet the cells by centrifugation. Aspirate off the supernatant.
2. Add 1 ml of TRIzol reagent per 1×10^7 cells in a polypropylene tube. Using a syringe and a 25-gage needle, aspirate the cells and TRIzol repeatedly in order to lyse the cells (seven or eight times is usually sufficient). At this point the sample may be transferred to a 1.5-mL microcentrifuge tube if the required volume of TRIzol is 1 mL or less.
3. Incubate the lysed cells in TRIzol for 5 min at room temperature (15–30°C).
4. Add 0.2 mL of chloroform/mL of TRIzol and shake the tubes in order to mix the contents thoroughly. Incubate at room temperature for 2 to 3 min. Centrifuge at 4000 rpm for 30 min at 4°C.
5. Aspirate off the upper aqueous phase and transfer to a clean tube. Avoid disturbing the interface because this may result in contamination of the RNA preparation by DNA.
6. Add isopropanol to the aqueous phase (use 0.5 mL of isopropanol/mL of TRIzol used in step 2). Mix and incubate at room temperature for 10 min. Centrifuge at 4000 rpm for 30 min at 4°C. The precipitated RNA should form a clear pellet at the bottom of the tube.
7. Aspirate off the supernatant and wash with 75% ethanol (use 1 mL of ethanol/1 mL of TRIzol used in step 2). Briefly vortex to expose the pellet to ethanol, and centrifuge at 4000 rpm for 10 min.
8. Remove the supernatant and air-dry the RNA pellet for 10 min to allow any remaining ethanol to evaporate. Dissolve the pellet in an appropriate volume of RNase-free water; incubating the solution in a 55°C water bath for 10 min will facilitate this.
9. Determine the concentration of RNA in solution using a spectrophotometer at A_{260}. One A_{260} unit of single-stranded RNA corresponds to a concentration of 40 mg/mL. Pure RNA preparations should have an A_{260}:A_{280} ratio of 2.0. RNA should be stored at –70°C to prevent degradation.

First-strand cDNA Synthesis

1. Add 1 mL random hexamers 1 mg/mL of (pd(N)$_6$ to an RNase-free 500-mL microcentrifuge tube together with a volume of RNA constituting between 3 and 5 mg (to a maximum volume of 11.5 mL). Add RNase-free water to bring the total volume to 12.5 mL.
2. Incubate at 70°C for 10 min. Quench the reaction on ice for 2 min. Briefly spin and set back on ice.
3. To each tube, add 5 mL first-strand buffer, 2 mL of 0.1 *M* DTT, 1 mL of 25 m*M* dNTPs, 0.5 mL of RNasin (40 U/mL), 1 mL of single-strand DNA-binding protein (0.5 mg/mL), and 1.5 mL of RNase-free water.
4. Add 1.5 mL of SuperScript II RNase H-Reverse Transcriptase (200 U/mL) to each tube, and incubate at 37°C for 1 h. The total reaction volume should equal 25 mL.
5. Inactivate the enzymes by heating to 65°C for 10 min.
6. Store synthesized cDNA at –20°C.

Analysis of Genomic DNA for Genotype Determination by ASPCR

ASPCR for G6PD and p55 genotyping consists of two rounds of PCR.

1. In the first round, aliquot the following into a sterile 200-mL tube for each PCR reaction (total volume of 50 μL) 1–10 μL of genomic DNA, 5 μL of 10X PCR buffer II, 2 m*M* $MgCl_2$, 0.2 m*M* dNTPs, 25 pmol of forward primer (6J-p55 or 7g-G6PD), 25 pmol of reverse primer (8gR-p55 or 9gR-G6PD), 1 U of *Taq* polymerase, and sterile distilled water to give a final volume of 50 μL.
2. Pipet 50 μL of mineral oil taking care not to puncture the layer. Cap the tube.
3. Perform PCR amplification in a Perkin-Elmer 9600 thermocycling machine using the following conditions: initial denaturation step at 95°C for 1 min, followed by 35 cycles of PCR at 94°C for 40 s, 62°C for 1 min, and 72°C for 1 min.
4. Visualize amplified PCR product in all reactions by agarose gel electrophoresis. Use a 1% agarose gel and 1X TAE running buffer. Load 5 mL of PCR product plus 1 mL of 10X gel-loading dye and include a lane containing a *Hin*dIII marker in order to assess the size of the product. Run at 90 V until the dark blue dye front is approximately two-thirds down the gel.
5. Stain the gel with ethidium bromide. Visualize the DNA on an ultraviolet (UV) transilluminator and photograph the gel.

6. In the second round (a sample from the first round is used as a template), aliquot the following into a sterile 200-mL tube for each PCR reaction (total volume of 50 μL) 5 μL of first-round products, 5 μL of 10X PCR buffer II, 1.5 m*M* $MgCl_2$, 0.2 m*M* dNTPs, 10 pmol of allele-specific primer as forward primer (e.g., 1gT or 3gG for p55/3C, or T4 for G6PD) and the same reverse primer as that used in the first round of PCR (8gR-p55 or 9gR-G6PD), 1 U of *Taq* polymerase, and sterile distilled water to give a final volume of 50 μL.
7. Pipet 50 μL of mineral oil taking care not to puncture the layer. Cap the tube.
8. Perform PCR amplification in a Perkin-Elmer 9600 thermocycling machine using the following conditions: initial denaturation step at 95°C for 1 min, followed by five cycles of PCR at 94°C for 30 s, 64°C for 1 min, and 72°C for 1 min.
9. Visualize 15 μL of amplified PCR products (from each second-round PCR) in all reactions on 1% agarose gels. Genomic DNA from homozygote individuals will generate second-round allele-specific products in only one well. Genomic DNA from heterozygote individuals will generate second-round allele-specific products in both wells.

Analysis of cDNA for Determination of Clonality by ASPCR

For rapid determination of clonality, the template for the first round of PCR is cDNA synthesized from total RNA by reverse transcription. Second-round PCR is conducted in an identical fashion as with genomic DNA. Clonal samples (using cDNA from heterozygous patients) will generate second-round allele-specific products in only one well. Nonclonal samples (using cDNA from heterozygous patients) will generate second-round allele-specific products in both wells.

Notes

1. A limitation of G6PD, p55, and recently introduced IDS assay is that only 76% of Caucasian females, 62% of African-American females, and even lower proportion of Asian females are heterozygous for at least one of these assays and thus suitable for clonality analysis. However, these limitations are now being overcome by assays currently under development.
2. The first-round products always should be visualized under UV light as the same high molecular weight band on first- and second-round agarose gels, and thus serve as an internal control.

6

Centrosome in Cancer

Recent studies have demonstrated that centrosome abnormalities are a common feature of most cancers. *Centrosome amplification* in cancer contributes to the loss of cell and tissue architecture (i.e., anaplasia) and has been implicated in the origin of chromosome instability leading to aneuploidy. The centrosome is a fascinating organelle that resides near the cell center, hence its name. It functions in the maintenance of cytoplasmic architecture through the nucleation and organization of microtubule arrays in interphase and mitotic cells. In addition to its fundamental role in microtubule organization, the centrosome may provide an important structural context for coordinating cell cycle regulation.

Centrosome Structure

Understanding of the molecular basis for these diverse cellular functions is beginning to emerge through the careful analysis of centrosome genes and proteins and centrosome formation, structure, and organization in early embryo development in model systems such as *Drosophila*, yeast, and the nematode and in mammalian somatic cells. Centrosomes consist of three fundamental components: a core structure consisting of a pair of *centrioles* that serve as a centrosomal organizer, a surrounding protein lattice or matrix called *pericentriolar material* (PCM) that serves as a framework to anchor microtubule nucleation sites; and *γ-tubulin complexes* that are responsible for the nucleation of microtubules.

Centrioles are small barrel-shaped organelles (~ 200 nm in diameter and 400 nm in length) consisting of a cylindric array of nine triplet microtubules. Once during each cell cycle the centrosome doubles from one to two in a process that is initiated with centriole duplication. The centriole pair embodies an intrinsic counting mechanism that establishes the number of centrosome equivalents in the cell so that a pair of centrioles equals one and two pairs of centrioles equal two centrosome equivalents. Studies suggest that centrosome size and organization of PCM depends on centriolar integrity.

The PCM is structurally complex and consists of a matrix of coiled-coil proteins, including pericentrin, Cep135, AKAP-450, and ninein. Several of these coiled-coil proteins act as anchors for other essential centrosome proteins and for key regulators of centrosome function. For example, γ-tubulin complexes are anchored to the centrosome by pericentrin, and protein kinase A is anchored by both pericentrin and the proteinkinase- A–anchoring protein—AKAP-450. The centriole pair duplicates during late G1 phase of the cell cycle, and centrosomes increase in size through the recruitment of additional PCM. The two centrosomes of G2/M cells show a dramatic increase in microtubule nucleating activity as they begin to function as spindle poles during mitosis.

Centrosome Cycle

The centrosome is duplicated once, and only once, during a normal cell cycle to yield two centrosomes that function as the spindle poles of the dividing cell. The process is most clearly illustrated by the duplication of the centrioles themselves. In early G1 phase of the cell cycle the two centrioles, which originated in previous cell cycles, usually are oriented in a characteristic orthogonal arrangement relative to one another. As cells pass the G1 restriction point and commit to *deoxyribonucleic acid* (DNA) replication and subsequent cell division, the two centrioles separate and move a short distance away from one another (centriole disjunction) and nascent *procentrioles* form at the proximal end and orthogonal to each preexisting centriole.

During G2/M phase of the cell cycle, centrosome duplication is completed through a maturation process involving the recruitment of additional PCM protein, and each new centrosome, containing one old and one new centriole, functions as a spindle pole during mitosis. The presence of only two centrosomes in the cell as it enters mitosis ensures the equal segregation of sister chromatids to each daughter cell. Mitotic spindle poles also play a role in determining the position and orientation of the cleavage furrow and in exit from cytokinesis. Although centriole duplication occurs in a semiconservative fashion in most cells, as described earlier, during development, and in certain cells under special experimental circumstances, centrioles can arise *de novo*.

Coordination of the Centrosome, DNA, and Cell Cycles

Progress in understanding the centrosome duplication cycle has accelerated. Several emerging lines of evidence suggest that, in addition to its function as a microtubule-organizing center, the centrosome may be a focal point for the convergence of cell cycle pathways implicating this organelle in the control of cell cycle progression. Centrosome duplication is strictly coordinated with the process of DNA replication, mitosis, and cell division. The control of centrosome duplication is tightly coupled to cell cycle progression through two pathways of regulation. The first of these regulatory pathways operates through activity of the G1/S and G2/M cell cycle regulators, including *cyclin-dependent kinase* (CDK) cyclin A and E, which coordinate the cell, centrosome, and DNA cycles. The second control pathway involves the p53-mediated G1/S and G2/M cell cycle checkpoints that monitor DNA integrity and arrest centrosome duplication through the induction of $p21^{waf1}$ synthesis and consequent inhibition of the CDK/cyclins.

The key stages of cell cycle progression are governed by the subcellular location and periodic activation and subsequent inactivation of the serine/threonine cyclin-dependent protein kinases (CDKs). Evidence suggesting a direct role for the CDKs in regulating the mitotic activity of centrosomes first came to light from studies on the localization of cyclin B and CDK1 ($p34^{cdc2}$) at the centrosome during G2/M phase and from experiments using *Xenopus* cell free extracts that implicated cyclins A and B in the control of microtubule dynamics. More recently, the direct involvement of CDK2 activity in regulation of centrosome duplication was established. Both centrosome duplication and DNA replication are dependent on CDK2 activation and are blocked by the CDK2 inhibitors butyrolactone I and roscovitine.

CDK2/cyclin E activity was subsequently identified as a key regulator of the centrosome cycle because centrosome duplication was blocked by the small protein inhibitors of CDK2, $p21^{waf1}$, or p27, or by immuno-depletion of CDK2 or cyclin E, and centrosome duplication was restored by excess purified CDK2/cyclin E. Separation of the centriole pair (centriole disjunction), an early event in the centrosome duplication cycle, was shown to be dependent on CDK2/cyclin E activity, suggesting that a CDK-mediated phosphorylation event regulates centriole pair cohesion. Additional protein phosphorylation events play key roles in controlling centrosome behavior and function during the cell cycle. Centrosome protein phosphorylation increases dramatically at the onset of mitosis and falls precipitously at the metaphase/anaphase transition. It is important to note that several centrosome-associated kinases and target substrates implicated in the regulation of the centrosome cycle become altered during the development of centrosome amplification in cancer. Finally, centrosome duplication also depends on the phosphorylation status of retinoblastoma tumor suppressor *retinoblastoma* (Rb), which governs the availability of the E2F transcription factor to promote S-phase progression. Taken together these findings establish two mechanisms by which DNA replication and centrosome duplication are coordinated during the cell cycle: Both DNA replication and centrosome duplication are controlled by the Rb pathway and depend on downstream transcriptional consequences of E2F activity, and both processes require CDK2/cyclin activation.

Centrosome and DNA Cycles Can Be Uncoupled

In certain cycling cells, multiple rounds of centrosome duplication can occur when DNA replication is blocked; thus, the centrosome cycle is not strictly dependent on DNA replication *per se*. However, recent evidence suggests that uncoupling of the centrosome and DNA cycles can occur only in cells that are defective in G1/S checkpoint controls. Several studies show that loss of p53 function and certain gain-of-function p53 mutations result in deregulation of centrosome duplication and lead to functionally amplified centrosomes. The tumor suppressor protein p53 is involved in the control of centrosome duplication through activation of the G1/S checkpoint and transcriptional regulation of several downstream targets including the CDK inhibitor $p21^{Waf1}$. This inhibitor blocks centrosome duplication through inhibition of CDK2/cyclin E activity. Moreover, reduced activity of $p21^{waf1}$ by antisense expression in human cell lines resulted in centrosome amplification. Although introduction of wild-type p53 into $p53^{-/-}$ mouse embryonic fibroblasts reestablished centrosome homeostasis, overexpression of $p21^{waf1}$ only partially restored control of centrosome duplication in p53-null fibroblasts.

Other control pathways and downstream targets of p53 may also play a role in the control of centrosome homeostasis. For example, p53 mutations and cyclin E overexpression act synergistically to further increase the frequency of centrosome amplification in cultured cells and in tumors. Taken together, these observations suggest that an imbalance between negative and positive cell cycle regulators could accelerate centrosome defects seen in the development of cancer.

It is important to emphasize that during cancer progression, centrosome amplification and genomic instability can also develop independently of loss of p53 function, suggesting the presence of alternative mechanisms leading to disregulation of centrosome homeostasis. Mutations in the *BRCA1* and *BRCA2* tumor-suppressor genes associated with the development of familial breast and ovarian cancers also have been implicated in the loss of checkpoint control of the centrosome cycle. The BRCA1 protein localizes at the centrosome during mitosis, and the hypophosphorylated form of BRCA1 coimmunoprecipitates with γ-tubulin, a centrosomal component essential for nucleation of microtubules. Mouse embryo fibroblasts carrying genetargeted deletions in *BRCA1* or *BRCA2* showed a defective G2/M checkpoint function, amplified centrosomes, aberrant mitoses, and aneuploidy. The *GADD45* gene, a downstream transcriptional product of the p53 pathway, has also been implicated in both DNA damage repair and activation of the G2/M checkpoint. Cells lacking *GADD45* expression show centrosome amplification, mitotic spindle defects, and chromosomal instability. These studies show that centrosome amplification can develop through alternative pathways that converge on G1/S and G2/M checkpoint regulators.

Evidence for a Centrosome-Based Cell Cycle Checkpoint

Studies suggest that these regulatory mechanisms may reside at the centrosome itself. This concept is based on several independent observations. The first is that ablation of centrosomes by microsurgery or laser treatment resulted in cell cycle arrest at G1 prior to the onset of DNA replication; the second is that signaling-kinase anchoring motifs are present in proteins of PCM; and the third is key cell cycle regulators, including the tumor suppressor proteins p53, BRCA-1 and -2, the cyclin/CDKs, and the anaphase-promoting complex/cyclosome, localize (albeit, some only transiently) within centrosome PCM. To summarize, centrosome ablation arrests the cell cycle and many important regulators of cell cycle progression reside in the centrosome. These observations suggest a mechanism by which key regulators may act locally within the structural context of the centrosome to coordinate steps critical for cell cycle progression and together suggest the existence of a centrosome-based cell cycle checkpoint.

Centrosome Amplification in Cancer

Centrosome defects have been implicated in the origin of mitotic abnormalities and the development of aneuploidy in cancer. Recent studies implicate centrosome defects in the origin of chromosomal instability and the pathogenesis of cancer. Centrosome defects (i.e., centrosome amplification) are characteristic of many solid tumors. The term "*centrosome amplification*" designates centrosomes that contain more than four centrioles (i.e., "*supernumerary centrioles*"), centrosomes that appear significantly larger than normal as defined by the staining of structural centrosome components in excess of that seen in the corresponding normal tissue or cell type, and/or when more than two centrosomes are present within a cell.

In addition, amplified centrosomes also show protein hyper-phosphorylation and altered functional properties such as an increased microtubule-nucleating capacity. These centrosome abnormalities have been implicated as a potential cause for the loss of cell and tissue architecture seen in cancer (i.e., anaplasia) through altered centrosome function in microtubule nucleation and organization and to result in chromosome missegregation during mitosis as a consequence of an increased rate of multipolar spindle formation.

Centrosome Amplification, Aneuploidy, and Chromosomal Instability

A key question: Does centrosome amplification lead to chromosomal instability and aneuploidy, or is centrosome amplification a consequence of aneuploidy? Aneuploidy is characterized as the *state* of an abnormal karyotype, having gains and/or losses of whole chromosomes. Aneuploidy occurs early in the development of many tumor types, suggesting that it may play a role in both tumorigenesis and tumor progression. Indeed, aneuploidy is present in the great majority of malignant tumors, in contrast to benign tumors, which are most often diploid. Aneuploidy can be distinguished from the persistent generation of chromosomal variations, termed "*chromosomal instability*" (CIN), which reflects the rate of change in karyotype.

Quantitative analysis of CIN can be determined as the percentage of cells with a chromosome number different from the modal chromosome number. Thus, tumors may show either "*stable aneuploidy*" (low CIN) or "*unstable aneuploidy*" (high CIN). Unstable karyotypes may lead to phenotypic heterogeneity in cancer, reflecting the persistent generation of new chromosomal variations.

The development of aneuploidy may be a consequence of centrosome amplification, which can lead to the formation of multipolar spindles and mis-segregate sister chromatids during mitosis (and, as a result, lead to high CIN). Chromosomal instability occurs exclusively in aneuploid tumors and tumor-derived cell lines, in contrast to diploid tumors, which contain centrosomes that are functionally and structurally normal. The degree of genomic instability in aneuploid tumors parallels the degree of centrosome abnormalities in cell lines from breast, pancreas, prostate, colon, and cervix tumors; from short-term culture of mouse mammary tumors; and from SV40 ST overexpressing fibroblasts. When tissues were examined, centrosome abnormalities were higher in high-grade prostate tumors and high-grade cervical tumors than in low-grade tumors. In prostate cancer, centrosome amplification has been implicated in the development of abnormal mitoses and CIN facilitating progression to advanced stages of the disease.

Strong support for a direct mechanistic link between centrosome amplification and CIN is suggested by the significant linear correlation between centrosome amplification and the rate of change in karyotype (CIN) seen in human breast tumors. Although such correlation alone does not necessarily imply cause and effect, these observations have led many authors to propose the hypothesis that centrosome amplification is the primary cause of genomic instability observed in most tumors. As discussed earlier, Boveri (1914) first recognized these features of cancer cells nearly a century ago and proposed that centrosome defects could lead to mitotic and subsequent chromosomal abnormalities. An alternative hypothesis has been proposed that claims chromosomal instability seen in cancer cells is caused by aneuploidy, i.e., that aneuploidy itself destabilizes the karyotype and thus initiates CIN leading to widespread heterogeneity in tumor cell phenotypes.

Several independent lines of evidence support the proposition that centrosome abnormalities drive genomic instability. In a study of human breast tumors, all specimens of ductal carcinoma *in situ* examined showed significant centrosome amplification, suggesting that centrosome amplification is an early event that occurs prior to invasion in breast tumors. Furthermore, cells transfected to express the *human papilloma virus* (HPV) E7 oncoprotein undergo centrosome amplification before developing nuclear morphology associated with aneuploidy. Finally, in a xenograft model of pancreatic cancer, metastatic foci showed a higher incidence of centrosome amplification than did the primary xenograft, and abnormal centrosome numbers were accompanied by a higher frequency of abnormal mitoses.

Taken together, these studies underscore the importance of proper coordination of the centrosome and cell cycles and illustrate the potential for severe consequences of failure of proper regulation of these processes. They also suggest that centrosome amplification may be an early event in tumorigenesis that can drive CIN and lead to genotypic and phenotypic diversity of cells within a tumor. The following sections present methods used in our laboratories to assess structural and functional centrosome characteristics that accompany centrosome amplification in cancer.

METHODS FOR ANALYSIS OF CENTROSOME AMPLIFICATION IN CANCER

Sample Procurement

Human tumor tissues should be collected according to an Institutional Review Board–approved protocol. It is useful to recruit a pathologist as a collaborator who can review all of the specimens in your study to confirm specific pathologies and to ensure consistent grading of the specimens. Prior exposure to chemotherapeutic or radiation therapy before surgery should be noted because these treatments themselves may cause centrosome anomalies. Tissue specimens are frozen in liquid nitrogen immediately after surgery and stored at −70°C until use or formalin fixed and paraffin embedded for later sectioning. Cultured cells should be seeded onto clean sterile glass coverslips, and cultured for 48 hr.

Morphological and Structural Methods

Centrosome size and number in tissue sections

Centrosome size can be determined in paraffin or frozen tissue sections using immunofluorescence labeling and confocal microscopy for measurements. The advantage of using tissue sections is that most tissues contain fibroblasts, which, as will be detailed later, can be used to normalize centrosome size so that meaningful comparisons can be made between tissue preparations and different slides. Antibodies against γ-tubulin, centrin, and pericentrin work well in cold methanol-fixed frozen sections, and anti-γ-tubulin works consistently in formalin-fixed paraffin sections.

Protocol for immunolabeling

1. Incubate sections in blocking buffer (phosphate buffer saline [PBS], pH 7.2, 5% normal goat serum, 1% glycerol, 0.1% bovine serum albumin [BSA], 1% fish skin gelatin, and 0.04% sodium azide) for 30 min.
2. Incubate sections for 60 min in primary antibodies labeled with Zenon probes according to the manufacturer's instructions.
3. Wash with PBS 3× for 5 min each.

4. Frozen section only (paraffin sections proceed to Step 5) postfix with 4% formaldehyde for 3 min, and wash with PBS 2× for 3 min each.
5. Stain nuclei with Hoechst 33342 (1 μg/ml) for 5 min.
6. Water rinse.
7. Air-dry for 5 min.
8. Mount coverslip with Prolong antifade medium.

For paraffin sections, once the slides are deparaffinated, antigen retrieval using pH 6 ethylenediamine tetra-acetic acid (EDTA) in a vegetable steamer for 30 min precedes Step 1 above. After the mountant has set, usually overnight, the slides can be observed and analyzed using a Zeiss LSM 510 or equivalent confocal microscope using a 100X high N.A. objective lens.

Protocol for confocal analysis of centrosome size and number

1. Configure the lasers and detectors for excitation and detection of Hoechst 33342 (364 excitation, blue emission) and Alexafluor 448 (448 excitation, green emission) and/or Alexafluor 568 (568 excitation, red emission).
2. Select pinholes equal to 1 Airey unit for each optical path.
3. Set up for Z stack collection of 3–9 optical sections spaced at 0.5 μm intervals. The number of sections depends on the thickness of the tissue section but should be kept constant for a given experiment.
4. Place the slide on the microscope and focus on a fibroblast centrosome.
5. Set the digital zoom at 2X and the line averaging at 4.
6. Set laser power and detection parameters so that the resulting signal is saturated or nearly saturated only at the centrosome. (*Note:* Because this procedure is designed to measure area rather than signal intensity, saturated or nearly saturated signal is optimal.)
7. Collect a Z stack and make a maximum intensity projection of the stack.
8. Open the brightness and contrast window, select the color of the centrosome signal, and maximize both brightness and contrast to create a pseudobinary image of the centrosome. No other labeling should be seen with these settings. If other labeling is present, go back to the detection settings and decrease detector gain slightly before collecting the image again. You may need to select a fresh fibroblast centrosome if photo-bleaching has occurred during these setup steps.

9. Open the measurement window and select area measurement.
10. Select the channel in which the centrosome signal was collected and adjust the slider down slightly so that everything but the centrosome signal is masked out.
11. Using the overlay function, draw a circle 3 μm diameter around the centrosome.
12. Select the area button to obtain the area of the centrosome signal inside the circle. It should be between 0.3 and 1.3 μm^2. If the value is less than 0.3 μm^2, return to the collection parameters in Step 6 and increase the detector gain and/or amplitude and repeat the process. If the value is greater than 1.3 μm^2, repeat the collection parameters in Step 6 and decrease the detector gain and/or amplitude and repeat the process. Once a value within the correct range is obtained, copy and paste the value into a spreadsheet. These steps establish the correct collection parameters for the particular slide under observation. From this point onward, do not alter the settings. You are now ready to use identical parameters to measure 4 additional fibroblast centrosomes, and then proceed to measure centrosomes in normal epithelial and tumor cells.
13. Focus on epithelial cells of interest.
14. Set the digital zoom at 2X.
15. Collect a Z stack and make a maximum intensity projection of the stack.
16. Open the brightness and contrast window, select the color of the centrosome signal, and maximize both brightness and contrast to create a pseudobinary image of the centrosome.
17. Open the histogram window and select area measurement.
18. Select the channel in which the centrosome signal was collected and adjust the low threshold slider down slightly so that everything but the centrosome signal is masked out.
19. Using the overlay function, draw a circle ~3 μm diameter around the first centrosome in the image. The diameter of the circle is not critical; just make sure that it includes the entire centrosome signal and excludes any autofluorescence your sample may have.
20. Select the area button to obtain the area of the centrosome signal inside the circle.
21. Copy and paste the value into a spreadsheet.
22. Repeat Steps 19–21 for each centrosome in the image.

23. Count the number of the nuclei in the field and enter the number in the spreadsheet.
24. Repeat Steps 13–23 until at least 50 nuclei have been counted for that tissue section.
25. Repeat Steps 1–24 for each new tissue section.

Once the measurements have been collected, you should have a spreadsheet for each tissue analyzed. For each tissue, calculate the average and standard deviation of the fibroblast centrosome size. A standard deviation less than 15% of the average value is indicative of adequate specimen preparation and signal collection. Divide 1 by the average value to get a normalization factor. Determine the average value for the epithelial cell centrosomes and multiply it by the normalization factor to determine the normalized value. This normalized value can then be compared to normalized values from other tissues. This analysis assumes that fibroblast centrosome size is consistent between tissues.

Centrosome number in tissues and cultured cells

A much simpler analysis using only a subset of the steps described earlier can be used to calculate the number of centrosomes per cell. In cultured cells, this analysis can also be used to categorize centrosomes labeled for γ-tubulin according to the number of γ-tubulin spots per cell and the spacing of paired spots. Proceed with "*Immunolabeling Protocol*," as described earlier. In the "*Confocal Analysis Protocol*," follow Steps 1–7, except use a digital zoom of 1 instead of 2. Collect representative images with a total of at least 50 nuclei per sample. For tissues, count the number of centrosomes in each image and the number of nuclei in each field to determine the average number of centrosomes per nucleus. For cultured cells, the number of labeled centrosomes can be counted for each individual cell and each centrosome can be scored as follows: (1) a single normal-sized spot, (2) a separated normal pair, (3) a single amplified spot, or (4) multiple spots. This scoring method is difficult to apply to tissue sections because it is not always possible to assign each centrosome to a nucleus; nevertheless, it is useful for the analysis of centrosome characteristics and for comparison with cell cycle kinetics established in parallel experiments.

Functional Assay for Microtubule Nucleation and Growth

Live cell microtubule regrowth assay

This assay assesses an important parameter of centrosome functional in living cultured cells—their ability to regrow *microtubules*

(MTs) after MT depolymerization. Native MTs are first depolymerized by cold treatment, then the specimen is returned to a temperature that supports MT polymerization, and the number and length of newly polymerized MTs are measured at intervals after recovery. The resulting MT asters are also characterized. Cells are cultured on sterile 12-mm-diameter glass coverslips placed in the wells of 24-well tissue culture dishes. Let the cells grow to 80% confluence before starting the following protocol.

Protocol for MT regrowth

1. Aspirate the growth medium from each well and rinse with microtubule stabilizing buffer (MTSB: 1% Triton X-100, 10 mM Pipes, pH 7.2, 2 mM EGTA, 1 mM $MgSO_4$).
2. Aspirate the MTSB and add cold growth medium diluted with one part cold MTSB. Place culture dishes on ice and store for 30 min in the refrigerator. For the control, proceed directly to Step 5.
3. Aspirate cold solution from each well and replace with warm medium/MTSB filling the well half full. Start timing the regrowth immediately after adding the warm solution for each time point. Place plates in a 25°C incubator.
4. At each time point, aspirate the liquid and replace with 0.1% of Triton (prewarmed at 25°C). Incubate for *exactly* 1 min at room temperature.
5. Aspirate Triton and add -20°C methanol to the top of the wells. Place in the freezer for 10 min.
6. Remove the coverslips from the culture dishes and place them cell side up on a paper towel.
7. Let air-dry for at least 10 min.
8. Proceed with the "*Protocol for Immunolabeling*," using primary antibodies against γ-tubulin and α-tubulin.

Protocol for confocal analysis of MT regrowth

1. Follow Steps 1–5 of the "Protocol for Confocal Analysis of Centrosome Size and Number," with the exception of taking single optical sections instead of Z sections.
2. Image cells for γ-tubulin labeled centrosomes and α-tubulin–labeled MTs.
3. Using the overlay function, draw a circle centered on the centrosome and extend the circle's perimeter to the end of the longest unbroken MT of the MT aster.

4. Display the circumference of the circle and enter that value into a spreadsheet. Convert the circumference to radius to determine the length of the longest MT.
5. Count the number of MTs in the aster.
6. Score the aster as organized (MTs radiating from the center in relatively straight paths) or unorganized (MTs criss-crossing each other in a helter-skelter fashion).
7. Score the cell as having single or multiple asters.

Abnormal mitoses

Analysis of mitotic structure is a surrogate for centrosome function in mitosis. Cells or tissue sections can be scored for the number of abnormal mitoses as a percentage of total mitoses. This can be done on paraffin sections stained *hematoxylin and eosin* (H&E) or stained by immunohistochemistry for Ki-67. It can also be done on cultured cells whose nuclear morphology has been adequately preserved by formaldehyde fixation and stained with Hoechst 33342 or DAPI. The first 50–100 mitotic nuclei are counted and scored for mitotic stage (prophase, prometaphase, metaphase, anaphase, telophase, or unknown) and categorized as normal bipolar or abnormal multipolar. Centrosome abnormalities are sometimes manifested as a prolongation of the time spent in prometaphase and metaphase, so a comparison of the distribution of mitotic stages between cell populations is an important part of the overall analysis of mitotic abnormalities.

In conclusion, in this chapter we have reviewed centrosome dynamics and regulation in normal cells and the origin and consequences of centrosome amplification in cancer. Methods for the quantitative assessment of amplification of centrosome structure and function in human tumors and in cultured tumor cells were also presented. These methods can serve as a starting point for investigators who are interested in persuing the role of centrosome behavior and the origin of chromosomal instability and anaplasia in the development of cancer.

7

DNA Damage and DNA Repair

DNA in human cells is continuously subject to damage. It is in most cases appropriately repaired, leaving relatively few permanent changes. The various kinds of damage comprise chemical modification or loss of DNA bases, single strand or double strand breaks as well as intra- and interstrand crosslinks. Each type of damage can lead to mutations. An important source of mutations are DNA replication and recombination. DNA replication is a particular critical phase, during which misincorporation of nucleotides, DNA polymerase slippage or stalling of replication forks may occur. A further source of mutations are physiological recombination processes that go astray, e.g. in germ cells or lymphocytes.

In addition to endogenous processes such as oxidative stress and spontaneous reactions of DNA such as cytosine deamination, diverse exogenous physical and chemical carcinogens cause DNA damage. Some carcinogens cause specific point mutations while others induce strand-breaks or various types of alterations. Carcinogens that induce strand-breaks may act as '*clastogens*', i.e. induce structural chromosomal aberrations. The involvement of specifically acting carcinogens is in some cases detectable by the kind of mutation found in a cancer.

Tumor viruses can be mutagenic by insertion, by causing rearrangements or loss of chromosomes, or indirectly through viral proteins, which interfere with the cellular systems that control genomic integrity. The various DNA repair systems in human cells are tailored towards the different types of DNA damage. They share components such as DNA polymerases and DNA ligases, but each employ additional specific proteins.

Specialized glycosylases remove damaged bases. AP (apurinic/apyrimidinic) endonucleases prepare sites lacking bases for short patch or long patch base excision repair. More problematic alterations such as carcinogen adducts and pyrimidine dimers caused by UV light are removed by nucleotide excision repair systems. Mismatched base pairs in DNA caused by mutagens or mistakes during DNA replication are the target of two interlinked mismatch repair systems. Double strand breaks pose a major challenge to cell survival and genomic integrity. They are recognized and handled by several different repair systems employing homologous or non-homologous recombination to avoid or minimize permanent damage. Still another repair system employs the FANC proteins to prepare cross-linked DNA for repair by recombination.

Inborn errors in these DNA repair systems underlie syndromes associated with developmental defects, neurological disease and cancer. For instance, excision repair is defective in xeroderma pigmentosum, mismatch repair in HNPCC (hereditary non-poliposis carcinoma coli), double strand repair in ataxia telangiectasia, and cross-link repair in Fanconi anemia, respectively. While each of these syndromes is rare, polymorphisms in DNA repair genes likely modulate cancer risk in the general population.

A second layer of protective mechanisms helps to avoid DNA damage. Reactive mutagens are intercepted by low molecular protective compounds such as glutathione or by proteins such as metallothioneins or glutathione transferases. Specific mechanisms protect against reactive oxygen species and against radiation. Genetic polymorphisms again, but also diet and other environmental factors influence the efficiency of these mechanisms in individual humans.

DNA damage can activate cellular checkpoints which prevent cell cycle progression and stop DNA synthesis and mitosis, or activate apoptotic cell death. Double-strand breaks elicit a particularly strong signal. Stress signals can also be activated by radiation or reactive oxygen species, through specialized signaling pathways. Infection by viruses also activates cellular checkpoints and stress signals.

DNA Damage during Replication: Base Excision and Nucleotide Excision Repair

The mutations and chromosomal alterations found in cancer cells represent only a small fraction of those that arise during the life-time of a human, because the great majority are removed by one of several repair mechanisms. These are excellently tuned to the various types of DNA damage that might cause mutations. Moreover, cells with substantially damaged DNA or aneuploid genomes are normally eliminated or at least prevented from proliferation. Therefore, cancer cells displaying genomic instability need to inactivate the systems responsible for this surveillance. Accordingly, defects in DNA repair systems and cellular surveillance mechanisms are an important, if not even necessary factor in the development of human cancers. Such defects may be inherited or acquired.

Damage to DNA can result from endogenous as well as exogenous sources. DNA replication is a particularly critical process, with an increased potential for spontaneous mutations and an increased sensitivity towards induced damage. Proliferating cells are therefore more susceptible to neoplastic transformation. Problems that may arise during DNA replication comprise misincorporation of bases, slippage of the replisome in tandem repeat sequences, single-strand breaks being converted into double-strand breaks by replication, stalling of the replisome at 'difficult' sequences or at bases modified by chemical reactions with exogenous carcinogens or endogenous proteins.

Replication of nuclear DNA is extremely precise with a nucleotide misincorporation rate of 10^{-7}-10^{-6}, since eukaryotic replication DNA polymerases discrimate well between the various nucleotides and the main replicase possesses a 3'-5' exonuclease proof-reading function. This level of precision is not always achieved by repair polymerases. In spite of the excellent fidelity of the replication proteins, in a genome of $>3 \times 10^9$ bp, several hundred mistakes are expected during each replication. Most misincorporations are corrected by base mismatch repair systems, leaving an estimated number of 1×10^{-10} base changes per cell division.

Base misincorporation is, however, only one of several problems that can occur during replication. *Mismatch repair* (MMR) systems also take care of single strand loops in replicated DNA that result from slippage of DNA in repeat sequences. Typically, slippage occurs in microsatellites which consist of tandem repeats of 1-4 bp repeats. Defects in mismatch repair therefore result in an increased frequency of base misincorporations, but also lead to microsatellite expansions or contractions. Even with fully functional mismatch repair, microsatellites are subject to a somewhat higher mutation rate than the average of the genome, which is one reason why they are normally polymorphic.

Another source of base misincorporation are mesomeric isoforms of the DNA bases that can mispair. The mesomeric isoforms of the standard four bases are shortlived, but some are stabilized by chemical modification. For instance, hydroxylation of guanine at the 8 position stabilizes a G:A mismatch. Most mismatches caused from frequent mispairing events such as OH-G:A are recognized by specific proteins that activate the mismatch repair system.

The precision of DNA replication also depends on the nucleotide precursor pools. Disparities in the relative levels of the deoxy-nucleotide triphosphates decrease the fidelity of base incorporation. As biochemistry textbooks discuss in detail, nucleotide biosynthetic pathways contain several cross-regulatory and feedback mechanisms to minimize such disparities. In addition, deregulation of precursor pools, in particular of guanine nucleotides, activates cellular checkpoints through the TP53 protein. Next to dGTP, dTTP may be most critical, because DNA polymerases also accept dUTP. In normal cells, dUTP levels are maintained low by enzymatic hydrolysis. In cells with suboptimal thymidine biosynthesis, e.g. as a consequence of low folate levels or of chemotherapy with methotrexate, significant levels of uracil bases are incorporated. These, like the rarer ones in normal cells, are removed by a specialized hydrolyase, *uracil-N-glycohydrolase* (UNG). This removal, however, induces abasic sites and strand breaks in DNA.

Spontaneous chemical reactions by DNA bases, outside of or during replication, represent a second type of problem. Hydrolytic cytosine deamination yields uridine which is foreign to DNA. It is recognized as such and removed by the uracil glycohydrolyase. The capacity of this enzyme is more than sufficient to remove the estimated ≈1000 uracils that are spontaneously generated in each cell per day. The rate of cytosine deamination can be increased by exogenous and endogenous compounds. For instance, nitrosation at the amino group leads to deamination of cytosine. Similarly efficient, another specialized glycosylase eliminates hypoxanthin arising from purine base deamination. Hydrolysis of methylcytosine, which constitutes 3-5% of cytosines in human cells, is more of a problem, since it yields thymidine upon deamination. A specialized enzyme, G-T mismatch glycosylase, removes the thymine from such mismatches. Still, the mutation rate at methylated CpG dinucleotides, at which methylcytosine is almost exclusively found in human cells, is higher than elsewhere in the genome, and mutations are usually C→T (or G→A). Deamination of methylcytosine is enhanced by oxidation of the methyl group towards hydroxy-methyl-cytosine. This yields hydroxymethyl-thymidine upon hydrolysis. This modified base can also be generated directly from thymidine by reactive oxygen species. In either case, it is removed by another specialized glycosylase.

Next to the amino group of cytosine, guanine presents the most sensitive base target for chemical reactions on DNA. Many electrophiles react rather spontaneously at its N7 or O6 positions. An important endogenous electrophile is S-adenosylmethionine, the standard carrier for biological methylation reactions. Methylation of guanine can lead to mispairing and methyl groups are therefore removed by a specialized enzyme. The methyl-guanine methyltransferase MGMT has a broader specificity and also removes other alkyl groups by transfer to its own cysteine groups, inactivating itself in the course of the reaction. Guanine is also a major site for alkylation by exogenous compounds including several cytostatic drugs and major carcinogens. Again, MGMT acts protectively. Down-regulation of the enzyme by epigenetic mechanisms is found in some cancers. It is an important factor in their responsiveness to chemotherapy, but likely also increases the rate of mutations in general.

Guanine is also the base most susceptible to reactive oxygen species. The most important product is 8-oxo-guanine (or 8-hydroxy-guanine, depending on which mesomeric form is considered). This base also mispairs and is removed by specialized glycosylases, prominently oxoguanine glycosylase 1 (OGG1). Since OGG1 is polymorphic in man, individuals may differ in their capacity of removing this type of damage.

As their designation indicates, base glycosylases in general hydrolyse the N-glycosidic bond between modified bases and deoxyribose, leaving abasic sites in DNA. Such sites also arise from spontaneous or induced hydrolysis of the N-glycosidic bonds of normal bases or of chemically modified bases. Purines are about 20-fold more susceptible to spontaneous loss from DNA than pyrimidines and >20,000 purine bases are estimated to be lost in a human cell each day.

Abasic sites having arisen spontaneously, been induced, or originated through enzyme action are filled in by short-patch repair. This is initiated by the action of one of several endonucleases, such as APE1 and APEXL2, which belong to a larger family of apurinic/apyrimidinic endonucleases (AP-endonucleases). They cleave the DNA strand with the missing base to provide a free 3'-hydroxyl group for DNA polymerase β. This enzyme removes the deoxyribose and replaces it with the correct nucleotide. DNA ligase III closes the strand break. The action of the polymerase and the ligase is coordinated by XRCC1. While only one base is replaced by short-patch repair, an alternative mode, '*long-patch repair*' replaces several nucleotides. This repair system involves the FEN endonuclease, DNA polymerase δ, PCNA, and DNA ligase I. It is one of several back-up systems to single-base repair.

The type of DNA repair resulting from the combined action of glycosylases, AP-endonucleases, DNA polymerases and DNA ligases is called '*base excision repair*'. By comparison, the mismatch repair mechanism taking care of mismatched bases and enzyme slipping during DNA replication is one kind of '*nucleotide excision repair*'. Similar to base excision repair, it involves the steps of damage recognition, incision, removal of a short stretch of nucleotides, resynthesis and ligation. Many, but not all components of this system are known in man. Damage recognition is achieved by different proteins depending on the type of damage.

Mismatched bases are recognized by the MSH2 and MSH6 proteins, whereas insertion or deletion loops resulting from slippage are recognized by MSH3 and MSH2. In either case, PMS2 and MLH1 are recruited. It is not clear whether any endonuclease is involved in DNA mismatch repair in humans. It seems that mismatch repair during DNA replication starts at existing single strand breaks and uses components of the DNA replisome plus the EXO1 exonuclease. All are coordinated by the PCNA subunit of the replisome.

An evident dilemma during mismatch repair is how to decide which of the unmatched bases is to be excised or, likewise, whether a single-strand loop constitutes a deletion or an insertion. In some prokaryotes, this decision is facilitated, since the parental strand is methylated, but the daughter strand is methylated only later on. For instance, E. coli uses adenine (*dam*) methylation at GATC sites for this distinction. In humans DNA is post-replicatively methylated at cytosines, but this modification does not seem to serve the same purpose. More likely, newly synthesized strands are distinguished by the presence of single-strand breaks that serve as the starting points for nucleotide excision.

Inherited mutations in components of the mismatch repair system carry a strong hereditary predisposition to certain cancers. Since in the affected individuals cancers in the colon and rectum are most conspicuous, with a life-time risk of up to 80%, these syndromes are summarized under the heading of HNPCC, for '*hereditary nonpolyposis colorectal cancer*'. They are genetically heterogeneous, since one or the other component of the mismatch repair can be defective. HNPCC is a dominant-autosomally inherited cancer syndrome. Cancers in families affected by HNPCC may also present in the endometrium, stomach, ovaries, hepatobiliary system and the upper urinary tract, in this approximate order of decreasing incidence. Mutations in at least 5 different genes can underlie the syndrome. Most frequently, one allele of *MSH2* and *MLH1* is mutated in the germ-line; mutations in *PMS2*, *MSH6*, and *PMS1* are less prevalent. Further candidates are *MBD4*, encoding a methylcytosine binding protein also involved in DNA repair, and *MYH* encoding a protein recognizing adenine-oxo-guanine mismatches.

The dominant mode of inheritance in HNPCC is not due to a dominant effect of the mutated gene product. Instead, the one remaining functional allele is generally sufficient for mismatch repair. However, cancers arise when the second, intact allele of the affected mismatch repair gene is accidentially mutated or exchanged by recombination with the first mutated allele in somatic cells. During DNA replication, these cells then accumulate mutations at an increased rate.

Some of these mutations may be irrelevant, such as those in the length of microsatellite repeats which are not repaired after slippage. Others, however, lead to inactivation of genes crucial for the control of cell proliferation, because single base mutations arise from unrepaired mismatches or slippage in base repeats within coding regions are not amended. For instance, the *MSH3* and *MSH6* genes *6* each themselves contain cytidine and adenosine hexanucleotide stretches which tend to expand or contract in cells with defective mismatch repair. Since they occur regularly, microsatellite expansions and contractions, which are collectively called '*microsatellite instability*' (MSI), can be used to diagnose cancers arising from defective mismatch repair. For this purpose, a standard set of five microsatellites that are most susceptible has been defined.

Cancers with microsatellite instability (MSI) are not restricted to HNPCC families, but also arise in sporadic (i.e. non-familial) cases. Overall, up to 15% of all colon cancers may belong to the MSI group, but only a few percent of all colon cancers arise in HNPCC families. The cause of '*sporadic MSI*' is mutation, deletion or epigenetic silencing of mismatch repair genes. The most frequent cause of MSI in sporadic cancers may be silencing of *MLH1* by promoter hypermethylation.

Nucleotide Excision Repair and Crosslink Repair

Processes like the hydrolytic deamination of cytosine or the oxidation of guanine lead to altered bases with an increased potential for mispairing. However, neither change interferes principally with DNA replication or transcription. This is different for some other types of damage inflicted on DNA. Ultraviolet radiation (UV) causes chemical reactions in DNA. UV radiation with wavelengths in the absorption maximum of DNA cannot penetrate into the body, but the UVB range from 280-320 nm can and just reaches into the absorption spectrum of DNA. This type of UV induces mainly reactions between adjacent pyrimidine bases such as thyminethymine cyclobutane dimers and thymine-cytosine (or cytosine-cytosine) 6-4 photoproducts. These intra-strand dimers present obstacles to transcription and replication of DNA.

Likewise, chemical reactions of endogenous compounds and activated chemical carcinogens can lead to modified bases that are too bulky to fit into a double helix and cannot be recognized by polymerases. Adducts of aflatoxin or benzopyrene at guanines are important examples. Even proteins can become covalently linked to DNA bases. Transcription and replication are also prevented, when opposite DNA strands in the double helix are crosslinked. This is exploited in cancer therapy by compounds like cis-platinum and mitomycin C.

Photoproducts and bulky adducts are removed by *nucleotide excision repair* (NER). Two interlinked systems are known in man, called '*global-genome*' and '*transcription-coupled*' repair. Transcription-coupled repair is more rapid, but is restricted to regions of the genome transcribed by RNA polymerase II. When the transcription polymerase encounters a bulky adduct or a cyclobutane photoproduct that prevents further progress, it activates repair through its associated TFIIH complex. This complex contains ≈10 proteins, including Cyclin H. This cyclin regulates kinases that normally phosphorylate and activate PolII, but also the DNA helicases XPB and XPD (also known as ERCC2 and ERCC3) which are involved in NER. The complex successively binds the CSB and CSA proteins which start the actual repair sequence.

The actual repair mechanism appears to be identical in transcription-coupled and in global-genome repair. However, recognition of lesions in global-genome repair does not involve the RNA polymerase, but is performed by the XPC and HHR23 proteins. It does also not require the CSA and CSB proteins. Global-genome repair is slower than transcription-coupled repair and has a broader specificity. Following lesion recognition, however, both repair systems use TFIIH components such as XPB and XPD, as well as the single-strand binding protein RPA and the XPA protein to fully unwind and mark the lesion in an ATP-dependent manner. The damaged segment of DNA is excised as a 18-24 nt single strand through 5'-incision by the ERCC1/XPF endonuclease and 3'-incision by the XPG (also ERCC5) endonuclease. The DNA gap is filled by DNA polymerases δ or ε supported by PCNA and RFC and sealed by a DNA ligase, presumably DNA ligase I.

Independent of nucleotide excision repair, photoproducts and other lesions encountered by the replisome can be bypassed through '*translesional repair*' which makes use of DNA polymerase η, a more robust enzyme: It it capable of replicating DNA with very different types of damage, but at the price of a higher error rate than during replication by standard polymerases like Pol δ.

Mutations in genes involved in nucleotide excision repair underlie the diseases xeroderma pigmentosum, Cockayne syndrome, and trichothiodistrophy. These rare diseases are inherited in a recessive fashion. Patients with Cockayne syndrome and trichothiodistrophy suffer from growth defects and progressive mental retardation. Specific and less specific skin defects are apparent, in particular scaly skin (ichthyosis) and brittle hair and nails which are diagnostic for trichothiodistrophy. The patients do not seem to be particularly prone to cancers, but show some symptoms of premature aging and their life expectancy is diminished.

In contrast, patients with xeroderma pigmentosum usually do not display growth defects and mental retardation, except for those in a subgroup overlapping with Cockayne syndrome. Instead, they suffer from extreme photosensitivity of the skin, with abnormal pigmentation. UV-exposed parts of the eyes are also subject to damage. The main clinical problem in these patients is a huge increase in skin cancer risk, estimated as ≈2000-fold. Almost all xeroderma pigmentosum patients develop multiple skin cancers in sun-exposed areas before the age of 30, and often already during their first decade of life. All types of skin cancers are increased, basal cell carcinoma, squamous carcinoma, and melanoma. Other cancer types may also occur at an increased frequency.

Typical Cockayne syndrome is caused by homozygous mutations in the *CSA* or *CSB* genes (hence the designation CS). Xeroderma pigmentosum is caused by mutations in *XPA* – *XPG* genes (now officially called *ERCC* genes), and likely in others. Some remain unidentified, but mutations in the gene encoding DNA polymerase η are responsible for a subgroup of the disease, XP-V. The very rare trichothiodistrophy syndrome is sometimes caused by mutations in a specific gene (*TTD-A*), but more often by certain mutations in *XPB* or *XPD*. Specific *XPD* mutations also account for most cases of combined xeroderma pigmentosum/Cockayne syndrome.

Mutations in Cockayne syndrome cause defects specifically in transcription-coupled repair which impair growth in general and the function of specific tissues such as the brain, since they diminish the efficiency of transcription. Apparently, other repair systems including global-genome repair are not fast enough to prevent this, but remove DNA damage eventually, at least preventing a large increase in cancer risk. In contrast, most defects in XP genes will compromise transcription-coupled as well as global-genome repair leading, in particular, to an increased sensitivity towards UV in exposed tissues. In the case of XPC, the defect is restricted to global-genome repair, with transcription-coupled repair apparently intact: It is not entirely clear, why defects in other XP genes do not regularly lead to impaired growth and neuronal degeneration. Neither is it obvious, why different mutations in the XPB and XPD genes lead to very different, in some respects even complementary phenotypes such as trichothiodistrophy and xeroderma pigmentosum.

Crosslinks between DNA strands are a still more severe impediment to transcription and DNA replication. Their repair is often only possible by sacrificing a fragment of DNA. The mechanisms involved in this type of repair are only partly understood. As in nucleotide excision repair, the actual mechanism may vary depending on when exactly the DNA modification is recognized, i.e. before, during or after DNA replication.

In non-replicating cells, several mechanisms may in principle be used. They range from outright deletion of the blocked double-stranded segment followed by non-homologous end-joining through error-prone excision/bypass-repair by components from the nucleotide excision repair arsenal to essentially error-free repair by homologous recombination with the homologous sister chromatid in G2 cells. How they proceed exactly and how they are chosen, is still being investigated.

Similarly to the mechanism used in G2 cells, the presence of a second homologous sequence can be exploited in a still diploid cell, when crosslinks are encountered at a DNA replication fork. Here, an excision is made behind the lesion, likely by XPF/ERCC1. A gap is created by resection, one strand is filled in using the homologous sequence as a template and the resulting structure is resolved by recombination. The second strand is synthesized following excision of the cross-linked fragment. Most of these mechanisms use components of strand break repair systems discussed below and are crucially dependent on FANC proteins.

Mutations in either of >7 genes encoding FANC proteins cause the recessively inherited disease Fanconi anemia (hence: FANC proteins). Patients with Fanconi anemia are small of height and display an assortment of malformations in different organ systems. Most typical are malformations of the lower arm (radius) and thumb. Further parts of the skeleton may be affected as well as the genitourinary system, the gastrointestinal tract, the heart and the central nervous system. '*Cafe au lait*' spots on the skin are an additional diagnostic sign.

The most problematic symptom in this pleiotropic disease is a diminished function of the hematopoetic system, often resulting in diminished production of all cell types (pancytopenia) which develops gradually during childhood. Malfunction of hematopoesis leads to bleeding, anemia, and susceptibility towards infections. Conversely, the patients often suffer from the preneoplastic '*myelodysplastic syndrome*', which is prone to progression into outright leukemias, typically AML (*acute myeloic leukemia*). When challenged with DNA crosslinking compounds like mitomycin C or diepoxybutane, cells from Fanconi anemia patients prove hypersensitive and typically arrest in G2. This assay provides a much clearer margin towards other diseases than the increased rate of spontaneous chromosomal breakage per se, which is more variable and is also enhanced in other diseases.

The hypersensitivity towards DNA cross-linkers in Fanconi anemia underlines the importance of the FANC proteins in crosslink repair. However, it hardly accounts for the full phenotype of the patients. It is therefore thought that the FANC proteins have additional functions, e.g. in the regulation of cytokine synthesis and action or of apoptosis. FANCC, in particular, is implicated in the cellular defense against oxidative stress. The most clear-cut evidence points to a wider role of FANC proteins in DNA repair and signaling of DNA damage. In normal cells, several FANC proteins A, C, E, F, and G co-operate in the nucleus to mono-ubiquitinate FANCD2. The induction of this mono-ubiquitination by cross-linking agents is the basis of a biochemical assay for Fanconi anemia.

Ubiquitinated FANCD2 appears to activate '*repair foci*' containing several proteins involved in homologous recombination repair of DNA. This type of recombination is not only used in crosslink repair, but also one of several alternatives for strand-break repair. Among the components of the homologous recombination protein complex are the BRCA1 and BRCA2 proteins. Inherited mutations in these genes – even in heterozygotes - predispose to breast and ovarian cancers. In fact, homozygous mutations in *BRCA2* lead to Fanconi anemia, and *BRCA2* is the *FANCD1* gene. Like BRCA2, BRCA1 also influences the FANC protein complex, regulating its interaction with BRCA2 and its ability to activate checkpoints. Conversely, certain mutations in other *FANC* genes may predispose to breast and brain cancers.

The function of FANC proteins in signaling of DNA damage and activation of homologous recombination repair, and likely other systems, explains why cells from Fanconi anemia patients show a decreased ability to correctly repair double-strand DNA breaks in general, not only after cross-linking. This regulatory function may also relate to some of the defects in hematopoesis, since maturation of B- and T-cells involves gene rearrangements requiring joining of double-strand breaks introduced by the lymphocyte-specific recombinases. Indeed, these rearrangements have been found to be compromised and to be more imprecise in Fanconi anemia patients.

Finally, several commonly used cytostatic drugs are DNA crosslinkers. For instance, cis-platinum is an essential component in many cancer chemotherapy formulas and has proven something like a miracle drug in the treatment of testicular cancer. There is mounting evidence that whether individual cancers respond to such drugs may depend on their expression level of FANC proteins.

Strand-break Repair

Repair of damaged DNA bases is a permanent process in living cells. It is only one of several processes, including chemical reactions and enzymatic actions, that generate single-strand breaks in DNA. These are therefore common, and it is estimated that 100,000 DNA single-breaks occur per cell each day. In the most simple case, single-strand breaks are repaired by DNA ligase, but components from the short- and long-patch base excision repair or nucleotide excision repair systems may be needed, when severe base damage or chemical modification of the sugar are associated with the loss of a base.

Like mismatch repair during DNA replication, repair of DNA strand-breaks goes on rather '*quietly*'. However, this changes dramatically, when DNA double-strand breaks are generated. These can arise by physiological and non-physiological mechanisms, endogenous processes and exogenous mutagens. During DNA replication, a double-strand break can result from a single-strand break, if this is not repaired, before it is encountered by the replisome. Sometimes two single-strand breaks may by chance occur closely together leading to a double-strand break. Other double-strand breaks are caused by exogenous agents. Some viruses encode enzymes that cut DNA in a similar fashion as restriction enzymes, e.g. retroviral integrases. Ionizing radiation can generate single- as well as double-strand DNA breaks as do several chemical carcinogens and some drugs used in chemotherapy. Bleomycin, e.g., cuts DNA directly, and topoisomerase inhibitors generate strand breaks by inhibition of these enzymes. Repair of DNA crosslinks also involves the generation of double-strand breaks.

Double-strand breaks are also created, in a controlled fashion, during physiological recombinations. Important processes of this kind are meiotic recombination and generation of functional *T-cell receptor* (TCR) and *immunoglobulin* (IG) genes in lymphocytes, which yield occasionally errors. Unequal recombination in germ cells is an important cause of inherited disease including cancer. Aberrant joining of genes encoding the T-cell receptor or immunoglobulins to other genes such as *MYC* is a frequent source of chromosomal translocations in lymphomas. Other translocations and deletions in cancers of the lymphoid lineage can result when the lymphocyte-specific recombination system acts accidentially at sites outside the TCR and IG gene clusters.

Independent of how they arise, double-strand breaks are dangerous as long as they exist, especially to a proliferating cell. They separate a fragment of DNA from the centromere, predisposing it to loss during mitosis. Moreover, the open ends can recombine with other parts of the genome, starting a chain reaction of recombinations and chromosome alterations that can lead to cell death or transformation. Double-strand repair therefore involves blocking of the open DNA ends in addition to actually mending the break. In addition, activation of double-strand DNA break repair is usually associated with the activation of cellular checkpoints that prevent the cell from entering or proceeding through S-phase and mitosis. Specifically, unrepaired DNA double-strand breaks in normal cells often elicit apoptosis. This mechanism provides another level of protection against carcinogenesis, in addition to DNA repair itself. Several repair systems in human cells deal with double-strand breaks. They can be classified into non-homologous and homologous repair systems.

Non-homologous end-joining (NHEJ) is an imprecise mechanism which is nevertheless most often used in human cells. Double-strand breaks are protected by the KU70/KU80 protein heterodimer, and bound by the 'MRN' complex consisting of the MRE11, RAD50, and NBS1 (Nibrin) proteins. These proteins prevent them from illegitimate recombination and attempt to align them. Compatible ends may become ligated, but in many cases the ends are processed. Processing can involve filling in 5'-overhangs and degrading 3'-overhangs. MRE11 possesses nuclease activity. In addition the FEN1 nuclease may be involved as well as the WRN protein which may also supply helicase activity additional to that of the KU70/KU80 proteins. Apparently, processing, unwinding and alignment of the strands proceeds until short complementary base stretches are found which can be used to hybridize the two ends. Remaining overhangs are processed, gaps are filled in and the sugar-phosphate backbone is religated by DNA ligase IV/ XRCC4. The end product of the repair process is a restored DNA double helix with a deletion, which is normally kept at a minimum. A distinct characteristic of sequences repaired by NHEJ are micro-homologies, i.e. short stretches of 1-12 bp which were identical in the original sequences at both ends of the deletion. These stretches of homology are much longer when deletions arise by illegitimate homologous recombination. In some cases, NHEJ repair leads to the insertion of a few additional nucleotides, as during V(D)J joining in lymphocytes. This may help to anneal sequences.

When NHEJ begins, it elicits signals that activate cellular checkpoints. The KU proteins constitute the regulatory subunits of DNA-dependent protein kinase (DNA-PK), which is essential for proper DNA repair. Its catalytic subunit phosphorylates not only itself and other proteins directly involved in repair, but also activates the TP53 protein, which is one of the most important regulators of cellular checkpoints. The phosphorylation of TP53 by DNA-PK and/or further enyzmes such as the ATM and ATR kinases elicits cell cycle arrest or even apoptosis. The NHEJ protein complex itself is regulated by ATM and other proteins. Within the MRN complex, Nibrin seems to exert the major control. It is phosphorylated and activated by the ATM protein kinase and in turn interacts with BRCA proteins.

In contrast to NHEJ, *homologous recombination repair* (HRR) can be performed in an error-free fashion, at least in principle. In human cells, it is the mechanism of choice in the G2 phase of the cell cycle when a second sequence identical to the damaged one is available in the sister chromatid. NHEJ, in contrast, appears to be the predominant mechanism in G1 cells. HRR may also constitute the preferred method for the repair of double-strand breaks that arise when breaks in one DNA strand are extended into double-strand breaks during replication and the replisome has stalled. In this situation, the BLM helicase may be crucially involved. Demarcation of the double-strand lesion in all other cases is likely performed by the RAD52 protein. As a clear-cut difference towards NHEJ, the KU proteins are not involved. The double strand break is then processed to yield a 3'-overhanging single strand of several 100 bases. In this processing the MRE11/RAD50/NBS1 (MRN) complex is again involved together with additional, less well characterized components. With the help of the recombination protein RAD51, the single strands invade the intact homologous double-strand DNA forming D-loop structures ('D' for '*displacement*'). The 3'-hydroxyls of the single-strands are then extended and a structure with two Holliday junctions forms. This is resolved by endonuclease action. There are several possible outcomes, depending on how the Holliday junctions are resolved. In one alternative, both original sequences are restored, in the other a crossover takes places. This does not result in a change of sequence when the sister chromatid is used. However, if a homologous sequence from a different chromosome was involved, gene conversion can happen.

Not all parts of the HRR mechanism are well understood, as for NHEJ repair. However, some components have been identified with certainty, because they are mutated in human inherited diseases. Homozygous mutations in the *NBS1* gene that compromise the function of Nibrin underlie the Nijmegen breakage syndrome. This very rare syndrome presents with mental retardation, immunodeficiency, and, tellingly, chromosomal instability and cancer susceptibility. Homozygous mutations in the *WRN* gene encoding a helicase/nuclease involved in double-strand break repair and telomere maintenance also increase the susceptibility to various types of cancer, particularly in soft tissues. However, the resulting Werner syndrome impresses primarily as a premature aging disease manifesting typically around puberty.

The most prevalent syndrome in this context is the recessively inherited *ataxia telangiectasia* (AT). It is caused by homozygous mutations in the gene encoding the ATM protein kinase that regulates DNA double-strand break repair. Like NBS patients, AT patients are prone to infections and chromosomal aberrations. They have a ≈100-fold increased risk of cancers, mostly of leukemias and lymphomas.

Both syndromes share, in particular, a hypersensitivity towards ionizing radiation. However, AT patients are not usually mentally retarded. Instead, they develop a gradual decline of the function of the cerebellum, which progressively impedes movements, speech and sight. This very specific ataxia led to the name along with the diagnostic telangiectasias which are aggregates of small dilated blood vessel appearing in unusual places such as the conjunctiva of the eye. They are thought to be caused by inappropriate angiogenesis. The chain of events leading to these lesions may involve lack of ATM function leading to incomplete function of TP53 alleviating suppression of angiogenesis induced by hypoxia. Other aspects of the pleiotropic ATM phenotype are less understood, including an elevation of the fetal albumin homologue α-fetoprotein that is useful for the diagnosis of the disease.

In contrast, the chromosomal instability and hypersensitivity towards ionizing radiation in the syndrome fit well with the known function of ATM as a central coordinator of double-strand break repair. DNA double-strand breaks caused by physiological recombination, by viral or retrotransposon enzymes, by ionizing radiation or chemicals, or by oxidative stress all appear to activate ATM. Likely, this occurs by different routes. The protein may itself sense damage to some extent, but the MRN complex through NBS1 certainly plays a part. A variant histone, H2AX, accumulates within 1 min at double-strand breaks to become phosphorylated by ATM; this could well be another sensor protein. H2AX can alternatively be phosphorylated by DNA-PK. Further candidates for damage sensors are RAD9 and RAD17 which are also ATM substrates.

Following its activation, ATM goes on to phosphorylate further proteins involved in DNA repair such as FANCD2, BRCA1, and RPA. Significantly, it also activates checkpoints that block the cell from further proliferation. Phosphorylation by ATM activates the TP53 protein, whereas it prevents the TP53 inhibitor protein HDM2 from binding to TP53. Together these actions lead to cell cycle arrest at the G1/S checkpoint via induction of the $p21^{CIP1}$ cell cycle inhibitor and at the G2/M checkpoint by other mediators. DNA replication can be arrested via phosphorylation of CHK2 (checkpoint kinase 2) and Nibrin, while phosphorylation of TP53 and BRCA1 also activates the G2/M checkpoint.

Some aspects of ATM function can also be provided by other protein kinases such as CHK2, ABL, and ATR. Severe damage by UV radiation, e.g., is signaled by the ATR protein kinase in an otherwise quite similar fashion, including phosphorylation of TP53 and CHK1 (instead of CHK2). The somewhat complementary functions of ATM and ATR are the likely explanation why AT patients and their cells are sensitive to ionizing radiation, but not to UV.

A public debate has developed on the issue of whether heterozygosity for ATM mutations leads to an increased cancer risk. This is a particular concern, since several methods commonly used in cancer screening and diagnosis employ ionizing radiation. The results of different investigations vary. It is possible that the cancer risk of heterozygous carriers of the disease may depend on which mutation is present. Some mutations may completely inactivate the affected allele. Others may show some degree of a dominant-negative phenotype, i.e. an altered protein product is formed which does not function in repair, but inhibits the function of the protein produced by the normal allele. In the case of the ATM protein, this is conceivable, since the protein normally exists as a dimer and its activation involves cross-phosphorylation between the subunits. So, dysfunctional subunits may inactivate some of the functional subunits as well.

Defects in DNA Repair and Cancer Susceptibility

It is clear from the previous sections that inherited defects in DNA repair are an important source of susceptibility to cancer. A number of syndromes related to DNA repair carry an increased risk of cancers. Homozygous mutations in the *ATM*, *NBS1*, *WRN*, *FANC*, and *XP/ERCC* genes underlie recessively inherited diseases, which confer an increased risk for cancers in the context of syndrome with a wider range of afflictions. Heterozygous mutations in MMR genes and in the *BRCAs* and perhaps certain ATM mutations lead to cancer predisposition in a dominantly inherited fashion. As a rule, no other consistent symptoms are associated with these mutations. With either type of predisposition, cancers develop at an increased rate as a consequence of an enhanced rate of mutations, either point mutations in MMR deficiency and XP, or chromosomal aberrations in the others. Also typically, in these diseases, cancers appear at an unusually early age.

Obviously, the question arises to what extent defects in DNA repair are involved in sporadic cancers (the great majority) which arise in people not carrying mutations in any of the above genes. In other words, since defective DNA repair is sufficient for cancer development, is it also necessary? Or can cancers arise in the course of the relatively long human lifetime just by accumulation of rare alterations that have occurred in spite of functional DNA repair? The answers to these questions are open.

One also has to consider in this regard that many genes involved in DNA repair are polymorphic. Several of these polymorphisms have been linked to an increased risk for one of the major cancers. Typically, the increases in cancer risk conferred by these polymorphisms to each individual are small compared to those resulting from mutations that lead to the full inactivation of a DNA repair system. However, frequent polymorphic forms of such genes could be important determinants of cancer frequency in the whole population.

In addition to inherited mutations or polymorphisms, acquired mutations inactivate DNA repair genes in many cancers or they become silenced by epigenetic mechanisms. This is documented in the case of certain MSI cancers arising through inactivation of MMR genes. It is not known precisely, to what extent chromosomal instability in other cancers is caused by inactivation of *ATM*, *NBS1*, *WRN*, *FANC* or *BRCA* genes through somatic mutations. Overall, such cases appear to be rare.

In contrast, a failure of cell cycle checkpoints activated by DNA damage is detectable in many, if not most cancers. Therefore, defects in DNA repair as such may not be required for cancer development, but defective signaling to checkpoints, e.g. by loss of checkpoint kinase or of TP53 function, could be necessary. Defective checkpoint activation allows cell proliferation to continue in spite of DNA damage, with the consequence that some defects become permanent and are propagated by the following cell generations.

Finally, it is possible that through a human lifetime those occasional DNA defects that have escaped repair accumulate, and perhaps DNA repair becomes less efficient during aging. In addition, telomere dysfunction in aging cells may provide a new challenge to DNA repair systems which they cannot always master.

Cell Protection Mechanisms in Cancer

Exogenous carcinogens and potential mutagens arising from endogenous processes are often prevented from encountering DNA by specific cellular protections mechanisms. These highly diverse mechanisms serve as a further tier of cancer prevention in addition to DNA repair and apoptosis. Often, they protect not only DNA, but cells in general from damage. Some of these mechanisms are very specific and some are very general. In the context of cancer, they are particularly important during two very different phases, viz. (1) during carcinogenesis and (2) during cancer therapy.

A number of low molecular weight compounds are employed in the cell to stabilize macromolecules and membranes, protect against altered osmolarity, buffer the redox state, and quench radicals and specifically reactive oxygen species. These chemically diverse compounds comprise polyamines, amino acids like taurine, the tripeptide glutathione, and the lipophilic and hydrophilic vitamins E and C, i.e. tocopherol and ascorbic acid. Glutathione, γ-glutamyl-cysteinyl-glycine (GSH), is part of a cellular redox buffer system and its thiol group also reacts readily with radicals. The normal oxidized form of glutathione is its disulfide GSSG, from which GSH can be recovered by glutathione reductase, which uses NADPH as the cosubstrate. GSH is also used in enzymatically catalyzed reactions for similar purposes. So, the selenium-containing enzyme glutathione peroxidase removes hydrogen peroxide generating GSSG. Lack of this enzyme may be one reason why selenium deficiency may increase the risk of cancer. Glutathione also reacts spontaneously with reactive electrophilic compounds, including activated carcinogens. These reactions are strongly accelerated by glutathione transferases (GSTs). The various isoenzymes in this family all catalyze the reaction of glutathione with several substrates, but each enzyme recognizes a different range of compounds. In most cases, carcinogens are inactivated by conjugation with glutathione. The conjugates are further metabolized and eventually excreted.

It is clear from this short description why polymorphisms in GST enzymes catalyzing reactions of glutathione modulate the risk of various cancers. In addition, the level of glutathione itself and the ratio of GSSG:GSH are also relevant. However, these same reactions are also relevant in the context of cancer therapy. Cytotoxic cancer drugs also react with DNA and some act by inducing reactive oxygen species. So, both reaction with glutathione catalyzed by GSTs and the quenching of reactive oxygen species by GSH and other radical catchers diminish the efficacy of such drugs in cancer cells, while they protect normal cells. In fact, GSTP1, one isoenzyme of the family, is often over-expressed in cancers becoming resistant to therapy, in some cases as a consequence of gene amplification. Paradoxically, the same enzyme is down-regulated in a few selected cancers such as prostate carcinoma.

A similar argument can be made for ionizing radiation. The effects of ionizing radiation on normal cells are mitigated by cellular protection mechanisms, in addition to DNA repair. For instance, polyamines stabilize cellular macromolecules such as DNA and structural RNAs. Tocopherol, ascorbate, carotenoids, and glutathione can all act to quench the effect of hydroxyl radicals and other reactive oxygen species. Therefore, it may in some cases be helpful to deplete such compounds prior to therapy.

GSTs and glutathione peroxidase (abbreviated GPx) are examples of cell-protective enzymes that modulate the effects of many different exogenous and endogenous agents. Others are more tailored towards specific compounds. For instance, metallothioneins are a group of small proteins protecting against toxic metal ions. They contain multiple thiol groups which are highly reactive towards potentially carcinogenic metal ions including cadmium and nickel. However, while they may prevent carcinogenesis by these and other substances, they may also contribute to resistance against chemotherapy that uses metallo-organic compounds, and specifically against the widely employed platinum complexes. Moreover, these proteins as well react with radicals induced by cancer treatments.

It is important to realize that the efficiency of the cellular protection mechanisms discussed here and of others less well understood appears to be determined by an interaction of genetic and environmental factors. On the genetic side, polymorphisms in a large number of genes in this context are expected to modulate the risk of cancers, but also the responses to therapies. On the environmental side, the type of exposure is, of course, relevant, but also factors like diet and immune status which affect the levels of low molecular weight compounds as well as of proteins involved in cell protection. Genetic and environmental factors may, in particular, synergize with each other. There is evidence for this type of interaction in a wide variety of human cancers.

8

Fingerprinting in Cancer

The *polymerase chain reaction* (PCR) has revolutionized the isolation and analysis of nucleic acid fragments from a wide variety of sources. PCR-based methods for nucleic acid detection and fingerprinting have become vital to modern molecular genetics, whether for the analysis of populations of organisms to determine population structure of an ecosystem, sampling a set of DNA sequences to infer evolutionary history, sampling genetic loci to build a map, or sampling differentially expressed genes to identify phenotypic markers.

PCR can be used to generate high resolution genetic maps of human and comparative genomes. Compared with Southern blot analysis, which detects *restriction fragment length polymorphisms* (RFLPs) and hypervariable minisatellite loci, PCR is faster, less labor-intensive, less expensive, and requires relatively small amounts of DNA. Additionally, PCR may be a more practical approach for large-scale mapping projects.

The classic approach to DNA fingerprinting utilizes *variable number tandem repeat* (VNTR) polymorphism in which alleles differ by a variable number of tandem repeats. Although the term *VNTR* could, in theory, encompass a wide range of repeat lengths, in practice the term is usually reserved for moderately large arrays of a repeat unit that is typically in the 5- to 64-bp region. If the VNTR locus is a member of a repeated DNA family, the use of a VNTR probe will produce a complex polymorphic band pattern on hybridization. The hybridizing bands appear on the filter as a ladder of bands, referred to as the *DNA fingerprint*, which visually resembles the bar-codes used by stores to identify and price merchandise.

ARBITRARILY PRIMED PCR

The arbitrary primer-based DNA amplification technique recently has been proposed as an alternative targeting tool for genetic typing and mapping. This strategy uses randomly generated primers to initiate amplification of discrete but arbitrary portions of the genome. It has been called by a plethora of terms such as random amplified polymorphic DNA, DNA amplification fingerprinting, multiple arbitrarily amplicon profiling, and arbitrarily primed PCR (AP-PCR).

AP-PCR is one of the fingerprinting techniques described by Welsh and McClelland in 1990. It was originally used to distinguish strains of *Staphylococcus* sp. and *Streptococcus* sp. by comparing polymorphisms in AP-PCR genomic fingerprints using PCR-length primers (18–32 nucleotides). This technique is a modification of PCR, a method that is widely used to copy sections of DNA for identifying gene structure or matching tissue specimens.

PCR conventionally uses two primers whose complementary sequences flank the desired sequence to amplify a region of DNA. The primers usually have specific nucleotide sequences that bind to previously identified segments of DNA. They bind to specific sites on opposing strands of the double-stranded DNA and, with successive cycles of PCR, make millions of copies of the intervening stretch of DNA. Normally, the primers are annealed to the template DNA at relatively high stringency. High stringency during the primer-annealing step ensures that the primers do not interact with the template DNA at positions where they do not match completely.

By contrast, AP-PCR allows the detection of polymorphisms without prior knowledge of nucleotide sequence. It is based on the selective amplification of genomic sequences that, by chance, are flanked by adequate matches to an arbitrarily chosen primer. The method utilizes short primers of arbitrary nucleotide sequence (10–20 bases) that are annealed in the first few cycles of PCR at low stringency. The low stringency of the early cycles ensures the generation of products by allowing priming with fortuitous matches or near matches between primers and template. This approach results in a high number of products having the original primer sequence at both ends.

After a few low-stringency cycles, the annealing temperature is raised and the reaction is allowed to continue under standard, high-stringency PCR conditions. This step will amplify a discrete number of sequences among those initially targeted and permits the unbiased analysis of the cell genome. Alternatively, an intermediate stringency primer-annealing step may be used throughout the PCR to achieve the same outcome. AP-PCR products are resolved on polyacrylamide gels and detected by autoradiography. If two template genomic DNA sequences are different, their AP-PCR products display different banding patterns. Such differences can be exploited in ways largely analogous to the uses of RFLP, including genetic mapping, taxonomy, phylogenetics, and the detection of mutations.

AP-PCR has three advantages when compared with classic DNA fingerprinting. First, minor amounts of template DNA are sufficient for analysis (50 ng of genomic DNA for AP-PCR vs 5–10 μg for Southern blotting). Second, somatic mutations detected in tumor fingerprints can, by chance, directly reflect a mutation in a coding sequence. Third, the possibility of reamplification, cloning, and sequencing of polymorphic bands enables the rapid identification of the sequences probably linked to tumor progression.

Applications of AP-PCR

Because no laborious cloning, nucleotide sequencing, or Southern blot hybridization is required, AP-PCR permits the rapid and cost-effective detection of polymorphisms and genetic markers in a variety of plants and animals. The most frequent use of AP-PCR has been for the detection of dominant polymorphic markers in genetic mapping experiments. Welsh and McClelland applied the technique of AP-PCR to genetic mapping in the mouse. They noted that AP-PCR is, in many respects, dramatically easier and faster than established methods for genetic mapping. Polymorphisms detected by AP-PCR also can be used as taxonomic markers in population studies of a wide variety of organisms. It has been applied extensively in plant breeding studies and in the differentiation of the strains of microorganisms. DNA fingerprinting of different strains has shown polymorphic sequences that can be used to identify the different genomes.

The reproducible and semiquantitative amplification of multiple sequences provides a powerful tool to study somatic genetic alterations in tumorigenesis. Peinado et al. showed the ability of AP-PCR to detect both qualitatively and quantitatively and to isolate, in a single step, DNA sequences representing two of the genetic alterations that underlie the aneuploidy of colorectal cancer cells: losses of heterozygosity and chromosomal gains. Moreover, they confirmed that AP-PCR could yield information on the overall chromosomal composition of the cell. The intensities of the bands derived from single-copy sequences were proportional to the concentration of the target sequences. The outstanding result using AP-PCR fingerprinting in the field of cancer research was the discovery of the microsatellite mutator phenotype mechanism for carcinogenesis in sporadic and hereditary colon cancers. AP-PCR is also useful for the detection and isolation of DNA sequences to levels well below the minimum levels required by other available methods, and the products can be used to clone or hybridize back to digested genomic DNA. In addition, AP-PCR can be applied to RNA to detect differentially expressed genes in a technique called RNA-AP-PCR.

Interspersed Repetitive Element PCR (Alu-PCR) DNA Fingerprinting

A major limitation of the standard PCR regime is that it allows amplification of a DNA sequence flanked between two convergent primers, each of which primes DNA chain extension in the direction of the other primer. Often, however, it is desirable to be able to access uncharacterized DNA sequences flanking a region for which sequence information is available. *Interspersed repetitive element* (IRE)-based PCR strategies have been used as a tool since 1989, and, they have had a major impact on human genome research.

Developed mainly around the primate-specific, simple-interspersed, nuclear-repeat element Alu, IRE-PCR has made it possible to amplify human genomic sequences from complex mixtures such as that encountered with a monochromosomal somatic cell hybrid. This application has now encompassed analysis and screening of large cloned DNA fragments such as yeast artificial chromosomes and bacterial atificial chromosomes.

Employing primers specific for the Alu repeat element was seen as an alternative to using arbitrarily designed 10-mers. The mammalian genome contains approx 10^6 copies of the Alu repeat element representing 7% of the total DNA per cell. The highly ubiquitous distribution of the Alu repeat means that the coverage of the genome afforded by Alu sequence-primed amplification could potentially be of high resolution. Additionally, rearrangements of genes at translocation breakpoints and recombination "*hot spots*" often have been often attributable to interspersed DNA elements.

By using the restriction enzymes to predigest the genomic template in this approach, it is analogous to the preparation of "*representations*" of the tester DNA by PCR in representational difference analysis. Both approaches are necessary to define a subpopulation of fragments that may be more readily analyzed. Additionally, varying the restriction enzyme used in the predigestion defined the spectrum of band sizes obtained in subsequent amplifications with the same Alu-specific primer. Therefore, we have two variable parameters to achieve multiple fingerprint profiles from the same DNA samples if we also apply primers specific to different regions of the Alu repeat element.

Our group applied the Alu-PCR fingerprinting technique to DNA from pancreatic cancer and paired normal samples to isolate and identify fragments of genomic DNA rearranged in malignant cells. Abnormalities were detectable in about 8.5% of the genomic fragments sampled in this analysis. Clearly, only a fraction of the genome is sampled in each Alu primer/restriction digest combination, and some are more useful than others. Because the digests use a single primer in the PCR reaction, only sequences lying between repeats in inverted orientation to one another will be amplified, and because their orientation is essentially random, this could result in about 30% of the inter-Alu sequences being potential templates in each case. Like the alternative genome-scanning technique of respresentational difference analysis, there is a bias toward the generation of smaller fragments, partly owing to the predigestion of the template DNA and partly because of the kinetics of PCR amplification. However, these are tags that enable the subsequent isolation of larger rearranged fragments by hybridization.

Alu-PCR: Advantageous in Screening for Tumor-Specific Lesions

Because Alu repeats contain runs of deoxyadenosine residues, they are often involved as targets for such ubiquitous somatic mutations, so that about onethird have deletion mutations in replication error phenotype (RER^+) cancers. Interestingly, Alu repeats can even be involved in the genesis of inactivating mutations; for instance, one of the most common germline mutations in the DNA mismatch repair gene *MLH1* is a 3.5-kb genomic deletion that appears to result from Alu-mediated recombination. Alu elements are also involved in the production of oncogenes as a result of chromosomal translocation events joining the *BCR* and *ABL* loci and the *LCK* and *TCRB* loci. Hence, the approach of using Alu sequences as the priming sites for the amplification of fingerprints from genomic DNA may have an advantage compared to AP-PCR if such regions are particularly affected by the cancer-associated rearrangements. However, it is likely that most rearrangements at repeat sequences are not significant to tumorigenesis. It may be possible to exploit other high-abundance repetitive elements in the human genome to similar ends, such as the L1 and MER families.

In conclusion, the Alu-specific PCR genomic fingerprinting technique allows the scanning of the human genome for genetic rearrangements associated with a cancer phenotype. With the generation of sequence tags for these rearrangements, their use as molecular probes may facilitate the isolation of gene sequences involved. Further analysis of such genes associated with these rearrangements may lead to the mutational mechanism and its contribution to the molecular pathology of cancers.

MATERIALS

Arbitrarily Primed PCR

1. Thermocycler (e.g., Peltier Thermal Cycler, model PTC-100).
2. Sequencing gel electrophoresis apparatus (40 cm long, 30 cm wide, 0.4 mm thick).
3. Gel dryer.
4. X-Ray film and exposure cassette.
5. Stocks of all four dNTPs (5 m*M*).
6. Stock of arbitrary primer (100 μM).
7. Radioisotope ([α-^{32}P] or [γ-^{33}P]) dATP (>2500 Ci/mmol).
8. *Taq* polymerase (5 U/μL).
9. Formamide dye solution: 96% formamide, 0.1% bromophenol blue, 0.1% xylene cyanol, 10 m*M* EDTA.
10. 10X Tris-borate-EDTA (TBE) buffer: 90 m*M* Tris-borate, 20 m*M* Na_2EDTA, pH 8.3.
11. Acrylamide stock solution (40% acrylamide:*bis*-acrylamide [29:1]).

Alu-Polymerase Chain Reaction

1. Thermocycler (e.g., Peltier Thermal Cycler, model PTC-100).
2. Sequencing gel electrophoresis apparatus (40 cm long, 30 cm wide, 0.4 mm thick).
3. Gel dryer.
4. X-Ray film and exposure cassette.
5. Stocks of all four dNTPs (5 m*M*).
6. Stock of Alu primer (100 μM).
7. (α-^{32}P) dATP (3000 Ci/mmol).
8. Restriction enzyme *AluI* (8 U/μL).
9. *Taq* polymerase (5 U/μL).

10. Formamide dye solution: 96% formamide, 0.1% bromophenol blue, 0.1% xylene cyanol, 10 mM EDTA.
11. 10X TBE buffer: 90 m*M* Tris-borate, 20 m*M* Na_2EDTA, pH 8.3.
12. Acrylamide stock solution (40% acrylamide:*bis*-acrylamide [29:1]).

Methods

Arbitrarily Primed PCR

1. Mix template DNA (100–200 ng) with reaction mixture for a 25-μL final reaction containing arbitrary primer, 1 to 2 Ci of [α-^{32}P]dATP or [γ-^{33}P]dATP, 0.2 m*M* of each dNTP, 10 m*M* Tris-HCl, pH 9.2, 3.5 m*M* $MgCl_2$, 75 m*M* KCl, and 0.5 U of *Taq* polymerase in a final volume of 25 μL.
2. Perform thermocycling using 5 cycles of 94°C for 1 min, 45°C for 5 min, and 72°C for 5 min; then 35 cycles of 94°C for 1 min, 60°C for 1 min, 72°C for 2 min. Add a final chase cycle of 72°C for 5 min to allow complete elongation of all products.
3. Mix amplification products with 5 μL of formamide dye solution, denature at 95°C for 3 min, and load 5 μL onto a 8% nondenaturing acrylamide gel mix prepared in 1X TBE buffer. Perform electrophoresis using a sequencing apparatus at 12 W overnight.
4. After electrophoresis, transfer the gel to Whatman 3MM paper, and dry under vacuum.
5. Autoradiograph the dried gel using an X-ray film at room temperature for 12 h.

Alu Polymerase Chain Reaction

1. Perform restriction digests of DNA samples at 37°C overnight. Use 10 U of restriction enzyme *Alu*I in a 20-μL reaction volume containing 1–5 μg of DNA.
2. Standardize the conditions for PCR amplification as follows: 50 m*M* KCl, 10 m*M* Tris-HCl, pH 8.3, 1.5 m*M* $MgCl_2$, 0.1% Triton X-100, 0.2 m*M* dNTPs, 1 U of *Taq* polymerase in a 50-μL reaction volume. The Alu primer concentration is a little higher (at 2 μ*M*) than normally used in an attempt to favor annealing of the primer to the repeat elements by displacing any rapidly forming duplexes in the template by virtue of this high concentration.
3. Perform thermocycling using 94°C for 3 min; then 10–15 cycles of 57°C for 30 s, 72°C for 1 min, 94°C for 45 s. Add a final chase cycle of 72°C for 5 min to allow complete elongation of all products.

4. Achieve radioactive labeling of PCR products by the addition of 1 to 2 Ci of [α-^{32}P]ATP (and the reduction of the unlabeled dATP in the buffer to 0.01 m*M*) followed by 20 more cycles of the above parameters.
5. Mix amplification products with 5 μL of formamide dye solution, denature at 95°C for 3 min, and load 5 μL onto a 6% nondenaturing acrylamide gel mix prepared in 1X TBE buffer. Perform electrophoresis using a sequencing apparatus at 12 W overnight.
6. After electrophoresis, mount the gel wet on a piece of old X-ray film or Whatman 3MM paper covered with Saran wrap, and then expose to an X-ray film within a cassette at –70°C overnight.

9

ONCOGENES

The first group of oncogenes to have been discovered form parts of the genomes of acutely transforming retroviruses, which cause hematological or soft tissue cancers in their avian or mammalian hosts. They act in a dominant manner and confer altered growth properties and morphology on specific target cells in mesenchymal tissues or the hematopoetic system. A second group of oncogenes consists of host proto-oncogenes that become activated when the insertion of slowly transforming retroviruses disrupts their regulation.

Retroviral insertion is only one of several mechanisms that can activate cellular proto-oncogenes to dominantly acting oncogenes. Other mechanisms include chromosomal translocation, gene amplification and point mutations. These mechanisms alter the regulation and/or function of cellular genes, which are thereby activated from proto-oncogenes towards oncogenes. As a consequence of these alterations, their protein products become overexpressed or deregulated and/or become overactive or mislocalized in the cell.

The oncogenes of acutely transforming retroviruses are in fact also derived from host genes, and have become deregulated and overactive by expression from the retroviral long terminal repeat and by mutations. Several genes such as NRAS, KRAS, ERBB1, and MYC orthologous to viral oncogenes have turned out to be overexpressed or mutated in human cancers. The cellular orthologs of other retroviral oncogenes are more subtly involved in human cancers.

Many cellular proto-oncogenes regulate cell proliferation, differentiation and survival also in their normal state. Some act as extracellular growth factors, some as their receptors and some as juxtamembrane adaptors or transducers in signaling cascades emanating from growth factor receptors or other membrane receptors. A large class of proto-oncogene products are protein kinases. They include growth factor receptors with a crucial tyrosine kinase activity. Other kinases are located in the cytoplasm. A further large group of protooncogenes consists of transcription factors acting in the nucleus. So, oncogenes can be categorized according to their cellular localization and/or their biochemical function. Indeed, a surprisingly large number of proto-oncogenes functions within or interacts with a single signaling network. At its core is the mitogenic '*MAP kinase*' cascade which links growth factor signaling to transcription in the nucleus and to the cell cycle, but also influences protein synthesis and the cytoskeleton.

Growth factor signaling and the MAPK cascade are tightly regulated in normal cells by feedback regulation and by short half-lifes of activated states. Oncogenic mutations make oncogene proteins independent of input signals, disrupt feedback regulation or prolong their active state. There are very few cases in which a single oncogene is sufficient to fully transform a cell towards malignancy. Rather, a single oncogene confers some aspects of the malignant phenotype and cooperates with others or with defects in tumor suppressors for complete transformation. This relationship is illustrated in cellular assay systems such as rat embryo fibroblasts, in which two different types of oncogenes are required for transformation.

Human cancers accumulate many genetic and epigenetic alterations during their progression. In a typical cancer many genes are overexpressed and many gene products are overactive. A fraction of these may indeed be necessary for the survival and sustained growth of the cancer. So, they might be regarded as oncogenes as well. A more strictly defined oncogene exhibits these same properties, but its overexpression or overactivity is caused by substantial changes in the gene, i.e. mutations or amplifications.

Retroviral Oncogenes

Several different types of viruses are involved in the development of cancers in humans and animals. In humans, predominantly DNA viruses are implicated. Among the retroviruses, only HTLV1 (*human T-lymphotropic virus*) and HIV are involved in carcinogenesis, but in a very roundabout fashion. In animals, in contrast, several retroviruses have been documented to directly cause cancers, by two different mechanisms, which can be categorized as '*acute*' and '*slow*'. Alternatively, they can be designated as '*transducing*' or '*cis-acting*'.

Acute transforming retroviruses such as ALV (*avian leukosis virus*) or RSV (*Rous sarcoma virus*) elicit leukemias, lymphomas or sarcomas rapidly after infection of their hosts. In fact, avian acute transforming retroviruses were often identified during epidemics that ravaged fowl farms. They were shown to be capable of transforming their target cells in a dominant fashion, without any apparent requirement for a co-carcinogen. Very early after their discovery at the begin of the 20th century, it was predicted that they carried genes which caused cell transformation and were accordingly termed oncogenes. The existence of these genes was formally and physically demonstrated in the second half of the 20th century and the first oncogene protein, v-src from RSV, was biochemically characterized in the late 1970's.

The v-src protein is a protein kinase located at the inside of the plasma membrane. While most protein kinases phosphorylate serine or threonine residues in their substrates, v-src phosphorylates tyrosine (which came as a surprise at the time of discovery). In the RSV genome, v-src is carried as an additional gene 3' to the standard gag, pol, and env gene complement. This is unusual for acutely transforming retroviruses. In most of them, one or two oncogenes replace parts of standard genes. Typically, oncogenes replace the pol and part of the gag gene and the oncogenic protein is expressed as a gag-fusion protein at very high levels. This high expression level contributes to the dominant mode of action of retroviral oncogenes. Of course, the replacement of pol or other viral genes by an oncogene sequence obliterates the ability of the virus to replicate autonomously, rendering it '*defective*'. For replication and propagation, defective retroviruses need intact replication-competent helper viruses that supply the proteins required for reverse transcription, integration, packaging and maturation. This requirement may explain why acutely transforming retroviruses are (fortunately) rare. Conversely, the unique ability of RSV to replicate autonomously may have contributed to its early isolation already one century ago.

Meanwhile, more than two dozen oncogenes have been isolated from retroviruses and have been biochemically characterized. Several points can be noted in this compilation. (1) Some oncogenes appear to be similar. In some cases this is due only to the nomenclature: v-myb and v-myc are not overtly similar beyond being transcription factors, but have both been discovered in retroviruses causing myeloid leukemias. In contrast, Ki-ras and Ha-ras are indeed highly similar proteins. This points to the existence of oncogene families. (2) The products of retroviral oncogenes appear to cover a relatively limited range of biochemical functions. Protein kinases like v-erbB, v-src and v-raf and transcriptional activators like v-fos, v-jun, v-myb and v-myc comprise the majority. Others are receptors, like v-erbB or v-fms, or proteins transducing signals from receptors, like the ras proteins. A limited number of other functions constitute the remainder. (3) Some oncogenic retroviruses carry two oncogenes which cooperate during transformation. For instance, the erythroblastosis virus contains two oncogenes, v-erbA and v-erbB. The first of these is a transcriptional repressor protein and the second a constitutively active cell membrane tyrosine protein kinase. Their cooperation likely results from v-erbA blocking differentiation of erythrocyte precursors and v-erbB stimulating proliferation and supporting survival of these cells to cause erythroblastosis.

Slow-acting Transforming Retroviruses

Slow-acting transforming retroviruses are as a rule replication-competent and do not transduce oncogenes. Instead, they cause transformation by integrating within or in the vicinity of cellular genes and altering their expression. In this fashion they convert cellular genes from proto-oncogenes into oncogenes in a cis-acting manner.

Integration of a slow-acting retrovirus disrupts negative regulatory elements of the targeted gene and/or activates its transcription by the transcriptional regulatory sequences contained in the retroviral LTR. Several mechanisms are conceivable by which the viral regulatory sequences could cause gene overexpression. Overall, the predominant mechanism seems activation of the cellular gene promoter by the enhancer in the retroviral LTR. This mechanism is most effective, if the retrovirus integrates in inverse orientation upstream from the promoter.

This mode of activation is shown for the cellular myc gene (initially called c-myc). This gene consists of three exons and contains several negative regulatory elements upstream of its two transcriptional start sites and in the first intron. Transcription from a physiological start site proceeds into the first intron and pauses there until further signals arrive, similar as during transcriptional regulation by attenuation in bacteria or by the tat protein of HIV. A typical retroviral insertion of the myc gene disrupts this negative control mechanism (as well as others) and at the same time elicits strong transcription from an otherwise inactive ('*cryptic*') promoter near the end of intron 1. In this fashion, myc transcription becomes independent of extracellular signals. Specifically, the expression of the gene is not down-regulated in response to differentiation signals.

The c-myc gene activated by slowly transforming retroviruses is very similar to the oncogene carried by the myelocytomatosis virus. Apparently, the cellular gene is the precursor of the viral gene and has been picked up by an evolutionary precursor of the myelocytomatosis virus. This may have occured by recombination of the c-myc mRNA with the retroviral genomic mRNA followed by transduction. Even more likely, the recombination may have involved a retroviral genomic transcript and a transcript from a c-myc locus into which a retrovirus had inserted. In this fashion, slow-acting transforming retroviruses may give rise to the rarer acutely transforming types.

When a slowly transforming retrovirus integrates into the c-myc gene, the target gene becomes deregulated and over-expressed. The v-myc gene contained in the myelocytomatosis retrovirus is likewise strongly expressed. In addition, there are several changes in the amino acid sequence of v-myc compared to the avian c-myc gene. These are not random. For instance, a change in most viral strains removes a threonine which is required for inactivation of the myc protein, further enhancing its oncogenicity. So, in summary, the acutely transforming retrovirus overexpresses an altered cellular protein, whereas a slowly transforming retrovirus deregulates the endogenous protein, which may remain unchanged, at least initially.

As in the example of c-myc/v-myc, retroviral oncogenes are almost always altered compared to their cellular orthologs, from which they were derived. These alterations are often more severe than in the case of myc. They comprise truncation, mutation or fusion to viral proteins which increase the activity, affect the regulation and alter the localization of the oncoproteins within the cell. For instance, the v-erbB product is derived from the cellular erb-B1 gene which encodes a growth factor receptor, EGFR. This receptor is basically composed of three domains: an extracellular domain binding the growth factor ligands, a transmembrane domain, and a cytoplasmic tyrosine kinase domain, which is controlled by an autoinhibitory loop. The viral product lacks most of the extracellular domain, but contains a small gag segment which causes aggregration of the protein, as would normally be induced by the ligand. Furthermore, a point mutation and a C-terminal truncation in the cytoplasmic domain relieve auto- and feedback inhibition. So, in summary, the virus encodes and overexpresses a constitutively active protein.

The different time-courses of transformation by acutely and slow-transforming viruses may be accounted for by these additional alterations in the transduced oncogene. Further differences may also contribute.

Acutely transforming retroviruses transduce the activated oncogene into each cell they infect and thereby create a large pool of potentially transformed cells. In contrast, slowly transforming retroviruses integrate into many different sites in different infected cells and only rarely '*hit*' a cellular proto-oncogene, yielding only a few potentially transformed cells. One reason for the time lag in tumor development is thus the time required for expansion of a tumor cell clone.

There are likely two more reasons. The first is that transduction of an activated oncogene into a large number of cells is bound to have a substantial effect on their interaction with each other and host cells. For instance, it could significantly alter the levels of autocrine or paracrine cytokines secreted by these cells or overwhelm an antitumor immune response. The second reason is that a larger pool of cells containing an oncogene increases the probability of a second mutation that causes complete transformation and subsequent tumor progression. There is indeed very good evidence that transformation by slowly transforming retroviruses often requires a second hit. Occasionally, this is provided by insertion of a second retrovirus elsewhere in the genome. Some acutely transforming retroviruses also carry two oncogenes, thereby achieving the '*two hits*' at one stroke.

A comparison reveals that several of these genes – like c-myc – possess viral homologs. This is expected, if one assumes that acutely transforming viruses arose from slowly-acting precursors. However, many genes activated by viral insertion have never been observed to be transduced. In some cases, this may be due to the size than can be accomodated in a retrovirus, but functional limitations are also conceivable.

Importantly, there is a cellular homologue for each and every retroviral oncogene found so far. So, all retroviral oncogenes are thought to have evolved from cellular precursors. For instance, the homologue of the v-src gene of RSV is c-src, a protein kinase located at focal adhesion points, at which the actin cytoskeleton is attached to the cell membrane. The c-src kinase relays signals from cell adhesion to the cytoskeleton and to other kinases that control cell proliferation. Such signals may be mimicked by the viral oncoprotein, which is altered towards the cellular protein by several point mutations and the replacement of the C-terminal 17 amino acids by an unrelated peptide.

Approaches to the Identification of Human Oncogenes

No acutely transforming retroviruses have been observed in humans and even activation of cellular genes by retroviruses or related viruses such as HBV is exceptional. Two cases of iatrogenic oncogene activation may have happened when during attempted gene therapy of severely immunocompromised children retroviruses carrying a therapeutic gene integrated into the *MLO2* proto-oncogene locus.

While such cases are clearly exceptional, the elucidation of the mechanisms by which retroviruses cause cancers in animals has been very instructive for the understanding of human cancers. Even if genes in the human genome are almost never activated by retroviruses to become oncogenes, many genes orthologous to the viral and animal oncogenes can be activated by other mechanisms in humans. Following rapidly on the discovery of cellular oncogenes, many human cancers were also screened for oncogenic alterations in these genes. Indeed, a large number of genes are now implicated as oncogenes in human cancers. These candidates were obtained through several lines of research.

Analysis of Human Orthologs of Retroviral Oncogenes

An obvious approach was to investigate the human orthologs of viral oncogenes for their level of expression and for mutations in human cancers. A huge amount of literature has resulted from this type of research. In summary, several orthologs of viral oncogenes are also over-expressed or mutated in human cancers and are clearly involved in their development. For instance, the human ortholog of v-erbB, *ERBB1*, and the human v-myc orthologue *MYC* are over-expressed, mutated and causally involved in many human cancers. Other genes are only directly involved in a more restricted range of cancers, such as rel in selected lymphomas. On the other hand, many strong viral oncogenes have never turned up as dominant oncogenes in humans, prominently v-src and v-fos. Instead, the products of the corresponding human genes are more subtly involved in shaping the phenotype of human cancers. Of note, while *ERBB1* or *MYC* are overexpressed in a wide range of human cancers, this is not in each case caused by primary changes in their genes. In summary, human orthologs of almost all viral oncogenes contribute in some way to one or the other human cancer.

3T3 Cell Transformation Assay

Cell culture assays such as the 3T3 fibroblast focus formation assay developed for the identification of viral oncogenes have also been used to discover human oncogenes. In the original 3T3 assay, the immortalized mouse fibroblast cell line 3T3 was infected with an oncogene-carrying retrovirus and yielded foci of transformed cells with altered morphology that grow out of the monolayer at confluence. Foci can also be obtained by transfection of DNA from human tumor cells. From such foci the gene responsible for the altered phenotype can be isolated. This assay has led to the identification of several human oncogenes. The most dramatic result was that three human orthologs of the v-ras genes can act as oncogenes. In humans orthologs of both the Ki-ras (KRAS) and Ha-ras (HRAS) genes exist as well as a third relative, NRAS, which possess similar structures and functions. All three genes were recovered from 3T3 focus formation assays, in each case carrying point mutations at specific sites, i.e. codons 12, 13, or 61. Thus, some cellular genes like the RAS genes can be converted from proto-oncogenes to oncogenes by point mutation only. The 3T3 assay has also yielded several additional genes, as well as a number of biochemically interesting artifacts from genes rearranged during the transfection procedure.

Other Transformation Assays

The 3T3 assay is limited by a strong bias towards a certain type of oncogene that is '*ras-like*', while others, like the potent myc oncogene, do not score. This limitation arises from the fact that the assay selects for the ability of oncogenes to keep fibroblasts growing beyond confluence and to alter their morphology. Mutated *RAS* genes confer these properties, but not all oncogenes do. Therefore, further cellular assays were developed to identify oncogenes acting on other properties. The most famous among these may be the REF assay, in which primary rat embryo fibroblasts are infected with retroviruses or transfected with purified oncogene or tumor cell DNA. In this assay, two oncogenes are required for focus formation, one '*ras-type*' and one '*myc-type*' oncogene. This is another instance of oncogene cooperativity, as found during retroviral transformation in animals. The precise molecular basis of this cooperation is still under investigation, almost twenty years after its discovery. In short, '*myc-type*' genes immortalize rodent embryo fibroblasts and stimulate their proliferation, while '*ras-type*' genes elicit overgrowth and altered morphology. Obviously, in 3T3 cells, the first step has already happened.

Gene Amplification

Since overexpression is often required for oncogenic function, genes that are strongly overexpressed in specific human cancers are obvious candidates for oncogenes. Specifically, some cancers contain recurrent amplifications of specific chromosomal regions. These can be detected by cytogenetic techniques. For instance, the overexpression of MYC and ERBB1 in human cancers often results from amplification of their genes located at 8q24 and 17p12. Investigation of other amplified regions has revealed further oncogenes. A segment of chromosome 2p24 frequently amplified in neuroblastoma, but also in some carcinomas, contained a gene related to *MYC* that was named *MYCN* (N for neuroblastoma). Another related gene, *MYCL*, was found amplified and overexpressed in lung cancers. A different region originating from chromosome 17q11-12 amplified in breast cancer and other carcinomas yielded an overexpressed gene similar to ERBB1. This is now officially named ERBB2, but still doubles as HER-2 or NEU, the latter, because a mutated form was independently discovered in a chemically induced rat neuroblastoma.

Findings like these confirm that consistently amplified regions in the genome of cancer cells often contain oncogenes and that genes related to known oncogenes can be oncogenes. However, the identification of oncogenes from amplified regions is not always straight-forward, since amplified regions can encompass several Mbp. For instance, a region from 12q14 commonly amplified in human tumors contains the genes *GLI1*, *CDK4*, and *HDM2*. Each of these genes possesses properties which make it a good candidate for an oncogene. Perhaps, one or the other in different tumors or more than one could be relevant. A different kind of complication is that some amplifications are associated with gene silencing rather than overexpression.

Chromosomal Translocations

Another type of chromosomal aberration in human cancers are translocations. In hematological cancers, in particular, they activate genes at the translocation sites to become oncogenes. So, systematic investigation of recurrent translocations in hematological cancers by cytogenetic and molecular cloning techniques has revealed several oncogenes. To a lesser extent, characterization of translocations in soft tissue tumors and carcinomas has been productive. One gene activated by several translocations is MYC, emphasizing what a potent oncogene it is. A second oncogene identified at a recurrent site on 11q13 in different cancers was initially named PRAD1 or BCL1, but has now been renamed CCND1 since it encodes Cyclin D1, a crucial regulator of cell cycle progression through the G1 phase. Interestingly, the same gene is also overexpressed as a consequence of amplification in some carcinomas. Not untypical, several neighboring genes are often co-amplified with CCND1, including *GSTP1*, and a growth factor gene. The typical translocation in follicular lymphoma activates the BCL2 gene (for breakpoint cluster 2). This gene belongs to an entirely different functional class: the BCL2 protein is a direct regulator of apoptosis at the mitochondrion and the first member of a larger family to be identified.

Oncogene Families

Since oncogenes often seem to come in families, it is tempting to speculate that genes related to oncogenes might also be oncogenes. This idea has inspired a lot of research activities. The gist of their many results is that the idea is in some instances correct, but overall more rarely than was originally expected. In some cases, the reasons are obvious (with hindsight). For instance, the MYC family includes members like *MXI1* and *MAD* that are actually antagonists of the proto-oncogenes *MYC*, *MYCN*, and *MYCL,* while *MAX* encodes a heterodimerization partner for all members. It is less straightforward to understand, why *ERBB1* and *ERBB2* are often oncogenically activated, but two further members of the family, *ERBB3* and *ERBB4*, rarely. Similarly, the closest human ortholog of the viral v-raf, *RAF1*, does not seem to be activated in human tumors, but its homologue *BRAF* certainly is, e.g., in melanomas. So, homology to a proven oncogene is a good indication of importance, but does not allow firm conclusions on the oncogenic potential of a gene.

Another temptation is to regard every gene that is strongly overexpressed in a human tumor as an oncogene. As pointed out above, the significance of overexpression can be doubtful even for *bona fide* oncogenes like *MYC* and *ERBB1*. An observed overexpression of a gene in a human cancer is not always easy to interpret, since it can be difficult to test the functional implications of this overexpression. The distinction whether a gene is active as an oncogene as a consequence of overexpression or is overexpressed but not active as an oncogene is not only of intellectual interest, but also essential for the design of targeted therapy.

Cancer Pathways

The dilemma of how to test the functional importance of a gene in a human cancer has been partly alleviated by the recognition that oncogenes as well as tumor suppressor genes often interact in '*cancer pathways*'. If the product of a gene can be demonstrated to influence the activity of a '*cancer pathway*' important in a certain tumor type, its overexpression or mutation can be understood as oncogenic activation. This line of investigation has yielded sufficient data to regard genes like *MDM2/HDM2*, CTNNB1, or CDK4 as proto-oncogenes.

FUNCTIONS OF HUMAN ONCOGENES

The oncogenes of acutely transforming retroviruses as well as human oncogenes can be categorized according to their biochemical function or to the localization of their products. A sketch of these localizations suggests that this spatial distribution may be more than incidential. Indeed, many proven or suspected human oncogenes belong to a functional network which transmits signals for proliferation and survival from the exterior of the cell to the nucleus.

A normal cell proliferates in response to extracellular signals that are conferred by soluble growth factors and are modulated by signals elicited as a result of cell adhesion to the extracellular matrix and neighboring cells. The first group of presumed human oncogene products accordingly comprises peptide growth factors like TGFα (transforming growth factor alpha), FGF1 (*fibroblast growth factor*) or WNT1 (wingless/int-1) which are mitogens for epithelial and/or mesenchymal cells. These or related factors are overproduced by many carcinomas.

Peptide growth factors bind to and activate receptors at the cell membrane such as the EGFR (*epidermal growth factor receptor*), the product of the *ERBB1* gene, or one of several FGF receptors. ERBB1 is overexpressed in different carcinomas, often as a consequence of gene amplification. FGFR expression is also altered in many human tumors and the FGFR3 in particular is activated by point mutations in cancers of the bladder and the cervix. Further growth factor receptors such as ERBB2, MET, IGFR1, KIT, and RET are also crucial oncogenes in human cancers. These receptors share structures and the mechanism of signaling and are summarized as receptor tyrosine kinases (RTKs, also: TRKs). RTKs constitute one of the biggest classes of oncogenes. However, some oncogene products are receptors belonging to different classes, e.g. cytokine receptors.

Binding of a growth factor to the extracellular domain of a RTK leads to formation of receptor dimers or heterodimers, e.g. between ERBB1 and ERBB2. It also causes a conformational change by which a pseudosubstrate peptide loop in the intracellular domain of the receptor is removed from the active center of the intracellular tyrosine kinase domain. The tyrosine kinase becomes active and the receptor subunits phosphorylate each other in trans. Overexpression of RTKs in tumor cells favors dimer formation. Thereby, it sensitizes the cells to lower concentrations of ligand growth factors or even leading to growth factor-independent activation. Oncogenic point mutations typically occur in the inhibitory loop, thereby causing constitutive activation of the tyrosine kinase activity. Assembly of several receptor dimers to larger complexes in the cell membrane may occur followed by internalization into endosomes.

Cross- and auto-phosphorylation of RTKs provide phosphotyrosine for recognition by adaptor proteins containing SH2 domains which dock to the activated receptor. The SH2 domains in different proteins all bind phosphotyrosines, but recognize them in different peptide contexts. To various extents, RTKs also phosphorylate proteins other than themselves. Usually, multiple proteins bind to one receptor by recognizing different phosphotyrosines. In this fashion, one receptor can activate several different signaling pathways. For instance, activated EGFR binds the adaptor proteins GRB2 and SHC (which again binds GRB2), PLCγ (phospholipase C), the regulatory subunit of PI3K (phosphatidyl-inositol-3'-kinase), and GAP (GTPase activator protein).

Phosphotyrosines are substrates for tyrosine phosphatases and also serve as recognition sites for proteins which lead to internalization and degradation of the receptor, such as CBL proteins. Together, these help to limit the strength of growth factor signals in normal cells and ensure that the signals are transient.

The adaptor protein GRB2 in turn assembles a further protein named SOS to the complex, which interacts with and activates RAS proteins. All RAS proteins, HRAS, KRAS, or NRAS, are ≈21 kDa proteins and are linked to the inside of the cell membrane through their C-terminus which is posttranslationally modified by myristylation, farnesylation and methylation. They belong to a larger superfamily of small monomeric G proteins that can bind alternatively GTP or GDP. In the active state, GTP is bound. Hydrolysis of GTP to GDP by the combined action of RAS and a GTPase activator protein (i.e., GAP) restores the basal inactive state. Normally, activation of RAS depends on interaction with SOS which acts as a guanine nucleotide exchange factor (GEF), loading the RAS protein with GTP instead of GDP. The activated state of normal RAS proteins is short-lived, since RTKs in parallel to the SOS GEF activate GAPs that stimulate GTP hydrolysis. However, mutations in RAS amino acids 12, 13, or 61, which surround the GTP binding site, obstruct the access for the GAP protein and prolong the active state.

RAS is the next branching point in the signaling network described here, since activated RAS acts on several pathways which affect protein synthesis, the cytoskeleton and cell survival, notably the PI3K pathway.

The main route by which RAS relays a proliferation signal is via interaction with RAF proteins. The three RAF proteins in human cells are Ser/Thr protein kinases. Like many protein kinases, they contain a regulatory domain and a C-terminal catalytic domain. In the inactive state, the protein resides in the cytosol and the kinase activity is blocked by the regulatory domain. Activated RAS translocates RAF to the cell membrane and relieves the inhibition of the regulatory domain. Interestingly, RAF activity is also modulated by phosphorylation of the CR2 segment in its regulatory domain. A tyrosine in this domain is phosphorylated by SRC family kinases, and serine and threonine residues are phosphorylated by protein kinase C isozymes which can be activated indirectly by PLC. So, here are further links in the network. In some human cancers, BRAF is altered by specific point mutations to become overactive. Mutations in BRAF occur in the same tumor types as mutations in RAS genes, but alternately to them. Since RAS proteins act on several pathways, this finding is important in showing that signaling via RAF is indeed significant for transformation. Tellingly, the main modification in the retroviral v-raf oncogene is the inactivation of the regulatory domain of the cellular protein.

Activated RAF is the first one in a cascade of protein kinases that further comprises MEK and ERK proteins. Alternative names for these are MAPK (mitogen-activated protein kinase) for ERK and MAPKK for MEK; RAF proteins can therefore be counted as MAPKKK (or MEKK). There are several additional MEKKs in parallel pathways in human cells. Most human cells contain two MEK and two ERK protein kinases. MEK are highly specific and phosphorylate predominantly ERK proteins at a tyrosine and threonine each in a TEY sequence. Activated ERKs phosphorylate a variety of substrates to activate protein synthesis, alter the structure of the cytoskeleton, and induce gene expression. Interaction of MEKs, ERKs and MAPKKs is supported and its specificity is enhanced by scaffold proteins. Phosphorylation of MAPKKs, MEKs, and ERKs is removed by several specific and less specific protein phosphatases in order to terminate the signal. Some of these phospatases, like MKP1 (MAP kinase phosphatase 1), are themselves activated by MAPK signaling, while others may be constitutively active.

Increased protein synthesis and cytoskeletal changes elicited by MAPK signalling in the cytoplasm are important for cell growth and also necessary for cell migration. Stimulation of cell proliferation in addition requires an altered pattern of gene expression and activation of the cell cycle in the nucleus. The mitogenic signal from growth factors for altered transcription is to a large extent relayed by the MAPK signaling cascade. Activated ERKs phosphorylate several transcription factors directly or stimulate other protein kinases like $p90^{RSK1}$ to do so. This induces the transcription of a larger set of genes, which again are organized as a cascaded network in the nucleus.

The first set of genes induced upon activation of the MAPK pathway by growth factors in previously resting cells are the '*early-response*' genes. They are, e.g. induced by treatment of quiescent cells in cell culture with growth-factors or serum. Among them are several from the oncogene lists, such as FOS, JUN, MYB, and MYC. The most important one of these in the context of human cancers is MYC which is frequently activated by overexpression or deregulation and thereby becomes active independent of growth factor signaling. As a rule, FOS, JUN and MYB are necessary for the growth of human cancers, but do not usually seem to act as oncogenes, strictly spoken. It is not entirely clear, why this is so. Certainly, one obvious reason is that the viral counterparts of these genes are severely altered and over-expressed. Moreover, cells from long-lived humans may have better checks against tumor formation than cells of many animals. Indeed, overexpression of proteins like FOS or JUN can induce apoptosis in some human cells.

Following their induction, the products of the '*early response*' genes induce the expression of genes required for cell cycle progression, directly or indirectly. In normal cells, one of the most important proteins that links the mitogenic signal to cell cycle regulation is Cyclin D1, the product of the *CCND1* gene. Overexpression of Cyclin D1 caused by gene amplification or translocation of *CCDN1* is important in several different human cancers. Moreover, Cyclin D1 is often overexpressed without alterations in the gene itself, likely as a consequence of '*upstream*' mutations in the MAPK pathway. Its overexpression may (partly) mediate the oncogenic effect of these alterations. The related gene *CCDN2* is expressed in a more restricted range of tissues than *CCDN1*. Accordingly, overexpression and amplification of this gene occur in a more limited range of human tumors, e.g. prominently in testicular cancers. D-Cyclins activate the cyclindependent kinase 4 to promote progression through the cell cycle. Amplification and overexpression of CDK4 are also observed in human cancers, e.g. in gliomas and hepatomas.

Finally, physiological signaling for cell proliferation requires a parallel signal for cell survival, by the same growth factor and its receptor or by a complementing pathway. For instance, insulin-like growth factors also stimulate the MAPK cascade, but more strongly confer a survival signal, which is mediated through PI3K. Therefore, the overexpression of the insulin-like growth factors IGF1 and IGF2 as well as PI3K and its downstream kinase AKT must be considered as an oncogenic event in many human cancers. Alternatively, cell death by apoptosis as a consequence of inappropriate stimulation of cell proliferation can be prevented by oncogenic overexpression of proteins like BCL2. This is the crucial event in follicular lymphoma, but this change or equivalent ones are also found in other hematological cancers as well as many carcinomas. The synergism between oncogenes that stimulate cell proliferation and oncogenes that prevent apoptosis induced by this stimulation is evident in many human cancers, most transparently in certain lymphomas. This is another example of oncogene cooperation.

Since human cancers accumulate many genetic and epigenetic alterations during their progression, in a typical cancer many genes are overexpressed and many of their products are overactive, and some may show mutations. Many of these genes may well be functionally important and promote tumor growth. It is tempting to regard every gene of this kind as an oncogene, particularly, if it shows a fitting biochemical property such as a protein kinase activity or DNA binding. In the context of human cancers, however, caution is warranted. This is because many cancers have developed over a long period, with many displaying genomic instability and/or an increased rate of point mutations. As a consequence, there may be a larger number of genes with alterations in their sequence and dosage in the definitive tumor clone than absolutely required for its growth. To prove that a gene of this sort is an oncogene by a strict definition, one would have to show that the altered or overexpressed gene product indeed dominantly confers an essential property for the survival and sustained growth of the cancer, and that its overexpression and/or overactivity are caused by substantial changes in the gene itself, i.e. mutations or amplifications.

10

Cancer Pathways

Proliferation, differentiation, and survival of normal cells are regulated by a limited number of pathways, which are partly interlinked. They transmit and integrate signals from growth factors, hormones, cell-cell- and cell-matrix-interactions. The pathways turn into '*cancer pathways*' by deregulation. Inappropriate activation of '*cancer pathways*' in some cases and inactivation in others are crucial for the development and progression of human cancers. In particular, many proto-oncogenes and tumor suppressors act within or upon cancer pathways'.

MAP kinase pathways transduce signals from the cell membrane to the nucleus, but also to the translational machinery and to the cytoskeleton. The canonical MAPK pathway activated by receptor tyrosine kinases proceeds through RAS proteins, RAF, MEK, and ERK protein kinases. It typically promotes proliferation in response to growth factors. Its activity is modulated by other signals emanating, e.g., from adhesion molecules. Other MAPK pathways mediate stress responses and may alternatively elicit apoptosis. While the functions of the various MAPK pathways are overlapping, the ERK pathway is the most important one in the control of cell proliferation. Another frequent target of membrane receptors is phospholipase C, which activates PKC isoenzymes that can stimulate MAPK signaling and other cellular processes. The diverse PKC enzymes are also targets of other factors, including the tumor-promoting phorbol esters.

Many growth factors, through receptor tyrosine kinases and RAS proteins, activate PI3K, thereby triggering the PDK/PKB/AKT protein kinase cascade that increases cell survival, protein synthesis, and cell proliferation. The PTEN and TSC tumor suppressors are antagonists of this cascade. In many instances, the PI3K pathway acts synergistically with the canonical MAPK pathway.

MAPK signaling promotes progression of the cell cycle at several distinct steps leading ultimately to phosphorylation and temporary inactivation of RB1 by CDKs. CDKs, Cyclins, CDK phosphatases, and CDK inhibitor proteins form a multi-layered network which ensures orderly cell proliferation, integrates proliferative and inhibitory signals received by the cell, and responds to cellular checkpoints monitoring cell cycle progress and genomic integrity. In human cancers, inappropriate stimulation of the cell cycle by alterations in '*upstream*' pathways and/or mutations in immediate regulators of the cell cycle are essential for uncontrolled proliferation. Many signals from checkpoints of genomic integrity are channeled through TP53 which elicit cell cycle arrest, apoptosis, or replicative senescence. Inactivation or curtailment of TP53 function by one of various mechanisms is therefore a prerequisite for genomic instability in human cancers.

Another limit to the expansion of carcinomas is provided by TGFβ signaling. As a rule, TGFβ factors stimulate the proliferation of mesenchymal cells, but inhibit the proliferation of epithelial cells. In response to TGFβ receptor activation, SMAD transcription factors become phosphorylated and translocate to the nucleus where they stimulate the expression of genes encoding e.g. CDK inhibitors or proteins involved in formation and remodeling of the extracellular matrix. Other SMAD factors act as feedback inhibitors. Disruption of this pathway is important during the progression of many carcinomas. TGFβ synthesized by non-responsive carcinoma cells activates tumor stroma and inhibits immune cells.

Stimulation of cell proliferation by cytokines often proceeds via the JAK/STAT pathway in hematopoetic cells and lymphocytes, and to a lesser degree in epithelial cells. Overactivity of this pathway is responsible for increased proliferation in hematological cancers. Its role in carcinomas is more ambiguous. In some, it is even down-regulated. In this short pathway, JAK protein kinases recruited by cytokine receptors phosphorylate STAT transcription factors which translocate into the nucleus to activate transcription. The JAK/STAT pathway is autoregulated by SOCS proteins.

Signaling through NFκB also regulates activation and proliferation of immune cells. In epithelial cells, this pathway can protect against apoptosis during cellular stress. Its activation may therefore contribute to prevention of apoptosis in carcinoma cells.

The patterning of tissues during fetal development involves several specialized regulatory systems, in particular WNT, Hedgehog (SHH), and NOTCH ligands, receptors, and pathways. These pathways remain important in adult tissues for maintenance of stem cell compartments and the regulation of cell fate. Disturbances in these pathways are fundamental for the development of specific human cancers. Thus, colon cancers invariably display constitutive activation of the WNT pathway, basal cell carcinoma of the skin of the SHH pathway, and certain T-cell leukemias of the NOTCH pathway. The responsible alterations are alternatively mutations in proto-oncogenes or tumor suppressor genes.

Cancer Pathways

Since >250 different genes have been demonstrated to be causally involved in human cancers and many more are implicated, it would seem that a bewildering variety of mechanisms may cause human cancer. While this could still turn out be so, the great majority of currently known oncoproteins can be assigned to a limited number of pathways or at least be demonstrated to act on these. These '*cancer pathways*' are, of course, systems that regulate fate, survival, proliferation, differentiation, and function of normal cells as well. In cancer cells, they are accordingly overactive or inactivated to cause the characteristic properties of cancer cells such as uncontrolled proliferation, blocked differentiation, decreased apoptosis, altered tissue structure, etc. Some '*cancer pathways*' are rather specifically involved in particular cancers, whereas others play crucial roles in a broad range of malignant tumors. To avoid considering each and every cellular regulatory system as a cancer pathway, a working definition might be formulated as: A '*cancer pathway*' is a cellular regulatory system whose activation or inactivation by a genetic or epigenetic mutation is essential for the development of at least one human cancer. Typically, cancer pathways become evident by alterations in different components of the same regulatory system in individual cases of one cancer type or in distinct cancers.

By this latter criterion, several regulatory systems treated in the previous two chapters can be regarded as prototypic cancer pathways. These comprise the MAPK pathway, the TP53 regulatory system, and the cell cycle regulatory network centered around RB1. These pathways all interact with each other. Further pathways and proteins are also connected to them, such as the PI3K pathway, the PKC kinases, the STAT pathway, the NFκB pathway, and the TGFβ response pathway. A third group of cancer pathways comprises the WNT and Hedgehog response pathways and the NOTCH regulatory system. They are essential in regulating the shaping and differentiation of tissues during fetal development and remain important even in grown-up humans for the maintenance of tissue homeostasis, particularly in tissues that undergo rapid turnover or frequent regeneration. They are particularly important in specific cancers.

MAPK Signaling as a Cancer Pathway

Signaling through the MAPK pathway composed of RAF, MEK, and ERK proteins is required for the proliferation of normal cells as well as for many cancer cells. In normal cells, it typically relays signals *receptor tyrosine kinases* (RTKs) activated by growth factors to the nucleus, resulting in the activation of gene expression. It can also be activated by a range of other extra- and intracellular stimuli and it elicits effects besides altered gene expression. In tumor cells, MAPK signaling is often enhanced, e.g. as a consequence of oncogenic activation of RTKs or RAS. This MAPK pathway is therefore considered as the '*classical mitogenic cascade*' or as the '*canonical*' pathway

In reality, this pathway is one of about six similar modules which each consist of a MAP kinase (like ERK1/2), a MAPK kinase (like MEK1/2), and a MAP kinase kinase (like RAF1, ARAF, or BRAF). These other MAPK modules respond likewise to extracellular signals from growth factors, but also to signals from hormones and cytokines acting through G-proteins, to cell adhesion molecules, and stress signals generated in the cell or at the cell membrane. Like the canonical pathway, these modules can stimulate cell proliferation, but also apoptosis, cell differentiation, or specific cell functions. None of them, however, has been as straightforwardly implicated in the control of cell proliferation and in cancer as the canonical pathway.

The best studied of the parallel pathways involves MEKK1, MEK4, and JNK (JUN N-terminal kinase) leading to phosphorylation of the transcriptional activator JUN. This pathway is activated by RAS proteins, specifically in response to stress resulting from UV irradiation and heat, or to certain cytokines. Alternatively, other GTP-binding proteins such as RAC or CDC42, which respond to cell adhesion signals, activate the pathway through MEKK1, 2, or 3. The outcome of activation of this MAPK pathway is more usually a stop to cell proliferation than its stimulation. In some circumstances, it can induce apoptosis. Accordingly, the JNK pathway appears to be important in the progression of some cancers, but more often it is down-regulated than overactive in cancers. Specifically, its components do not seem to constitute a primary target of mutations in human cancers. Interestingly, there are several points of cross-talk between different MAPK pathways, e.g. at the level of MAPKKs. Moreover, JUN is phosphorylated as a consequence of activation of the JNK MAPK pathway, while the protein is transcriptionally induced by the ERK MAPK pathway. So, during normal cell proliferation, these two MAPK pathway synergize.

Both the ERK and the JNK MAPK pathways can be activated through RAS proteins. RAS-GTP acts directly at the level of the MEKKs by recruiting RAF proteins or MEKK1 to the cell membrane and relieving their autoinhibition. RAS proteins also act in an indirect manner on the G-protein RAC through activation of PI3K, a crucial component of a further cancer pathway. In addition to RAC, RAS proteins regulate further similar small G-proteins, such as RAL and RHO, by activating their *GTP-exchange factors* (GEF) or *GTPase activating proteins* (GAP). Through these routes, RAS is thought to elicit the changes in the cytoskeleton and consequently cell shape, adhesion, and migration which are commonly seen in cells with oncogenic RAS, e.g. in the 3T3 assay system.

Clearly, such changes are expected to also influence the behavior of a tumor cell in vivo. The action of RAS on the PI3K pathway may be particularly significant in those cancers in which that pathway is not autonomously activated. The high prevalence of RAS mutations in human cancers is thus well explained by its function as a nodal regulator of several pathways relevant to essential properties .of cancer cells. Among these various effects, the activation of the ERK MAPK pathway is likely most crucial for stimulation of cell proliferation in cancers with RAS mutations, as well as in those with oncogenic activation of receptor tyrosine kinases upstream of RAS. One of several arguments for this tenet are mutually exclusive mutations in *RAS* genes and *BRAF* in several cancers, prominently in melanoma.

The activation of the JNK MAPK pathway by RAS points to another facet in the pleitropic function of these proteins. Overactivity of RAS proteins in normal cells can induce growth arrest, apoptosis or replicative senescence. In some cell types, RAS activation may also induce differentiation. So, in addition to their effect on cell proliferation, RAS proteins in their active state also stimulate responses that eventually terminate their effects or under some circumstances evoke fail-safe reactions against hyperproliferation. Depending on the circumstances, the JNK MAPK pathway may act in this fashion.

Another mechanism of this kind is induction of *CDKN2A* with increased transcription of p14^{ARF1} and p16^{INK4A} that leads to stabilization of TP53 and slows phosphorylation of RB1. Still another fail-safe mechanism may be exerted through the RASSF1A protein. This protein is encoded by a complex locus on chromosome 3p21.3, binds to microtubuli and may block mitosis. Loss of 3p is a common finding in clear-cell renal carcinoma and many other carcinomas. Furthermore, *RASSF1A* is inactivated by promoter hypermethylation in a wide range of human cancers.

Since RAS proteins are almost invariably activated when signals emanate from active growth factor receptors, they mediate many effects of the physiological or oncogenic activation of receptor tyrosine kinases, specifically an activation of the MAPK pathway downstream of RAS proteins. In fact, RAS proteins mediate not only signals by receptor tyrosine kinases, but are also involved in cellular responses to cytokines and hormones acting through G-protein coupled serpentine receptors. Conversely, receptor tyrosine kinases and others modulate the activities of the MAPK, PI3K, and further cancer pathways not only through RAS, but also by diverse other mechanisms.

PI3K Pathway

The *PI3K pathway* functions in the control of cellular metabolism, particularly that of glucose transport and utilization, in the regulation of cell growth, particularly of protein biosynthesis, and it prevents apoptosis. The pathway is stimulated by RAS proteins and by active receptor tyrosine kinases, but it also feeds back into pathways downstream of RAS. It is distinguished as a cancer pathway, since its major inhibitory component, PTEN, is a classical tumor suppressor. Two other proteins affected in a human tumor syndrome, TSC1 and TSC2, modulate intermediate steps of the pathway. Moreover, in some instances PI3K is implicated as an oncogenic protein. For instance, its gene is amplified in ovarian cancers.

The abbreviation PI3K stands for phosphatidyl inositol phosphate kinase, since the enzyme phosphorylates the membrane phospholipids phosphatidyl inositol (PI), PI(4)P, and PI(4,5)P to yield PI3P, PI(3,4)P, and PI(3,4,5)P, respectively. Several different isoenzymes of PI3K exist, of which PI3Kα is the one most relevant in the context of cancer. PI3Kα also has protein kinase activity, but the substrates have not been well defined. It is a heterodimer consisting of a p110 catalytic subunit and a p85 regulatory subunit which in the basal state restricts the activity of the catalytic subunit.

Following receptor tyrosine kinase activation and autophosphorylation, the PI3K heterodimer binds to tyrosine phosphate via the SH2 domain of p85 leading to activation of the catalytic subunit. This is also - independently or synergistically - stimulated by direct interaction with RAS-GTP. Lipid phosphorylation generates PI(3,4,5)P at the inner face of the plasma membrane. This creates binding sites for proteins containing a *pleckstrin homology* (PH) domain, which in this way become relocated to the membrane. There are several such proteins, among them GEFs for RAC and other RAS-like proteins involved in the organization of the cytoskeleton.

The actual PI3K pathway proceeds through the protein kinases PDK1 and AKT, which is also known as PKB. PDK1 becomes directly activated by binding to PI(3,4,5)P, whereas AKT additionally needs to be phosphorylated by PDK1 to become active. PDK1 phosphorylates further protein kinases, including the PKC isoenzyme ζ and the $p70^{S6K}$, which is also a target of ERK MAP kinases. The main effector of the pathway, however, is the AKT protein kinase. Following its own activation by PDK1, it can phosphorylate a variety of proteins. One major substrate is mTOR, a protein kinase controlling the initiation of translation at the EIF4 step. So, the combined actions of PDK1 and AKT lead to an increase in protein synthesis. This effect is important in the anabolic action of insulin and *insulin-like growth factors* (IGFs) in many tissues, but it is also a prerequisite to cell proliferation and therefore central to tumor growth. AKT activity may be antagonized by CTMP (*C-terminal membrane protein*), a potential tumor suppressor.

The acronym mTOR stands for '*mammalian target of rapamycin*', since rapamycin inhibits this kinase specifically. Physiologically, mTOR is inhibited by the TSC1/TSC2 protein complex. TSC1 and TSC2 are also called *Tuberin* and *Hamartin*. Either protein is mutated in tuberous sclerosis, an autosomal dominant disorder affecting ≈1/6000 persons. The *TSC* genes, which are located at chromosomes 9q34 and 16p13, respectively, behave as classical tumor suppressors. Thus, in affected persons, one defective copy of a *TSC* gene is inherited. Mutation of the second allele leads to hamartomas, usually small benign tumors consisting of different connective tissue components which occur in several organs including brain, heart, lung and kidneys. Although carcinomas are not usually found in this syndrome, the *TSC1* gene may be involved in bladder and perhaps renal carcinomas. During growth, inhibition of mTOR by the TSC proteins is relieved by phosphorylation of the large TSC2 protein at Ser939 and Thr1462 by the AKT protein kinase. As loss of TSC function leads to overactivity of mTOR, rapamycin is now investigated for the treatment of this condition.

The tumor syndrome caused by mutation of *TSC* genes underlines the importance of activation of protein synthesis and stimulation of cell growth by the PI3K pathway. This pathway has, however, further functions. This is dramatically demonstrated by the hereditary Cowden tumor syndrome caused by mutations in the *PTEN* gene, located at 10q23.3. Its product is a lipid phosphatase and protein phosphatase, as PI3K is a lipid kinase and protein kinase. PTEN antagonizes PI3K by hydrolytically removing phosphates at position 3 of phosphatidyl inositols. Like mutations in the TSC genes, PTEN mutations in the germ-line predispose to multiple hamartomas, but unlike tuberous sclerosis, the Cowden syndrome carries a risk for major common cancers, such as colon and breast cancer. Deletions, mutations and inactivation of the *PTEN* gene are as well observed in many different sporadic cancers. The wide range of cancers in which its inactivation is prevalent points to PTEN as one of the most important tumor suppressors. Typically, in sporadic cancer loss of PTEN is associated with tumor progression and a more aggressive clinical course.

The AKT protein kinase not only stimulates protein synthesis but also cell survival and cell proliferation. Cell survival is promoted by several routes. Phosphorylation of forkhead transcription factors like FKHR-L1 prevents their transcriptional activation of proapoptotic and growth-inhibitory genes. Phosphorylation by AKT also inhibits the important apoptosis activator BAD. In either case, the proteins phosphorylated by AKT are recognized by 14-3-3 proteins. The protein complex is retained in the cytosol, preventing FKHR-L1 from entering the nucleus and BAD from interacting with mitochondrial proteins, respectively. Through the same mechanism, phosphorylation by AKT limits the activity of the $p27^{KIP1}$ cell cycle inhibitor. TP53 activity may also be diminished, since AKT appears to activate MDM2. Further effects on cell proliferation result from phosphorylation of *glycogen synthase kinase* 3 (GSK3) by AKT. As implied by its name, this enzyme is an important regulator of glucose metabolism, and a major target of insulin action. In addition, it regulates cell proliferation by phosphorylating and inhibiting Cyclin D1 and MYC. Perhaps its most important function is in the regulation of β-Catenin levels within the WNT pathway, which is particularly important in colon cancer.

In summary, during normal cell proliferation the PI3K pathway may be essential to complement the MAPK pathway. Somewhat simplified, the MAPK pathway mainly stimulates cell proliferation (i.e. DNA synthesis and mitosis), but requires additional signals through the PI3K pathway which provides the necessary stimulus for cell growth (including protein biosynthesis) and, importantly, counteracts the pro-apoptotic effects caused by isolated MAPK stimulation. Appropriate stimulation of cell proliferation by growth factors therefore involves a coordinated activation of these two pathways. Alternatively, certain growth factors preferentially stimulate the PI3K pathway, prominently members of the insulin family, such as IGF1 and IGF2, and act primarily as '*survival growth factors*'. They can in this fashion complement growth factors which act predominantly through the MAPK pathway. Accordingly, in tumor cells, mutations leading to the constitutive activation of the MAPK pathway can be complemented by increased activity of survival growth factors or by mutations in the PI3K pathway, e.g. those disabling PTEN function.

Regulation of the Cell Cycle by the MAPK and PI3K Pathways

Normal cell proliferation thus often involves the coordinate activation of MAPK and PI3K pathways. Together, these pathways elicit a panoply of changes, such as increased metabolism, enhanced protein synthesis, reorganization of the cytoskeleton, inhibition of proapoptotic signals, and, of course, stimulation of cell cycle progression from G1/G0 into S-phase. Several mechanisms synergize to achieve this last effect.

Following their translocation into the nucleus as a consequence of MAPK activation, activated ERK protein kinases phosphorylate several transcriptional activators involved in cell cycle progression. In addition, ERK kinases phosphorylate the $pp90^{RSK}$ kinases which then as well translocate to the nucleus to phosphorylate a further set of transcriptional activators. Among the more important targets are the SRF, ETS1, ELK1 and MYC factors, which are all stimulated by this type of phosphorylation, and, of course, the AP1 components FOS and JUN, which are also induced at the transcriptional level.

In many cells, an important consequence of these events is a stimulation of Cyclin D transcription. Accumulation of Cyclin D drives cell cycle progression during most of the G1 period. It is counteracted by degradation of the protein which is increased if Cyclin D is phosphorylated by GSK3. This inhibitory phosphorylation is blocked by phosphorylation of GSK3 by AKT. The coordinate activation of Cyclin D is thus an important point of synergy between the MAPK and PI3K pathways. Further genes activated as a consequence of MAPK pathway stimulation are CDC25A and – to a lesser extent - CDK4. Induction of the CDC25A phosphatase synergizes with Cyclin D accumulation to increase CDK4 activity, since the phosphatase removes the inhibitory threonine phosphate from CDK4, as well as from CDK2.

As the CDK4/Cyclin D holoenzyme accumulates, it binds more and more $p27^{KIP1}$, diverting it from CDK2. Since Cyclin E begins to accumulate at this stage of the cell cycle, the activity of the CDK2/Cyclin E enzyme increases consequentially. The Cyclin E gene promoter is activated by E2F1. So, as RB1 starts to become hyperphosphorylated and less capable of inhibiting E2F, more Cyclin E is produced leading to still higher activity of CDK2. This autocatalytic loop eventually leads to irreversible commitment to S-phase, but is limited by $p27^{KIP1}$.

For CDK2 to become fully active, the $p27^{KIP1}$ inhibitor must be removed. This occurs by successive phosphorylation, oligo-ubiquitination, and proteolytic degradation. In normal cells, the down-regulation of $p27^{KIP1}$ is a gradual process which accelerates when CDK2 becomes sufficiently active to phosphorylate some of the inhibitor protein, thereby liberating further CDK2 molecules to phosphorylate more $p27^{KIP1}$, in another autocatalytic loop. A crucial component in this process is MYC. MYC is induced by many growth factors, but its half-life and activity are also regulated by phosphorylation. ERK phosphorylation at Ser62 leads to increased stability and activity, whereas GSK phosphorylation at Thr58 has the opposite effect. So, again, the inhibitory phosphorylation of GSK by AKT synergizes with activation of the MAPK to activate MYC. Activation of MYC contributes to the increased transcription of Cyclin D1, CDK4, and CDC25A, and leads to a small decrease in transcription of $p27^{KIP1}$. Moreover, MYC induces CUL1, a component of the protein complex that ubiquitinates $p27^{KIP1}$. Still another mechanism involved is decreased translation of $p27^{KIP1}$, likely as a consequence of PI3K activation. So, regulation of MYC and $p27^{KIP1}$ are further points of synergy between the pathways.

The synergisms exerted on the regulation of the cell cycle by the concomitant activation of the MAPK and AKT pathways during normal cell proliferation are reflected in the alterations observed in cancers. Overactive receptor tyrosine kinases may be such potent oncogenes, since they are capable of activating both pathways. Oncogenic RAS may likewise activate both pathways, albeit less efficiently. Conversely, oncogenic MYC itself, while very efficient in promoting cell growth (also in a broader sense) and stimulating cell cycle progression, also tends to drive cells into apoptosis, which is again counteracted by factors that activate the PI3K pathway, such as IGF peptides or RAS mutations. This explains the cooperation of RAS-like and MYC-like oncogenes in rodent cell transformation assays. This cooperativity is also at work in many human cancers.

However, these combinations of alterations are probably not sufficient to cause human cancers, since they are counteracted by further fail-safe mechanisms. The most important one may be activation of TP53 by hyperproliferation signals and through accumulation of CDK inhibitors like $p16^{INK4A}$ and $p21^{CIP1}$ during continuous rapid growth of human cells. These fail-safe mechanisms lead to apoptosis in some cases, but more typically to replicative senescence. Thus, at some point in the development of human cancers, latest during progression, these mechanisms need to be inactivated. The most radical way for their inactivation is loss of both RB1 and TP53. Another frequent mechanism is deletion of the *CDKN2A* locus encoding $p16^{INK4A}$ and $p14^{ARF}$. Of note, while the prime significance of these alterations may be the inactivation of fail-safe mechanisms against hyperproliferation, they also decrease the dependence of tumor cells on external growth factors and increase their tolerance of genomic instability.

So, alterations that lead to an increased or constitutive activity of the MAPK and PI3K pathways may in some cases be self-limiting. At the least, they exert a strong selection pressure favoring further changes that lead to progression towards a more aggressive phenotype. This sort of progression is observed in many human cancers, in carcinomas as well as hematological cancers.

Modulators of the MAPK and PI3K Pathways

The MAPK and PI3K pathways have multiple effects in the cell, influencing a variety of protein kinases, transcription factors, cytoskeletal proteins, proteins acting at the ribosome, and apoptotic regulators. Conversely, they are activated not only by signals from receptor tyrosine kinases, but also modulated by many others. These emerge, e.g., from other types of receptors, such as cytokine receptors and G-protein coupled serpentine receptors, as well as from various cell adhesion molecules.

This part of intracellular signaling involves a number of additional protein kinases and other enzymes. Several have in fact been discovered in substantially altered form as retroviral oncogenes, but in human cancers they rarely appear as oncogenes or tumor suppressors fitting the strict definitions proposed at the ends. However, these proteins are clearly important in human cancers for the establishment of typical properties of tumor cells and as modulators of the MAPK and PI3K '*cancer pathways*'.

Most *receptor tyrosine kinases* (RTK) and some *G-protein coupled receptors* (GPCR) activate the MAPK cascade through RAS activation. Many GPCRs and some RTKs employ phospholipases in this activation, typically PLCβ in the case of GPCRs and PLCγ in the case of RTKs. These phospholipases cleave phosphatidyl inositol bisphosphate in the membrane to yield diacylglyerol and inositol triphosphate (IP_3). IP_3 is a second messenger molecule that regulates cytosolic Ca^{2+} levels, which again affect many different cellular functions, including metabolism, transcription, and the state of the cytoskeleton.

The diacylglycerol liberated by the PLC reaction is also a signal molecule which binds and activates protein kinases of a class named PKC. It comprises >10 members in humans, with different tissue distributions and specificities. The most widely distributed member is PKCα. This enzyme, like the '*classical*' PKCβ and PKCγ isoenzymes is activated synergistically by diacylglycerol and Ca^{2+}, other isoenzymes such as the likewise widely distributed PKCδ are independent of Ca^{2+} levels. Still another class represented by PKCζ are independent of both activators. The structure of the PKCs is modular like that of many other protein kinases. A distal catalytic domain containing the ATP and substrate binding site is normally inhibited by a pseudosubstrate in the proximal regulatory domain. In the classical PKC isoenzymes, the regulatory region contains binding sites for diacylglycerol and for calcium ions. Binding of both activators relieves the autoinhibition. Like RAF, PDK, and AKT, many PKCs are activated at the inner face of the plasma membrane.

The diacylglycerol binding site in PKCs also recognizes phorbol esters like *tetradecanoyl phorbol acetate* (TPA), which is also called *phorbol myristyl acetate* (PMA). This compound from plants is a strong irritant and stimulates the proliferation of some cells. In animal experiments, it promotes tumor growth in the skin, although it is not mutagenic. It is thus the prototype of a '*tumor promoter*'. However, the effect is dependent on the tissue and the species. This may relate to the type of PKC present and how important it is for the regulation of proliferation in a particular tissue. PKCs may also bind and react to other ligands.

PKCs are serine/threonine protein kinases with a (wide) range of their substrates, differing between the individual isoenzymes. Since

PKCs such as PKCα and PKCε can phosphorylate RAF, they can mediate a stimulation of the MAPK cascade independent of or synergistically with RAS. By phosphorylating cytoskeletal proteins like MARCKS, they affect the structure of the actin cytoskeleton. This influences cell motility and transport processes which are also directly regulated by PKCs. PKCs also phosphorylate nuclear receptors like the VDR. Last, not least PKCs can phosphorylate and regulate receptor tyrosine kinases, including the EGFR.

In effect, PKCs are typically used in the cell to relay signals from one activated pathway to others, i.e. in '*cross-talk*'. This may be more of a coordinating than a determining task, which could explain why they have not appeared as '*true*' oncogenes in spite of their close connection to the control of cell proliferation and motility. However, inhibition of PKCs does block the proliferation of some cancer cells and clearly, activation by phorbol esters can principally stimulate the proliferation of normal and particularly transformed cells. Moreover, PLCs and PKCs are apparently critical mediators of the effect of several oncogenes, including retroviral oncogenes like yes and cellular oncogenes like TRK that act in lymphoid cells. They may also be necessary in those (rarer) cases, where the proliferation of cancers is caused by G-coupled receptors.

PKCs are also participants in the cross-talk in the cell between cell adhesion molecules and growth-regulatory pathways. Signals emerge from cell-cell-adhesion as well as from cell adhesion to the substrate. Cell-cell-adhesion is often mediated by cadherins which are connected to the cytoskeleton and influence its activity. Different cadherins, to different extents, activate or inhibit cancer pathways. E-Cadherin, the major cadherin in many epithelia, binds β-Catenin and may thereby limit the activity of the WNT/β-Catenin pathway in some cell types. Likewise, E-Cadherin activates the PI3K pathway to yield a robust survival signal. Both signals are reasonable for a cell firmly integrated into a relatively quiescent epithelium. In some (but not all) invasive carcinomas, E-Cadherin is down-regulated or becomes replaced by other cadherins that activate different pathways.

Integrins mediate cell-matrix interactions by binding to extracellular fibronectin. At the inner surface of the cell membrane, they provide a focus to organize the attachment of the actin cytoskeleton at focal adhesion contacts. Focal adhesion contacts are the hub of a signaling network that influences the cytoskeleton, cell proliferation and survival. The integrin-linked kinase ILK regulates and signals the connection between integrins and the cytoskeleton. The focal adhesion kinase FAK then signals the establishment of the focal adhesions. It is autophosphorylated and can accordingly be recognized by SH2 domains in SRC protein kinases.

SRC kinases are the human orthologs of the v-src gene product of RSV. They are located to the inner face of the plasma membrane by a myristyl anchor. Upon binding to FAK they become activated and further phosphorylate this kinase in turn. Activated SRCs behave very similar to activated receptor tyrosine kinases, binding adaptor proteins like SHC/GRB2, phosphorylating and activating a number of proteins, including RAS as well as PLCs and consequentially PKCs, and leading to stimulation of the MAPK and PI3K pathways. Integrins are also capable of activating PKCs directly and of interacting with other small GTPases like RAC that regulate the structure of the cytoskeleton.

SRC kinases are often overexpressed and overactive in human cancers, although not mutated like their viral counterpart. It appears that the activation of these enzymes is often associated with advanced stages of carcinomas, where cells become highly invasive and migratory. Increased activity of FAK and ILK is also observed in such cancers. It is not entirely clear whether the increased activity of these enzymes is cause or effect of increased motility and altered attachment. However, in either case, the activation is likely to be necessary, as cell proliferation requires an attachment signal. Stimulation of proliferation without such a signal may lead to anoikis, a specific type of programmed cell death. In a cancer cell with altered attachment, activation of the signaling pathways from adhesion molecules may be needed to compensate. Like in their subversion of the TP53/RB1 checkpoint mechanisms, during their progression cancer cells appear to acquire the ability to circumvent this additional barrier against inappropriate proliferation.

TP53 Network

The TP53 protein is the central node in a network that is linked to several others both upstream and downstream of TP53. Upstream events that modulate TP53 function include prominently activation of protein kinases that sense DNA damage such as ATM and DNA-dependent protein kinase. They phosphorylate TP53 at its N-terminus, increasing its transcriptional activity and decreasing its sensitivity to inhibition by HDM2, in the process enhancing also its half-life. Other types of cellular stress, such as hypoxia or imbalances in nucleotide metabolism, e.g. following treatment with cytostatic antimetabolites, also activate TP53.

A further set of mechanisms controls the activation of TP53 upon inappropriate cell proliferation. The relationship is in fact intricate. In many cells that enter the cell cycle, the TP53 gene is more strongly transcribed. This may be regarded as a kind of precautionary measure providing sufficient TP53 for proper checkpoint function. The activity of TP53 is limited during normal cell cycles through phosphorylation of its C-terminal domain by G1 and G2 CDKs and by the cell-cycle dependent casein kinase II. Moreover, TP53 accumulation is prevented by transport out of the nucleus, poly-ubiquitination and degradation mediated by HDM2. Phosphorylation of TP53 as a consequence of DNA damage overcomes these restraints. Similarly, checkpoint failures, e.g. incomplete replication noticed at the G2→M boundary, activate checkpoint-dependent kinases such as CHK1 and CHK2 which also phosphorylate the TP53 N-terminus blocking HDM2 interaction and alleviating the effects of inhibitory phosphorylation. Defects in the RB1-dependent restriction point at the G1→S boundary, caused e.g. by oncogenic MYC or RAS, lead to increased transcription of $p14^{ARF1}$ which blocks HDM2 and thereby increases TP53 activity and concentration.

There are also several different pathways downstream of the TP53 node. TP53 induces cell cycle inhibitors, prominently $p21^{CIP1}$ in G1 and 14-3-3σ in G2 which block the cell cycle. The extent of TP53 activation is, of course, limited by its induction of HDM2. It seems that induction of apoptosis by TP53 through the intrinsic and extrinsic pathway is induced in a competitive fashion to cell cycle inhibition. So, the outcome of TP53 activation may not only depend on its extent, but also on the circumstances of a cell that determine whether cell cycle arrest or apoptosis are first in place, each preventing the other. One can imagine, e.g., that a cell with strong expression of apoptotic inhibitors like BCL2 may undergo cell cycle arrest, while a cell that is exposed to ligands of TNFRSF receptors which are induced by TP53 may undergo apoptosis. Importantly, cell cycle arrest induced by TP53 may often be irreversible and take the form of '*replicative senescence*'.

The fate of a cell in response to TP53 is also determined by the activity of several other '*cancer pathways*'. Many of these interactions are known, but not all are understood. So, increased activity of ERK and JNK MAPK pathways tends to activate TP53. Similar, increased activity of the WNT pathway in colon cancer and particularly in liver cancer appears to be incompatible with intact TP53 over a longer period. Conversely, activation of the PI3K and NFκB pathways in cancers tends to counteract the effects of TP53. In the case of the PI3K pathway, this may be due to the activation of HDM2/MDM2 by AKT and to increased '*survival signaling*' at large which may compensate for decreased signaling by survival factors caused by TP53. Among others, TP53 strongly induces IGFBP3, a secreted protein that binds and sequesters IGFs. As IGFs act largely through the PI3K pathway, autonomous activation of this pathway, e.g. by loss of PTEN function, will obliterate this branch of TP53 action. While this change will diminish the proapoptotic effect of TP53, AKT phosphorylation of $p21^{CIP1}$ moderates the influence of TP53 on growth arrest. So, overactivity of the PI3K pathway will limit the effects of TP53 activation on cell growth and survival. In comparison, overactivity of the NFκB pathway found in many cancers is expected to more selectively impede apoptosis induced by TP53. The induction of antiapoptotic proteins like BCL-X_L and IAPs may be a key element in this protective effect. AKT also phosphorylates and activates NFκB factors.

Finally, the targets of activated TP53 include genes involved in cellular metabolism, in the shaping of the extracellular matrix and of angiogenesis. This facet of TP53 action would be expected to counteract the effects that tumor cells exert on their environment.

The diverse effector functions of TP53 thus relate to typical aspects of the tumor phenotype, in a surprisingly consistent one-to-one fashion. Conversely, TP53 is activated as a consequence of a diverse set of aberrations which have the common denominator of potentially leading to cancer. These relationships explain why the TP53 network has such a strongly nodal character. As a consequence, loss of TP53 as such is the most common alteration in the network observed in human cancers and perhaps the most common alteration overall. Alterations in its immediate regulators like HDM2 and $p14^{ARF1}$ are still relatively frequent. Loss of function of the protein kinase activators which activate TP53 such as ATM or CHK1 is found in hereditary diseases associated with an increased predisposition to cancer, but more rarely in sporadic cancers. This may mean that the most crucial property of TP53 in established cancers is its ability to respond to hyperproliferation. Alterations in the effectors downstream of TP53 may not have the same impact as TP53 loss itself. Where they occur, they appear to target primarily effectors of TP53 induced apoptosis. So, mutations of BAX and promoter hypermethylation of APAF1 and other presumed apoptotic mediators of TP53 are found in some cancers. Hypermethylation also inactivates 14-3-3σ which is involved in G2 arrest induced by TP53, but this protein has additional functions.

Signaling by TGFβ Factors

The TGFβ superfamily of growth factors comprises ≈30 members with diverse functions. For instance, members of the family such as mullerian inhibitory factor or bone morphogenetic proteins (BMPs) shape tissues during development. In the context of cancer, TGFβ1 has drawn the main interest, as it is a potent growth inhibitory factor for epithelial cells and because mutations in the pathway that relays TGFβ signals in the cell are frequent during the progression of many carcinomas. TGFβ1 is also an inhibitory factor for many cells of the immune system. In contrast, it stimulates the proliferation of many mesenchymal cell types. This last property had originally led to the designation '*transforming growth factor*', because the EGF-like TGFα and TGFβ cooperate to stimulate anchorage-independent growth of mesenchymal cells in culture, which is an indication of a transformed phenotype.

In carcinoma tissues, not only the loss of response to TGFβ in the tumor cell, but also the effects on immune and mesenchymal cells are significant. TGFβ produced by carcinoma cells or liberated from preprotein forms bound to the extracellular matrix inhibits the immune response against the cancer, while stimulating stromal cells to proliferate and to lay down extracellular matrix on which the carcinoma can extend its growth. This relationship may explain why defective responses to TGFβ often portent the onset of invasion and metastasis in the course of carcinoma development. In particular, the ability of carcinoma cells to secrete or activate TGFβ for other cells while being themselves unresponsive to its growth-inhibitory effect helps to establish an environment favorable for the establishment and expansion of metastases, e.g. in prostate cancers.

The main intracellular pathway for TGFβ signaling is surprisingly straightforward. The growth factor associates with receptor type II at the cell membrane to form a trimeric complex with receptor type I. Receptor type I becomes phosphorylated and is itself activated as a serine/threonine kinase. It phosphorylates SMAD2 or SMAD3 proteins which are presented by the SARA protein at the inner face of the cell membrane. The phosphorylated SMADs are set free and heterodimerize with SMAD4. Together they are transported into the nucleus where they activate or repress various genes. SMAD factors are not very potent transactivators and their action is strongly dependent on the interaction with other transcription factors binding in their vicinity. This may partly explain why their action is context-dependent and different among various cell types. Activation of the pathway is counteracted by the inhibitory SMADs, SMAD6 and SMAD7. These are encoded by genes induced by TGFβ or BMP signaling, leading to a feedback inhibition. SMAD2 and SMAD3 are categorized as R-SMADs, 'R' denoting receptor-regulated. Further R-SMADS, SMAD1,5, and 8 are activated by distinct receptors for BMPs, which otherwise function in the same manner. Signaling through the pathway can be down-regulated by ERK and JNK kinases which phosphorylate R-SMADs. Conversely, MAPK pathways are also activated by some members of the TGFβ receptor family. Further cross-talk takes place between TGFβ signaling and the canonical WNT pathway. In general, these pathways tend to inhibit each other.

Loss of responsiveness to TGFβ in carcinomas can be brought about by alterations at several steps of the pathway. They include receptor mutations, loss of R-SMADs or Co-SMADs by deletions or their inactivation by mutation. Such alterations are, e.g., observed in invasive colon carcinomas or in metastatic prostate carcinomas.

Signaling Through STAT Factors

Signaling through STAT factors in human cancers can also have quite different consequences. As in SMAD factor signaling, this is partly due to varying and '*context-dependent*' effects of the >7 different STAT factors in different cell types. In cells of the hematopoetic system, STAT signaling pathway promotes cell proliferation in response to interleukins and other cell-type specific growth factors and cytokines, e.g. GM-CSF and erythropoetin. STAT signaling is also activated in epithelial cells as one of several pathway in the action of growth factors such as EGF and the cytokine IL-6 as wells as by protein kinases relaying adhesion signals, such as SRC, and of activated ABL kinase. STAT factors also mediate interferon effects. So, in hematological cancers, constitutive activation of STAT signaling is a common finding, e.g. in chronic myelogenic leukemia. Here, STAT5 is the major factor involved. In some carcinomas as well, activation of STAT pathways is found, e.g. in squamous cell carcinomas of the head and neck as a consequence of overexpression of the EGFR prevalent in this cancer type. Here, STAT3 may be the most relevant member of the family. In other carcinomas, STAT signaling appears to be actively repressed, likely in conjunction with the inhibition of the cellular response to interferons. The down-regulation mainly concerns STAT1.

The STAT signaling pathway is similarly straightforward as the SMAD pathway. Like R-SMADs, STATs are phosphorylated at the cell membrane and travel to the nucleus to act as transcriptional activators. Upon binding of their ligand, many cytokine receptors, e.g. the IL-6 receptor gp130, begin to recruit janus kinases (JAK1 or JAK2) which phosphorylate the receptor protein at tyrosine residues. These phosphotyrosines serve as the binding sites for the SH2-domain of the various STAT proteins, predominantly STAT1, STAT3, or STAT5. Upon binding to the receptor/JAK complex, the STAT factors also become activated by phosphorylation. The phosphorylated factors homo- or heterodimerize and travel to the nucleus to bind to specific recognition sites in gene promoters. A typical binding sequence for STAT factors is the GAS element mediating γ-interferon (IFNγ) responses; the slightly different ISRE elements respond to IFNα/β. Like SMAD factors, STAT proteins are not strong transcriptional activators and usually combine with other factors binding to neighboring sequences for efficient transcriptional activation. Among the STAT target genes are those encoding SOCS factors which act as JAK inhibitors and contribute to termination of STAT signals. This termination is supported by dephosphorylation through SHP protein phosphatases. The activity of STAT factors is moreover cross-regulated by protein kinases of the MAPK and PI3K pathways.

Constitutive activation of STAT pathways in hematological cancers is achieved by several mechanisms. In some leukemias STAT factors are part of fusion proteins, in others they are indirectly activated by other fusions events such as the formation of the BCR-ABL protein. Inactivation of SOCS genes, e.g. by promoter hypermethylation, may compound such changes. This change is accordingly also found in carcinomas with constitutive STAT activation resulting from receptor tyrosine kinase activation. In contrast, in some other carcinomas, expression of STAT factors, specifically STAT1, is down-regulated, perhaps as cells become unresponsive to the growth-inhibitory effects of interferons.

NFκB Pathway

Similar to the STAT pathway, the NFκB pathway is not unambiguously a pathway whose activation promotes cancer, and like the STAT pathway, it has different functions in hematopoetic compared to other cell types. The primary functions of the NFκB pathway are the regulation of activation of lymphoid cells, of inflammation and of apoptosis. However, in some cell types, it is also involved in the regulation of cell proliferation, specifically in response to cytokines.

The designation NFκB means nuclear factor regulating the expression of the Ig kappa chain in B cells. NFκB factors are heterodimeric transcription composed of a larger REL subunit and a smaller p50 or p52 subunit. The REL subunits comprise RELA, RELB and c-REL. RELA is the most abundant and widespread of these and therefore commonly known as p65. It is also the strongest transcriptional activator. RELA and c-REL form heterodimers with p50, which is derived from a larger p105 precursor. These heterodimers are normally retained in the cytoplasm by a protein inhibitor IκB. RELB associates with the precursor of the p52 subunit, p100, which also contains an inhibitory domain similar to IκBs. In this fashion, the RELB-pre-p52 complex is also retained in the cytoplasm.

Activation of the transcription can be elicited by different signals, including reactive oxygen species like singlet oxygen and other types of cellular stress, and in a more controlled fashion by cytokine receptors. In lymphoid cells, these would be receptors for interleukins or co-receptors for activation. In macrophages, they could be receptors for cytokines or bacterial lipopolysaccharides acting through toll-like-receptors. Activation of NFκB factors in many cell types is also typically elicited by receptors of the TNFRSF family which regulate apoptosis, and this activation modulates the efficiency of the response. Cytokine actions on epithelial cells also involve NFκB factors in addition to STAT factors and cross-talk with MAPK pathways.

The two different types of cytosolic complexes are activated by two similar mechanisms. A multiprotein complex which contains the IKK protein kinase phosphorylates the inhibitory subunit, which in the case of the p65/p50 complex permits immediately transport into the nucleus. In the case of RELB/p52, additional phosphorylation by the NIK protein kinase contained in the complex initiates the proteolytic removal of the inhibitory domain of the p52 pre-protein, and the complex can enter into the nucleus.

Four kinds of target genes of NFκB factors can be distinguished. (1) As in STAT and TGFβ responses, feedback inhibitors are induced, in this case IκB proteins. (2) A limited but illustrous set of regulators of cell proliferation are induced, prominently MYC and Cyclin D1. (3) A much larger set of proteins is induced that modulate apoptosis. Most, like BCL-X_L and FLIP are anti-apoptotic, while others like the FAS receptor and its ligand (CD95 and CD95L) are pro-apoptotic. (4) An even wider set of proteins is induced in immune cells, but also non-immune cells that relate to immune function and particularly inflammation. These comprise proteins for cell-cell communication, e.g. adhesion molecules, chemokines, and cytokines, but also factors involved in specific or unspecific immune responses. Specifically, NFκB factors are the main mediators of the induction of the inducible nitrogen oxide synthase (iNOS) and of cyclooxygenase 2 (COX2), which contribute to the burst in oxidative radicals in immune defense, but also in inflammation.

This last function of the NFκB pathway may perhaps be the most problematic during carcinogenesis. Activity of the pathway is a requirement for inflammation and specifically for chronic inflammation. So, overactivity of the pathway is crucial in the development of cancers associated with chronic inflammation, and in some cases, is relatively specifically elicited by the pathogenetic agent, such as *Helicobacter pylori* in the stomach. Consequentially, agents that block activation of the pathway can diminish the extent of inflammation and prevent such cancers. Some commonly used non-steroidal anti-inflammatory drugs (NSAIDs) like acetylsalicylic acid (aspirin) inhibit the IKK.

Obviously, the antiapoptotic effect of NFκB factors is also problematic, if the pathway becomes constitutively activated in cancer cells. Normally, this antiapoptotic effect appears to be employed to select and protect lymphoid cells during immune defenses. So, translocations and amplifications of REL genes in various human lymphomas may act through this mechanism, but in these cells the pathway also tends to stimulate proliferation. The retroviral orthologue of the REL genes, v-rel is a potent oncogene causing leukemias and lymphomas.

The effect of NFκB activation in carcinomas is less well understood. Certainly, its effect on apoptosis may be relevant. Even the induction of the FAS ligand by these factors may be employed by the carcinoma cells for a counterattack against the immune system. However, NFκB could also influence proliferation, particularly in metastases. Some cancers may establish metastases in certain organs by becoming responsive to local growth factors, including chemokines and cytokines. For instance, breast and prostate cancers metastasize preferentially to bone by a sort of mimicry in which they assume some properties of osteoblasts or osteoclasts, including responsiveness to growth factors for these cells that act partly through NFκB. This is, however, only one part of a much more complex interaction.

Finally, the pathway is implicated in a human dominant cancer syndrome. The rare disease cylindromatosis is caused by inherited mutations in the *CYLD* gene at chromosome 16q. It behaves like a classical tumor suppressor gene. Mutations in the second allele lead to tumors of the hair follicles and sweat glands. The protein encoded by the *CYLD* gene is a component of the IKK protein complex. It appears to regulate the duration of the NFκB pathway activation by cytokines like TNFα by de-ubiquitination of a regulatory subunit of the TNF receptor complex. Treatment of the disease and tumor prevention is now attempted by inhibitors of the NFκB pathway.

Developmental Regulatory Systems as Cancer Pathways

As in adult tissues, signaling through MAPK and other pathways is involved in the regulation of cell proliferation, cell differentiation and apoptosis during ontogenetic development. However, the development of an embryo is, of course, neither a homeostatic replacement nor a simple expansion, but involves many decisions on the developmental fates of individual cells and of cell populations.

From the pluripotent cells in the epiblast, some are developed into primordial germ cells, while others form the germ layers which interact further to form tissues and organs. This requires again cell fate decisions as well as an excellent coordination between the expansion of more or less committed precursor populations by cell proliferation and their differentiation into temporally quiescent or terminally differentiated cells.

In many developing tissues, cells are set aside to form stem cell or precursor populations that allow a continuous supply of differentiated cells exerting specific tissue functions or at least a replenishment of the differentiated cell compartments after tissue damage. Many growth factors and signaling pathways discussed in the preceding part of the chapter are also involved in these processes, but several additional pathways function specifically in cell fate decisions and in the establishment of tissue stem cells and their regulation in adult tissues. Three of them have also become notorious in the context of human cancers. They are the WNT, the Hedgehog/SHH and the NOTCH pathways.

More than 20 factors belong to the WNT growth factor family in humans. They are ≈40 kDa proteins with >30% homology towards each other. The proteins are secreted after being being glycosylated and covalent linkage of a lipophilic moiety. Accordingly, the factors bind well to the extracellular matrix and stick to cell membranes, which restricts their diffusion. Therefore, they are limited to acting as paracrine or autocrine factors. During development, WNT proteins drive the expansion and morphogenesis of many different tissues, in particular of tubular and ductular epithelial structures in the kidney and the gut. Of course, WNT factors and pathways interact with others, e.g. with Hedgehog-dependent pathways in the development of the limbs. Individual WNT factors remain involved in the homeostasis of adult tissue and specifically seem to control stem cell compartments, e.g. in the gastrointestinal tract.

WNT factors are normally recognized by Frizzled receptor proteins (FZD) at the cell surface. There are again several of these that respond to different WNT factors. They are supported by specific LRP proteins (LRP5 and LRP6) which seem to recognize the lipid part of the WNTs and are counteracted by *secreted Frizzled related proteins* (SFRP). The FZD receptors may not only differ with respect to which WNT they bind, but also with respect to which intracellular pathways they stimulate. At least three different pathways are known, but only one is really well characterized. The decisive step in this pathway is the accumulation and activation of β-Catenin which is prevented by the coordinated action of several proteins including APC, Axin and GSK3β. This particular pathway is therefore called the WNT/β-Catenin or '*canonical*' WNT pathway. Its constitutive activation is crucial in the development of colon cancer. It is also important in other cancers, e.g. in hepatocellular carcinoma. Its deregulation is alternatively brought about by loss of function of negative regulators, such as APC or Axin or by oncogenic mutations activating β-Catenin. *APC* and *CTNNB1* (encoding β-Catenin) therefore behave as tumor suppressor and oncogene, respectively.

The WNT/Ca^{2+}. pathway involves activation of classical PKCs and other Ca^{2+}-dependent protein kinases. Its function is largely undefined, but it may promote cellular differentiation to a greater extent than the '*canonical*' pathway. The WNT/polarity pathway involves the small GTP-binding protein RHO and acts on the polarization of the cytoskeleton. It also leads to phosphorylation of JNK1 kinase and thus to cross-talk with this MAPK pathway. These two other pathways are little studied so far in the context of human cancers. Likewise, the significance of altered expression of WNT factors, of FZD receptors and of SFRP1 in several different types of human cancers is still under study. However, at least one instance of WNT factor activation by a retroviral insertion has been documented.

Somewhat comfortingly, there are only three Hedgehog proteins in man. They are *Sonic Hedgehog* (SHH), *Desert hedgehog* (DHH), and *Indian Hedgehog* (IHH). Like WNT factors, they act in a paracrine fashion; and as for WNTs, their diffusion is limited by a lipophilic modification, in this case covalent attachement of cholesterol. Hedgehog factors are perhaps best studied for their role in limb development, but they are certainly also crucial for the development of many other organs, as diverse as the brain and the prostate. Also like WNTs, they contribute to tissue homeostasis in fully grown humans and, in fact, are also implicated in the maintenance of stem cell populations. The most important factor in adult tissues is SHH. Hedgehog factors bind to smoothened receptors such as SMO1 and initiate their own intracellular signaling pathway which ultimately leads to the activation of GLI transcriptional activators. Activation of SMO1 is prevented by PTCH1. Perhaps unsurpringly, there is accumulating evidence of cross-talk between the SHH and WNT pathways inside the cell.

Constitutive activation of SHH signaling appears to lie at the core of several cancers with a precursor cell phenotype such as small cell lung cancer and basal cell carcinoma of the skin. This activation can alternatively be brought about by mutations in activating components, such as point mutations in SMO1 or - perhaps - overexpression of GLI transcription factors, or by inactivation of a negative regulatory component, usually PTCH1. So, these have to be regarded as oncogenes and tumor suppressors, respectively.

Like the WNT and SHH pathways, the NOTCH pathway was first encountered in Drosophila and has been more extensively studied for its function in development in model organisms than in humans. It is now firmly established as a cancer pathway in man, and is also considered to factor in the neurological Alzheimer degenerative diseases. The emerging consensus is that both disruption and overactivity of the NOTCH pathway can promote cancer development. This ambiguity is not entirely unprecedented for cancer pathways, since the TGFβ and STAT pathways, e.g., act differently in different cell types. In the case of NOTCH signaling, its ambivalence is related to its pronounced dosage sensitivity which derives from its biological function.

Like the WNT and SHH pathways, the NOTCH pathway also controls stem and precursor cell compartments. More precisely, its characteristic function is the regulation of binary cell fate decisions. This includes the decision of whether a cell remains a tissue precursor or goes on to differentiate, such as in the basal layer of the epidermis. NOTCH signaling is also involved in decisions like whether a differentiating intestinal cell becomes an enterocyte or a secretory Paneth or goblet cell or whether a cell in the lymphocyte lineage enters the T-cell or B-cell sub-lineage. In system theory, this kind of decision is called a bifurcation and its control requires a metastable equilibrium which develops towards either of two opposite states upon slight perturbations, like a coin standing on its edge. This comparison describes the kind of function provided by the NOTCH signaling system.

Four different NOTCH receptors, NOTCH1-4, are known, and are expressed on the cell surface. They are activated by ligands expressed on the cell surface of neighboring cells. Two different kinds of ligands are known. In humans, they comprise the three '*delta-like*' DLL1, DLL3, and DLL4 and the '*jagged-like*' JAG1 and JAG2 ligands. These ligands differ somewhat in the response they elicit and more substantially in their sensitivity towards modification of NOTCH receptors by FRINGE glycosylases. These elongate glycosyl chains on NOTCH receptors that prevent binding of JAG, but not of DLL proteins.

Importantly, expression of NOTCH receptors and their ligands is each self-reinforcing and cross-inhibitory and therefore tends to become mutually exclusive. Thus within an organized tissue, different types of cells express either receptors or specific ligands. A precursor cell population, e.g., may express a receptor, while cells that have taken a step towards differentiation express a ligand, or the other way round. The latter situation is found, e.g., in human epidermis, where basal cells express NOTCH ligands and cells in upper, differentiated layers express NOTCH1.

NOTCH receptors are heterodimers formed by proteolytic cleavage from a single precursor. The protease involved is the γ-secretase presenilin whose dysfunction is one cause of Alzheimer disease. The extracellular domain of NOTCH binding the ligands on neighboring cells contains EGF-like repeats and a cystein-rich domain termed LN. The second subunit remains bound to it by a small extracellular domain, continues through the membrane into its larger intracellular segment. This segment contains ankyrin repeats, which mediate protein-protein interactions, a nuclear localization signal, a transcriptional transactivation domain, and a PEST sequence likely responsible for regulated proteolytic degradation.

Following activation by ligands, the intracellular NOTCH domain (sometimes called TAM) becomes free to move into the nucleus, where it replaces repressor proteins from the CBF1 transcription factor (also known by multiple other names such as CSL or RBJ1) to activate its target genes. Activation of NOTCH receptors additionally elicits CSL-independent events which are not as well elucidated. NOTCH target genes appear to be different in different cell types. Thus, in neuronal precursors NOTCH signaling inhibits expression of neuron-specific genes. In keratinocyte precursors, it induces differentiation markers and the p21^{CIP1} CDK inhibitor causing cell cycle arrest. NOTCH signaling often inhibits WNT/β-Catenin, SHH and AP1 signaling, and, conversely, supports NFκB activation.

As would be expected from its function in normal epidermis, NOTCH receptors appear to function as tumor suppressors in this organ. Down-regulation of NOTCH1 and NOTCH2 is a regular finding in basal cell carcinoma, although the extent to which it contributes to this tumor is debated. As NOTCH signaling inhibits the SHH pathway, its loss may exacerbate the overactivity of this pathway that causes this type of cancer. Similarly, loss of NOTCH function may be a prerequisite for formation of small cell lung cancers, which also show activation of the SHH pathway, likely by an autocrine mechanism. In this case, NOTCH activity appears to prevent the precursor cells from adopting the neuroendocrine, '*stem-cell like*' phenotype displayed by these cancers.

In other cancers, NOTCH proteins undoubtedly function as oncogenes. One type of T-cell acute leukemias (T-ALL) is characterized by a translocation between chromosome 7 and chromosome 9, t(7;9) (q34;q34.3), which leads to the overexpression of the cytoplasmic domain of NOTCH1 under the influence of the T-cell receptor β enhancer. Constitutively active NOTCH signaling appears to direct an inappropriately large fraction of lymphocyte precursors towards a T-cell fate where they become malignant by further mutations. In a similar fashion, NOTCH overactivity appears to cooperate with viral oncoproteins such as the SV40 T-antigen in mesothelioma and HPV E6 and E7 in genital cancers. Here, the inhibitory effect of NOTCH signaling on the cell cycle is abrogated by the viral oncoproteins whereas its precursor cell maintenance function remains active and contributes to expansion of the tumor.

11

Cancer of White Blood Cells

Leukemias and lymphomas are cancers arising from cells of the hematopoetic lineage (hence: *hematological cancers*). Leukemias originate from hematopoetic stem cells or cells at different stages of myeloid or erythroid differentiation which spread throughout the body. Lymphomas also develop from more differentiated lymphoid cells in lymphoid organs and may present as localized cell masses. Hematological cancers can be classified by their derivation from erythroid, myeloid, or lymphoid cells at specific stages of development as determined by their morphology and by protein markers.

Hematological cancers are also often characterized by recurrent chromosomal aberrations, which in their initial stages may represent the only evident genetic change. These aberrations also comprise chromosome gains and losses, but specific translocations are most distinctive. Translocations cause hematological cancers by either of two mechanisms. They activate a proto-oncogene by destroying its negative regulatory elements and/or by placing it under the influence of activating enhancers or they fuse two genes from the translocation sites that yield fusion proteins with novel properties. Either way, the gene product from the translocation site drives tumor development. During tumor progression, such as during the blast crisis of chronic myelogenous leukemias, further genetic and epigenetic changes accumulate, as commonly seen in carcinomas.

Chronic myelogenous leukemia (CML) is a disease of hematopoetic stem cells characterized by hyperproliferation of often immature cells of the myeloid, megakaryocytic and erythroid lineages. Its diagnostic chromosomal change is the '*Philadelphia chromosome*' resulting from a translocation between chromosomes 9 and 22 that creates the BCR-ABL fusion gene. The gene product is a fusion protein that retains the protein kinase activities of both original proteins, but is deregulated and mislocalized to the cytosol. There, the BCR-ABL protein activates several signaling pathways that promote cell proliferation, block apoptosis and decrease cell adhesion, thereby blocking maturation and causing release of immature cells into the blood. After several years, CML turns into blast crisis, a rapidly lethal disease resembling acute leukemias. This progression is promoted by interference of the BCR-ABL protein with the control of genomic stability. The acute phase of the disease is characterized by more pronounced chromosomal instability, with loss of tumor suppressors such as TP53 and $p16^{INK4A}$.

CML is treated by interferon therapy, chemotherapy and allogeneic stem cell transplantation. An important component of current therapy is a specific inhibitor of the ABL kinase, imatinib, which represents one of the great successes of molecular cancer research. Cytogenetic and molecular methods which detect the BCR-ABL translocation are helpful in diagnosis and in monitoring of treatment.

The efficacy of interferon therapy and allogeneic stem cell transplantation in CML have implications extending beyond this specific disease. They suggest that tumor cells can be recognized and kept under control through surveillance by the immune system. Highly sensitive molecular methods corroborate this assumption by proving the presence of Philadelphia chromosomes in healthy humans.

Burkitt lymphoma (BL) is an aggressive cancer derived from B-lymphocytes endemic in certain tropical areas of the world, and sporadically occuring in immuno-compromised individuals. These lymphomas have an extremely high proliferation rate which is not compensated by a high rate of apoptosis. Three alternative, diagnostic chromosomal aberrations invariably bring the *MYC* proto-oncogene on chromosome 8q24.1 under the influence of immunoglobulin gene enhancers from chromosome 14 (major translocation), 22, or 2 (minor translocations). Often, these translocations also destroy negative regulatory elements constraining this potent oncogene. MYC activity can be further augmented by point mutations.

Epstein Barr Virus (EBV), present in a few cells in most humans, but in the majority of BL clones, acts as a cofactor in this disease, perhaps by decreasing apoptosis. Additional genetic alteration in BL that diminish apoptosis severely aggravate the disease by counteracting the tendency of MYC to induce apoptosis in addition to cell growth. Beyond chemotherapy and stem cell transplantation, no specific treatment is available for BL.

In contrast, *promyelocytic leukemia* (PML), an *acute leukemia* (hence also: APL), is an example for successful targeted molecular therapy. It arises most often from a translocation involving chromosomes 15 and 17, t(15;17) (q22;q21), that creates a fusion protein from the nuclear coordinator PML and the retinoic acid receptor α (RARα). The fusion protein blocks differentiation and apoptosis of partially differentiated myeloid cells from which the tumor is derived. Unlike RARα, it does not respond to physiological levels of retinoic acid. Fortunately, pharmacological doses of retinoic acid activate the fusion protein, eliciting tumor differentiation and apoptosis. This '*differentiation therapy*' is not efficacious in cases of PML caused by fusion of RARα with the chromatin repressor PLZF. However, since PLZF acts by recruiting histone deacetylases, combined treatment with retinoids and histone deacetylase inhibitors may be possible. PML illustrates the importance of chromatin alterations in the development of human cancers and the therapeutic potential of understanding tumor pathophysiology at the molecular level.

Common Properties of Hematological Cancers

Hematological cancers comprise leukemias and lymphomas which arise from the hematopoetic lineage. All cells in this lineage originate from stem cells which in humans, after birth, are located in the bone marrow, after residing in the liver during the most of the fetal period. Here, stromal cells and an appropriate extracellular matrix support stem cell maintenance and help to regulate differentiation. Hematopoetic stem cells in the bone marrow and circulating in the blood can be identified by their expression of the surface antigen CD34.

The first step of differentiation of the rare pluripotent hematopoetic stem cells distinguishes the lymphoid lineage and the myeloid/erythroid lineage and leads to a larger population of '*committed*' progenitor cells. The lineages split further and lead to the various types of differentiated cells such as the B-cell and T-cell subtypes in the lymphoid branch, as well as the erythrocytes and platelets (*erythroid* and *megakaryocytic lineage*) and mast cells, granulocytes, monocytes and macrophages (myeloid lineage).

Proliferation and differentiation of hematopoetic cells are directed and controlled by a panoply of growth factors present in the bone marrow environment, and intracellularly by networks of lineage- and cell-type transcription factors. In each branch of the lineage, the options for differentiation are progressively restricted and cells become more and more committed towards a specific fate. In parallel, as a rule, their proliferative potential becomes more and more restricted, most obvious in case of erythrocytes which even lose their nuclei. Especially the later stages of differentiation in the myeloid and erythroid lineages are characterized by a tight coupling between differentiation and loss of proliferative potential, so that the number of cells produced is limited. For cancers to arise in this lineage, this dependency must be broken or the stimuli must be mimicked. Moreover, since differentiation diminishes proliferative potential, a carcinogenic change must block or at least substantially diminish the rate of cell differentiation.

The relationship between proliferation and differentiation is somewhat different in the lymphoid lineage since mature lymphocytes still remain competent for proliferation in response to infections. Their multiplication, however, is normally dependent on stimulation by antigens and by paracrine factors, mostly cytokines. Moreover, when an infection abates, lymphocyte numbers are restrained by apoptosis and only memory cells survive for longer periods. Controlled apoptosis is also involved in the selection procedure against self-reactive lymphocytes. Thus, cancers in the lymphoid lineage can arise not only in immature cells by failure along the path to differentiation, but also in differentiated cells by acquired independence of external proliferation stimuli or by evasion of apoptosis, or in the worst case both.

The phenotype of individual leukemias and lymphomas is therefore strongly dependent on which stage in which lineage is primarily affected. A hematological cancer may be derived from a stem cell such as in chronic myelogenous leukemia, a partially differentiated cell as in acute promyelocytic leukemia, or a cell at an advanced stage of differentiation as in multiple myeloma (a B-cell lymphoma). The many different subtypes of B-cells and T-cells, in particular, with different functions and tissue distributions, can give rise to a large variety of lymphomas.

The name of a hematological cancer often indicates the dominant cell type. Obviously, the cell of origin cannot always be straightforwardly identified, because cancer cells deviate from the original cell. In many types of leukemias and lymphomas, only the introduction of molecular markers in the last decades has allowed to determine their cell of origin and, in more than a few cases, to recognize morphologically similar diseases as different entities. Molecular markers used for this purpose comprise surface antigens characteristic for lineages and differentiation stages as well as typical chromosomal aberrations. An identification as precise as possible is, of course, necessary to predict prognosis and to choose appropriate treatments.

Genetic Aberrations in Leukemias and Lymphomas

On average, leukemias and lymphomas contain fewer genetic aberrations than carcinomas. Very often, their karyotype is near-diploid with few chromosomes altered. Those aberrations that are present, however, are characteristic for the particular type of leukemia or lymphoma. Although chromosomal losses and gains are also found, many hematological cancers are characterized by typical translocations.

In some hematological cancers, these translocations are so characteristic that they allow to classify the disease accordingly. So, >90% of chronic myeloid leukemias contain a characteristic translocation between the long arms of chromosomes 9 and 22, t(9;22) (q34;q11). On the other hand, apparently similar diseases may result from disparate translocations. So, the same t(9;22) translocation is found in 25% of acute lymphoblastic leukemias as well. However, in this group of diseases, a variety of other translocations are found.

Unlike deletions such as those of 6q or 13q found in some leukemias, translocations do not simply destroy genes and their functions, but alter them. Two mechanisms can be distinguished.

1. The coding region of the gene at the translocation site remains intact, but its regulation is altered, since the translocation removes some of its own regulatory regions and/or brings the gene under the influence of novel regulatory elements. In most cases, this leads to ectopic or deregulated expression of a gene product acting as an oncogenic protein. Burkitt lymphoma with its translocations activating the MYC gene is a case in point. Another frequent translocation t(14;18) (q32;q21) leads to deregulation and overexpression of the anti-apoptotic regulator protein BCL2 in follicular lymphoma. Here, the *BCL2* locus is brought under the control of a heavy-chain immunoglobulin enhancer.
2. The translocation creates a fusion protein expressed from a novel gene formed from the segments of two genes flanking the translocation sites. The fusion protein may have a different expression pattern, intracellular localization, regulation, and activity (or a combination of these properties) compared to the original components. Not infrequently, the destruction of one or both original

genes also matters. Two examples out of many for this mechanism are the BCR-ABL fusion protein in chronic myeloid leukemia and the retinoic acid receptor fusion proteins in acute promyelocytic leukemia.

The characteristic translocations are causally involved in the development of each specific cancer subtype. An impressive illustration of this relationship is found in *acute myeloid leukemia* (AML). Translocations in AML often interrupt the genes encoding transcription factors involved in the differentiation of myeloid cells, such as that encoding C/EBPα, and create fusion protein, which instead of activating target genes repress them. Some cases lack these characteristic translocations. In these, point mutations in the *CBPA* gene have been found which lead to a truncated protein that acts as a dominant-negative inhibitor of the protein expressed from the remaining intact allele.

AMLs belong to those hematological cancers that behave quite heterogeneously in the clinic. The course of the disease and the response to therapy can to a certain degree be predicted from the type of translocation (or *mutation*) present. In general, determining the characteristic translocations in a leukemia or lymphoma is very helpful in the diagnostis and treatment of the disease.

It is not entirely clear, which further genetic changes in addition to the typical translocations are present in the initial stages of leukemias and lymphomas and to what extent they are required for their development. Certainly, however, many leukemias and lymphomas progress to a state of more generalized genomic instability with aneuploid karyctypes, additional point mutations and changes in DNA methylation. Genes affected at this stage also comprise some of the oncogenes and tumor suppressors important in carcinomas, such as *RAS* genes, *S TP53*, *RB1*, *CDKN2A*, and also *CDKN2B*. This genomic instability not only confers a more aggressive character, but also presents a significant obstacle to chemotherapy by allowing the development of resistant cell clones, e.g. through point mutations or gene amplification.

Molecular Biology of Burkitt Lymphoma

Burkitt lymphoma (BL) is an aggressive malignancy consisting of highly proliferative B-cells which infiltrate lymph nodes and other organs. The tumor cells are distinguished as B-cells by their expression of IgM and κ or λ light chains and by specific surface markers such as CD19 and CD20. The high proliferative rate is obvious from numerous mitotic figures. Staining for markers such as Ki67 or PCNA, which are characteristic of cycling cells, shows that almost all tumor cells are participating in proliferation. The rapid proliferation in this cancer is only partly compensated by a high apoptotic rate, evident most straightforwardly from interspersed macrophages phagocytosing the apoptosed tumor cells.

BL was first described as a tumor in young people in equatorial Africa where it is endemic in some regions. It is much rarer in Europe and North America, although more frequent in the context of AIDS and in other immunocompromised patients. In tropical areas, most BLs harbor *Epstein-Barr virus* (EBV), which is not as consistently associated with the disease in countries of the temperate zones. Treatment by chemotherapy and stem cell transplantation12 can be successful in some cases.

The three characteristic translocations in BL all involve the *MYC* locus at 8q24.1. The most frequent, 'major' translocation joins the gene to the *IGH* locus at 14q32 which encodes the immunoglobulin heavy chain. The 'minor' translocations involve the *IGL* (Igλ) locus at 22q11 or the *IGK* (Igκ) locus at 2p12. These loci encode the two immunoglobulin light chains, either of which can be used in B cells. One of these three translocations is found in each case of BL. The diagnosis of BL therefore is made contingent on their presence. The converse is not true, i.e. these translocations are also found in other lymphomas, all of which are also aggressive.

In each translocation, the MYC gene is brought under the influence of an immunoglobulin gene enhancer which is strongly active at this stage of B-cell differentiation. BL is thus an important example of the gene activation mechanism by translocations. The translocations in BL result in deregulation and overexpression of a potent oncogene, which normally ought to become down-regulated in mature B-cells. While the overall result is the same, the mechanisms leading to deregulation differ in detail between the various translocations.

In most major translocations, the translocation breakpoint lies at some distance upstream of the *MYC* gene, which remains intact. The translocated *IGH* locus is *H* oriented in inverse orientation, with the enhancer positioned towards the *MYC* gene. This configuration appears to result in a '*classical*' enhancer activation mechanism, in which the strong enhancer activates the unchanged MYC promoters.

In some of the major translocations, the breakpoints are located in the first intron of the *MYC* gene, so that the first exon with the P1 and P2 promoters is removed. The gene is transcribed from the otherwise '*cryptic*' (i.e. unused) P3 promoter located in the first intron. In this configuration, all elements in the *MYC* upstream region controlling transcription are deleted. Specifically, the translocation inactivates an attenuation mechanism in the first intron which makes transcription of the gene contingent on continuous stimulation. In these translocations, the placement of the *IGH* enhancer next to the gene does not seem to be absolutely essential for *MYC* activation, but the presence of an active *IGH* gene is required, perhaps to guarantee an open chromatin structure.

In the minor translocations, the breakpoints are located downstream of the *MYC* gene, sometimes at a considerable distance (>100 kb). The regulatory regions of the *MYC* gene remain largely intact, with the possible exception of a negative regulatory element presumed to lie downstream of the gene. The light chain loci are located in inverse orientation with their downstream enhancers oriented towards MYC. These seem to be mainly responsible for driving MYC over-expression. In the *IGK* locus, further elements may contribute, including an intronic enhancer.

In all translocations, the translocated *MYC* gene becomes susceptible to mutations that augment the effects of the enhancers. In translocations retaining the *MYC* regulatory regions, point mutations are found which inactivate negative regulatory elements in exon 1 and the first intron, thereby exacerbating overexpression. In all translocations, mutations are also found in the N-terminal coding region of MYC. In general, these stabilize the protein. For instance, a common mutation in Thr58 prevents a regulatory phosphorylation that targets the gene for proteosomal degradation. Interestingly, an according mutation is also common in the v-myc oncogenes of retroviruses.

The genetic alterations at the *MYC* locus found in Burkitt lymphoma can be understood as accidents during the maturation of B-cells. During the differentiation of B-cells, V(D)J recombination of the *IGH* and either *IGL* or *IGK* immunoglobulin genes is employed to generate the antibody repertoire necessary for the immune response to many different antigens. Later, a further recombination event accompanies the switch from expression of IgM to that of IgG. Furthermore, in the germinal centers of the lymphoid organs, somatic hypermutation is directed to the rearranged immunoglobulin genes to generate additional antibody variants with higher affinities and improved specifity towards the encountered antigens. These processes are recognizable in BL, although deviant.

The RAG recombinases mediating V(D)J rearrangements recognize particular sequence motifs in the immunoglobulin genes which are found in the vicinity of the breakpoints in the translocated immunoglobulin genes, although not usually in the *MYC* gene. It is therefore possible that the translocations are initiated by the physiological introduction of double-strand breaks into the immunoglobulin genes by B-cell specific recombinases. By accident, these breaks are then wrongly connected to the *MYC* gene. Likewise, placement of the *MYC* gene into an immunoglobulin gene cluster may set it up as a target for somatic hypermutation. The accidents that initiate BL are likely to be very rare, even if favored by the unknown agents that cause endemic BL. However, activation of *MYC* provides a strong proliferation stimulus that may provide a large pool of cells from which the lymphoma arises, likely by further alterations that are less conspicuous than the translocations. Since BL is more frequent in immunocompromised individuals, an immune defense may exist which normally eliminates B cells with aberrantly rearranged immunoglobulin genes.

Activation of *MYC* to an oncogene accounts for many of the properties of BL cells. MYC stimulates many aspects of cell proliferation and cell growth. In particular, in many cell types overexpression of MYC is sufficient to maintain them active in the cell cycle, independent of growth factors. It may therefore account for the high proliferative fraction and rate in BL. MYC, through its action on telomerase, may also contribute to immortalization. Moreover, some proteins regulated by MYC are involved in cell adhesion, e.g. LFA-1 in lymphocytes. This may lead to altered interactions of BL cells with other immune cells.

The oncogenic potential of MYC is normally restrained by two factors. (1) The gene and the protein are tightly regulated by a variety of mechanisms which are subverted by the translocations and mutations in BL. (2) MYC is a strong inducer of apoptosis. This induction is, at least partly, mediated by induction of $p14^{ARF}$ by E2F1 which is a transcriptional target of MYC. $p14^{ARF}$ then blocks HDM2/MDM2 activating TP53 to elicit apoptosis. The high apoptotic rate found in BL suggests that a mechanism of this sort may indeed be active, but not sufficiently so as to compensate for the increase in proliferation.

It is therefore thought that the development of BL requires at least one further genetic alteration which limits apoptosis. Different recurrent genetic alterations, each observed in a fraction of BLs, may account for this requirement. About one third of all cases have mutations

Table 11.1. Effects of MYC on various cellular functions

Function	*Some proteins regulated by MYC*
Cell growth	↑ RNA polymerase, nucleolar proteins, ribosomal proteins, splice factors, eIF proteins, CAD, polyamine biosynthesis (ODC, spermidine synthase), chaperones,
Cell proliferation	↑ Cyclin D2, Cyclin B1, CDK4, CDC25A, E2F1, CUL1, hTERT ↓ $p21^{CIP1}$, $p27^{KIP1}$, MYC
Cell differentiation	↓ cell-type specific bHLH transcriptional activators, ID proteins
Metabolism	↑ LDH , PFK, enolase
Adhesion	↓ LFA1, PAI1
Apoptosis	↑ E2F1 ($p14^{ARF}$), BAX

in *TP53* and LOH at 17p, others have lost TP73, a related protein and a potential mediator of TP53-induced apoptosis. The *BCL6* gene at 3q27 is affected in BL, as well as in other B-cell lymphomas, by translocations and mutations, which may also stem from somatic hypermutation. The function of the transcriptional repressor BCL6 is probably specific to B-cells at a certain stage of differentiation in germinal centers. It is down-regulated during terminal differentiation. The various translocations, which are typically promoter substitutions, appear to keep the gene active beyond its time. Importantly, BCL6 does not stimulate cell proliferation, but influences the expression of specific B cell proteins and decreases apoptosis.

Since EBV is found in so many BL, it is tempting to speculate that this herpes virus may provide a complementary function to that of MYC in the development of this tumor. The relationship has, however, emerged as more roundabout. EBV occurs in >90% of all adults, but only in a fraction of B-cells. It is capable of immortalizing cells of this type. This ability is therefore used in the laboratory to generate permanent lymphoblastoid lines. The virus exists as an episome, whose maintenance and replication require minimally the expression of the EBNA-1 protein. In lymphoblastoid lines and in long-term infected cells *in vivo*, further genes are expressed which down-regulate apoptosis and help to avoid immune detection. These genes are obvious candidates for synergizing with MYC in BL, but most of them are more weakly expressed in the actual disease than normally. The EBER RNAs of the virus are also good candidates for cooperating with MYC. Conversely, there is evidence that strong MYC expression may support the maintenance of the virus.

Several alternative plausible explanations are therefore considered for the evident association of the virus with the disease. For instance, EBV-infected cells may be more susceptible to accidents during attempted V(D)J recombination or the BL cells may be initially protected from apoptosis and elimination by the immune system by EBV proteins, while later on the same functions would be provided by other alterations such as translocations or mutations of *BCL6*.

Molecular Biology of CML

Chronic myeloid leukemia (also: *chronic myelogeneous leukemia*, commonly abbreviated CML) is a moderately frequent leukemia occurring in adults, most often in their 40's or 50's. While its causes are in general unknown, it has been observed following exposure to high doses of ionizing radiation.

CML originates from hematopoetic stem cells. As a consequence, the production of many different cell types is increased overall and mature cells as well as progenitor cells of many or all hematopoetic lineages are present in the blood, prominently the myeloid cells for which the disease is named. Almost all cases are caused by one specific genetic alteration, a BCR-ABL fusion gene, usually present in an aberrant, smaller appearing chromosome 22 termed the Philadelphia chromosome.

If left untreated, CML continues over several years with rather unspecific symptoms, but then progresses through an accelerated phase into blast crisis in which highly aberrant leukemic cells kill the patient within months.

Until recently, CML was treated by chemotherapy and/or by interferon α (IFNα) which lead to hematological remission, i.e. a normalization of the cell distribution in blood, in about 70% of the cases. In 10% of the cases, '*cytogenetic*' remissions are achieved, i.e. no metaphases with Philadelphia chromosomes are detected in bone marrow aspirates. However, these treatments do not usually lead to a cure and the cancer recurs eventually.

A better chance of a cure is provided by allogeneic stem cell transplantation. Here, hematopoetic stem cells from an HLA-matched donor are transplanted. These provide normal cells necessary for function of the blood and immune system, but also generate an immune response towards the tumor. However, in some cases the immune cells from the bone marrow graft attack not only the tumor cells, but also normal tissues, leading to chronic or acute *graft-versus-host-disease* (GVHD), which can be lethal. Therefore, although better selection of donors supported by genotyping helps, stem cell transplantation remains risky.

Stimulation of an immune response against the tumor cells also appears to be responsible for the efficacy of IFNα in the treatment of CML. Like the increased incidence of Burkitt lymphoma in immunocompromised individuals, it points to a role of the immune system in prevention of cancer by some sort of immune surveillance. This effect can apparently be recruited for therapy in some cases. The evidence from CML for a tumor-specific immune surveillance is actually a bit stronger than that from BL, because a virus might be involved in the pathogenesis of the latter disease, so the immune response may actually be directed against an exogenous antigen. There is no evidence for an infectious agens in CML.

Many properties of CML can be explained as consequences of a single genetic change, i.e. the creation of the BCR-ABL gene by a translocation between chromosomes 9q34 and 22q11. The translocation creates a novel gene which expresses a fusion protein with properties different from those of the original genes.

In most cases of CML, the translocation is reciprocal and the resulting chromosomes 9q+ and 22q- (or Ph') are the only aberrations in the karyotype of many CML cells in the chronic phase. Of course, being balanced, the translocation creates two fusion genes, but for all we know only the *BCR-ABL* fusion is relevant. Here, the promoter of the *BCR* gene from chromosome 22 drives the expression of a fusion protein consisting of a large N-terminal region from BCR and most of the ABL protein originally encoded on chromosome 9. The breakpoints in *BCR* and *ABL* can be located in different exons leading to several different fusion genes and proteins of different molecular weights. They all, however, concur in retaining the serine/threonine kinase activity of BCR and the tyrosine kinase activity of ABL, while lacking domains that control the activities of these kinases in the original proteins. Moreover, the fusion proteins also localize primarily to the cytoplasm instead of to the nucleus. The functions of the normal BCR and ABL proteins are not overly well characterized. The ABL kinase is normally involved as a signaling molecule in DNA repair and apoptosis, interacting a.o with DNA-PK. Although the precise function is unclear, it is certainly not a growth-stimulatory protein. Of note, an abl gene has also been recruited by the Abelson leukemia virus as an oncogene. In this murine virus, the N-terminal domain of the cellular gene is replaced by a part of the viral gag protein.

The BCR-ABL fusion protein acts in a pleiotropic fashion changing the activity of several signaling pathways and protein complexes in the cell. It interferes with the control of proliferation, apoptosis, adhesion, and DNA repair. RAS is activated and the MAPK pathway stimulated by GRB/SOS binding to a phosphorylated tyrosine (Y177) in the BCR domain, which is generated by the activity of the ABL tyrosine kinase. This kinase also phosphorylates and activates JAK2 and thereby the STAT pathway which stimulates proliferation in the hematopoetic lineage. Phosphorylation of STAT5 may also contribute to inhibition of apoptosis. This effect may be enhanced by activation of PI3K which is otherwise inhibited by normal ABL.

An important factor in the pathogenesis of CML is decreased adhesion, which explains the appearance of hematopoetic precursors in blood. By being lost from their proper environment, the immature cells are removed from exposure to growth factors and interactions with the ECM of the bone marrow which guide their differentiation. Altered adhesion is caused by the misdirected activity of the ABL tyrosine kinase which in the cytosol is bound to actin and phosphorylates proteins that organize the cytoskeleton like paxillin and *focal adhesion kinase* (FAK). Integrin function is also impeded and CBL is activated leading to altered turnover of membrane proteins.

Moreover, there is evidence that BCR-ABL also interferes with DNA repair, acting largely in a fashion opposite to the normal ABL protein, i.e. down-regulating TP53 and ATM signaling. This last activity of the oncoprotein may tile the path towards progression of the disease to its accelerated phase and blast crisis.

If perhaps not the only genetic alteration in chronic phase CML, the formation of a *BCR-ABL* fusion gene is certainly a consistent event and likely obligatory. This is helpful in the diagnosis of the disease and even more for monitoring of its treatment. It also provides a clear target for therapeutic intervention.

Detection of BCR-ABL can be made by several techniques, with different sensitivities. Cytogenetically, the Ph' chromosome can be detected in metaphases or more sensitively by FISH (*fluorescence in situ hybridization*) showing a closed apposition of the normally separate genes in interphase nuclei. Molecular techniques are even more sensitive, especially detection of a fusion transcript by RT-PCR.

Prior to therapy, the billions of leukemia cells in the blood are obvious under the microscope. Following therapy, their number decreases and hematopoetic precursors disappear. This is called '*hematological remission*'. Unfortunately, it does not amount to a cure, because the cancer often recurs after some time, in CML after several years. Such patients harbor '*minimal residual disease*'. Indeed, cytogenetic methods often detect tumor cells in the bone marrow of patients with an apparent normalization of the cell numbers and composition in the blood. If this is not the case, one speaks of '*complete cytogenetic remission*'. However, even this does not signify a certain cure, because millions of descendents of the tumor stem cells in the bone marrow may remain hidden among the normal cells in the blood. Descendents of these cells are detectable by RT-PCR in peripheral blood samples. So, the notion of '*molecular remission*' has entered modern hematology denoting the situation in which even this sensitive method detects no more leukemia cells. CML patients with '*molecular remission*' are usually cured.

So, very sensitive methods have been developed which are capable of detecting very few cells with Ph' chromosomes. Surprisingly, they reveal their presence in persons without evidence of disease and no evidence of their numbers increasing. The interpretation of this finding is controversial. It may mean that a second genetic event is needed for CML development after all, or provide further evidence for successful immune surveillance.

The elucidation of the role of BCR-ABL in CML has also led to the development of a specific drug, an inhibitor of the ABL kinase, imatinib (STI-571, marketed under the name of '*Gleevec*' or '*Glivec*'). This drug has recently proven very efficacious against CML, inducing remissions even in blast crisis CML and used as first-line therapy in chronic phase patients. However, while remissions are long-lasting in a large proportion of chronic phase patients (the cure rate will only be ascertained after longer observation periods), resistant tumors develop in many acute phase patients. Importantly, the mechanisms underlying this resistance show that the target was well chosen. In some cases, the resistance is caused by point mutations in the ATP binding domain of the ABL kinase in the BCR-ABL fusion protein which diminishes the impact of the inhibitor. In other cases of resistance, the fusion gene has become amplified.

The different rates of resistance against imatinib in blast crisis patients vs. chronic phase patients illustrates the development of genomic instability during the progression of CML towards blast crisis. Blast crisis cells are aneuploid with multiple chromosomal aberrations including chromosomal losses, gains, further translocations and amplifications.

Among the genes affected by these changes are *RB1* and *TP53* as well as *CDKN2A* which are inactivated by gene loss, mutation or, in the case of *CDKN2A*, also by promoter hypermethylation. Loss of TP53 by mutation and deletion certainly contributes to resistance against chemotherapy in this disease, as in cancers in general. Another remarkable instance of hypermethylation is that of the remaining intact *ABL* gene, underlining the tumor suppressor function of the normal gene. In contrast, the *MYC* gene is over-expressed as a consequence of trisomy 8 or outright gene amplification in blast crisis, but not in the chronic phase.

Acute myeloid leukemias other than those developing from CML also display characteristic translocations that lead to fusion proteins. One of them is a t(3;21) event which creates the AML/EVI1 fusion gene and protein. This translocation is also prevalent in blast crisis leukemia developing from CML. Like MYC overexpression, it is thought to further stimulate proliferation, but also to exacerbate the block to differentiation, which is relatively weak in chronic CML. Finally, a typical indicator of the acceleration phase that precedes blast crisis is an increased copy number of the *BCR-ABL* gene itself, typically becoming evident as a duplication of the Ph' chromosome. Once again, this highlights the crucial importance of this genetic alteration in CML, even at its final stage.

Molecular Biology of Promyelocytic Leukemia

Promyelocytic leukemia is, like the final phase of CML, an acute leukemia and therefore alternatively abbreviated as APL or PML (or most systematically as AML M3). It is, however, not a disease of stem cells, but of cells from an intermediate stage of differentiation towards granulocytes, denoted promyelocytes. These cells are obviously arrested at this stage and continue to proliferate. Compared to CML, PML is a rare disease comprising only a fraction of all AML. Like CML, however, PML has become paradigmatic for the understanding of leukemias and beyond, primarily as an example of successful '*differentiation therapy*' and, more recently, of chromatin alterations in cancer.

A distinctive t(15;17) (q22;q21) translocation found in >90% of all PMLs fuses the *PML* gene at chromosome 15q22 to the *RARA* gene at 17q21. Variant translocations always include *RARA* as well, but fuse it to the *PLZF* (promyelocytic leukemia zinc finger) gene at 11q23, to the *NPM* (*nucleophosmin*) gene at 5q35, or *NUMA* (*nuclear matrix associated*) gene at 11q13.

This general involvement of the retinoic acid receptor RARα in PML translocations is striking, as already in the 1980's its ligand *all-trans retinoic acid* (ATRA) was found to induce often dramatic hematological remissions of PML. Responsiveness to ATRA is specific for PML, and not observed in other AMLs. PML also responds better to certain drugs which are more generally used in chemotherapy, such as anthracyclins. So, precise diagnosis is a prerequisite for optimal treatment of this disease. Moreover, as in CML, cytogenetic and molecular techniques are employed to monitor treatment, detect minimal residual disease and select patients for stem cell transplantation.

Both certain cytostatic drugs and ATRA are efficacious in PML, and are used in combination. Cytostatic drugs act through apoptosis and cell cycle arrest in PML, as in other leukemias. In contrast, ATRA relieves the block to differentiation in the disease, allowing terminal differentiation towards granulocytes, with a concomitant decrease in proliferation. Some degree of apoptosis also occurs. This type of treatment has therefore been called '*differentiation therapy*'.

The PML-RARα fusion protein in PML acts as an inhibitor of both proteins from which it originates. It may also have gained additional, novel functions. RARα, retinoic acid receptor α, belongs to a group of closely related receptors for retinoic acids which are part of the steroid hormone receptor superfamily. Retinoic acid is produced from vitamin A as a locally acting hormone regulating growth and differentiation of many tissues, prominently the skin, reproductive organs and some glands. Accordingly, the closely related RARβ and RARγ proteins are frequently inactivated in other cancers, e.g. RARβ in breast and prostate cancer.

The basic structure of RARα resembles that of steroid hormone receptors. An N-terminal transcriptional activation domain (AF-1) is followed by the DNA-binding domain, an hinge region, and the ligand binding domain (LBD) containing a second transcriptional activation function (AF-2), with a short C-terminal region. The LBD/AF-2 domain is the most crucial one in the protein, since the ligand bound in this region elicits heterodimerization and recruitment of transcriptional co-activators such as CBP in exchange for the co-repressor N-CoR/SMRT. The DNA-binding domain interacts with a specific recognition site in

DNA called RARE (*retinoic-acid responsive element*) which has the typical motif for steroid hormone receptor-like transcriptional activators, AGGTCA. RARE sites actually used consist of a direct repeat of this sequence separated by five arbitrary nucleotides. The second half-site is occupied by one of the more distantly related RXR receptors which form heterodimers with RARs, as they do with several other receptors of the superfamily. Binding of RAR to a gene promoter usually leads to opening of the chromatin structure by remodeling and histone acetylation as well as to transcriptional activation.

In hematopoesis, gene regulation by retinoic acid appears to be particularly important during granulopoesis at the stage of promyelocyte differentiation. At this differentiation step, growth-promoting genes such as *MYC* need to be down-regulated and inhibitors of the cell cycle such as $p21^{CIP1}$ must be up-regulated. The genes of transcription factors more specifically involved in myeloid differentiation such as C/EBPε and HOXA are also RARα targets. Most interestingly, the RARα gene is activated by its own product. This auto-regulatory loop may provide a crucial amplifying step for the signal that makes differentiation irreversible.

The PML protein, named after the disease, is normally localized in 10-30 '*PML nuclear bodies*', a subcompartment of the nucleus consisting of morphologically recognizable protein assemblies sized 0.2 - 1 μm. The assembly of ≈1,000,000 proteins in these nuclear bodies is dependent on PML which may be their principle organisator and regulator. The function of the nuclear bodies is not entirely clear.. Most likely, they act as a reservoir and interaction structure for proteins involved in response to cellular stress, DNA repair, apoptosis and chromatin structure. Proteins found to associate with PML and nuclear bodies include the proapoptotic DAXX protein, the Bloom syndrome helicase BLM, and TP53, but also the mRNA-cap-binding protein EIF-4E. Interestingly, formation and function of nuclear bodies may involve SUMOlation, i.e. covalent attachment of a SUMO protein to PML and other constituents. Another regulator of nuclear bodies is the JNK1 kinase. PML itself may then mediate the SUMOlation of other proteins, including TP53. The function of PML is reflected in its structure which contains several motifs involved in protein-protein interactions, such as a RING finger and a coiled domain.

The PML-RARα fusion protein retains most parts from both partners. PML mostly lacks its C-terminal Ser-Pro rich domain, while RARα lacks part of the AF-1 interaction domain. However, these changes suffice to turn the fusion protein into a transcriptional repressor at physiological concentrations of retinoic acids, and to destroy nuclear bodies and interfere with their function. Transcriptional repression may be aided by dimerization of the fusion protein which then binds to a dimeric RARE promoter site and recruits co-repressors to repress rather than activate genes crucial for myeloid differentiation.

Fortunately, the variant protein can still be turned into a transcriptional activator by micromolar concentrations of retinoic acid, i.e. at pharmacological concentrations, 100-1000-fold above the physiological level. In response to ATRA treatment, the co-repressors dissociate allowing transcription of the genes required for granulocyte differentiaton. The fusion protein itself is rapidly degraded following ATRA treatment, so transcription may also or even predominantly be promoted by normal RARα, which is itself induced during differentiation. Like the function of RARα, that of PML seems also to become restored as evidenced by reappearance of nuclear bodies.

The overall effect of ATRA treatment at the cellular level is differentiation towards a more mature granulocytic cell, with arrest of proliferation, but also significant apoptosis. Of note, the ensuing differentiated cells are no more cancerous, but are not normally functioning and can pose problems to the host. Moreover, retinoic acid at supraphysiological concentrations has some side-effects. So, while differentiation therapy is efficacious and may seem more elegant than chemotherapy, it is strenuous and dangerous to the patient.

Like the predominant type of PML caused by t(15;17) translocations, those with the variant t(5;17) and t(11q13;17) translocations respond to ATRA treatment. However, the rare t(11q23;17) translocation, which creates the PLZF- RARα fusion gene, does not. The difference lies in the fusion partner. PLZF is itself a transcriptional repressor capable of recruiting co-repressors and histone deacetylases. Therefore, in this fusion protein, not only is RARα locked in a repressor conformation, but also its fusion partner contributes to repression to at least the same extent. At least experimentally, however, it has been possible to still reactivate RARα by a combined treatment with ATRA and inhibitors of histone deacetylases. These may obliterate the repressor function of PZLF. As more and better such inhibitors become available, there seems to be a chance of successful treatment for patients with this translocation as well.

Finally, the obvious question is whether the RARα translocations are sufficient to induce PML. This cannot be definitely answered at present. Since vitamin A deficiency and other maladies that cause inefficient function of RARα only moderately affect granulopoesis, with at most a mild hyperplasia of promyelocytes, not only the loss of retinoic acid responsiveness, but the formation of the fusion protein is certainly crucial. Although the details are controversial, a function of PML in the regulation of apoptosis and replicative senescence is generally accepted. Moreover, the fusion protein obviously has a dominant-negative effect on at least some aspects of PML function. So, inhibition of differentiation and of apoptosis could well be oncogenic effects provided by the fusion protein. This leaves room for a genetic change that causes hyperproliferation. The best candidate for this is mutation of *FLT3*. The FLT3 protein is a receptor tyrosine kinase activated by the hematopoetic growth factor M-CSF which is particularly active in the myeloid lineage. Mutations in the *FLT3* gene are observed in several different subtypes of AML and in at least a third of PML patients.

Detection and Quantification of Leukemia-Specific Rearrangements

A number of leukemia-specific chromosomal translocations have been identified that have been cloned and are appropriate markers for molecular studies. In addition, leukemia nonspecific clonality markers, such as the junctional region of the rearranged immunoglobulin (Ig) and T-cell receptor (TCR) genes can be used for minimal residual disease studies. It is commonly accepted that the Ig heavy chain (IgH) gene junctional regions as well as the junctional regions of rearranged TCR-γ and TCR-δ can be used as targets for polymerase chain reaction (PCR) analysis. The detection and quantification of leukemia specific rearrangements will be explained on the example chronic myelogenous leukemia (CML), since this disease was the first human tumor associated with a specific chromosomal rearrangement and a specific fusion gene. The spectrum of molecular methods to detect fusion genes and their products has been established on CML during the last 15 years.

Chronic Myelogenous Leukemia

In many ways, CML serves as a paradigm for the utility of molecular methods to diagnose malignancy or to monitor patient response to therapy. CML is a clonal myeloproliferative disorder of the primitive hematopoietic stem cell an annual incidence of approx 1–2 per 100,000. The disease was described by Virchow in 1845, introducing the term *Weißes Blut*. CML constitutes a clinical model for molecular detection and therapy surveillance since this entity was

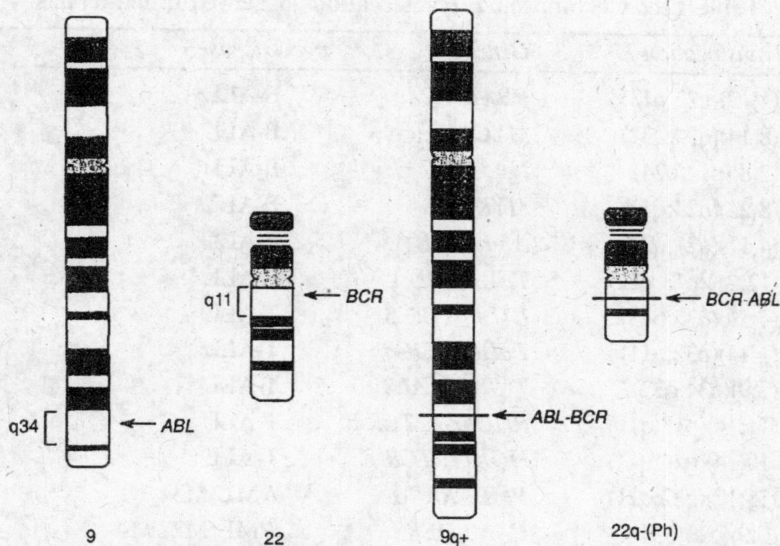

Fig. 11.1. Philadelphia (Ph) translocation. Reciprocal translocation of genomic material from the long arms of chromosomes 9 and 22.

the first leukemia known to be associated with a specific chromosomal rearrangement, the Philadelphia (Ph) translocation t(9;22)(q34;q11), and the presence of two chimeric genes, *BCR-ABL* on chromosome 22, and *ABL-BCR* on chromosome 9. *BCR-ABL* is transcribed to a specific BCR-ABL mRNA and encodes in most patients a 210-kDa chimeric protein with increased tyrosine kinase activity. The central role of BCR-ABL in several pathways that lead to uncontrolled proliferation has been shown in vitro and in vivo by transfection and transplantation experiments in mice. *ABL-BCR* is expressed in about 60% of patients with CML but lacks any biologic function.

Detection and Quantification of BCR-ABL-Positive Cells

Cytogenetic analysis of bone marrow metaphases

The degree of tumor load reduction is an important prognostic factor for patients with CML on therapy. Conventional cytogenetics is considered the "*gold standard*" for evaluating this response. This method, however, is limited by the requirement of mitotic cells. Insufficient metaphases are obtained in many cases on interferon-α (IFN-α) therapy. Furthermore, cytogenetic analysis is not applicable to patients with Ph-negative, BCR-ABL-positive disease.

Commonly, response is determined according to the Houston classification:

Table 11.2 Chromosomal translocations observed in leukemias

Translocation	*Genes*	*Disease*
t(1;19)(q23;p13)	*PBX1*, *E2A*	B-ALL
t(8;14)(q24;q32)	*MYC*, IgH	B-ALL
t(2;8)(p12;q24)	*Igκ*, *MYC*	B-ALL
t(8;22)(q24;q11)	*MYK*, *Igλ*	B-ALL
t(4;11)(q21;q23)	*AF4*, *MLL*	B-ALL
t(12;21)(p13;q22)	*TEL*, *AML* 1	B-ALL
t(7;19)(q35;p13)	*LYL1*, *TCR-β*	T-ALL
t(1;14)(p32;q11)	*TAL1*, *TCR-δ*	T-ALL
t(7;9)(q34;q32)	*TCR-β*, *TAL2*	T-ALL
t(11;14)(p13;q11)	*RHOM-2*, *TCR-δ*	T-ALL
t(10;14)(q24;q11)	*HOX11*, *TCR-δ*	T-ALL
t(15;17)(q22;q21)	*PML*, *RARα*	AML M3
t(6;9)(p23;q34)	*CAN*, *DEK*	AML M2, M4
t(8;21)(q22;q22)	*ETO*, *AML1*	AML M2
inv(16)(p13;q22)	*CBFβ*, *MYH11*	AML M4Eo
t(9;22)(q34;q11)	*c-ABL*, *BCR*	CML, ALL
t(8;13)(p11;q12)	*ZNF198*; *FGFR1*	8p11 MPD
t(9;12)(q34;p13)	*ABL*, *TEL*	Ph-negative CML, MDS
t(5;12)(q33;p13)	P*DGFR-β*, *TEL*	CMML

1. Complete response (0% Ph-positive metaphases).
2. Partial response (1–34% Ph-positive metaphases).
3. Minor response (35–94% Ph-positive metaphases).
4. Nonresponse (≥ 95% Ph-positive metaphases).

The Ph chromosome is present in about 90% of patients with a clinical picture consistent with CML. Three to five percent of patients show a normal chromosome 22 with molecular evidence of the *BCR-ABL* translocation. At presentation, cytogenetic analysis usually reveals the Ph chromosome in 100% of cells analyzed with standard 20- to 30-cell analysis.

Major drawbacks of cytogenetics are the requirement of bone marrow cells in mitosis, and the analysis of relatively small numbers of metaphases, resulting in significant sampling errors. The advantage of cytogenetics is the early detection of a cytogenetic evolution as a sign for acceleration of the disease.

The frequency of cytogenetic analysis can be reduced considerably if patients are monitored by other methods, such as quantitative Southern blot, *fluorescence in situ hybridization* (FISH), quantitative Western blot, or quantitative reverse transcription (RT)-PCR. Molecular methods can be performed on peripheral blood specimens and are therefore less invasive than conventional cytogenetic analysis of bone marrow metaphases. Furthermore, these techniques are applicable to Ph-negative, BCR-ABL-positive cases. Results obtained by Southern blotting, Western blotting, and FISH are readily quantifiable, but the sensitivity is not generally superior to that of cytogenetics.

Fluorescence in situ hybridization

FISH analysis is typically performed by cohybridization of a BCR and an ABL probe to denatured metaphase chromosomes or interphase nuclei. Probes are large genomic clones, such as cosmids or yeast artificial chromosomes, and are labeled with different fluorochromes.

Dual-color FISH using probes for *BCR* and *ABL* genes allows the specific detection of *BCR-ABL* gene fusion in interphase or metaphase nuclei. Most cells exhibit four distinct signals, two of each color corresponding to the two normal *BCR* and *ABL* alleles. CML cells are recognized by the juxta- or superposition of one of the *BCR* and *ABL* signals. FISH analysis does not depend on the presence of the Ph chromosome and will detect rare *BCR* and *ABL* variant fusions. The lineage of positive and negative cells can be determined in combination with conventional May-Grunwald staining or immunocytochemistry.

A limitation of the interphase FISH method is the background of a variant proportion of false positive cells, depending on the probe/ detection system used. In practice, the limit of detection of CML cells is typically 1–5% and depends, in part, on which probes are used, the size of the nucleus, the precise position of the breakpoint within the *ABL* gene, and the criteria used to define colocalization. The advantage of FISH over conventional cytogenetics is the analysis of a larger number of nuclei, resulting in smaller sampling errors. Therefore, FISH is applicable for quantification of residual disease in partial, minor, and nonresponders to IFN-α as well as for determination of the BCR-ABL positivity of individual cell colonies or the proportion of BCR-ABL-positive cells in small samples, such as highly enriched cell fractions.

The sensitivity of interphase FISH can be considerably increased by introducing a third probe that permits identification of both the Ph chromosome and the derivative 9 chromosome in Ph-positive cells, thus lowering the rate of false-positive cells, or by choosing breakpoint spanning probes that result in two fusion signals.

The development of a high-resolution quantitative procedure termed *hypermetaphase FISH* (HMF) should make it possible to distinguish different levels of Ph chromosome positivity at presentation. In HMF, FISH is coupled with procedures for increasing the number of bone marrow cells that can be analyzed. When readings can be obtained on 500 cells, one can reliably estimate parameters that characterize *minimal residual disease* (MRD). However, HMF evaluates only cycling cells and cannot count Ph-positive cells that do not enter division.

Southern blot analysis

Southern blotting exploits the fact that the breakpoint within the *BCR* gene generally falls in a very limited area, the 5.8-kb major breakpoint cluster region (M-bcr). Genomic DNA extracted from leukocytes from a patient is digested by a set of appropriate restriction enzymes (*Bgl*II, *Xba*I, *Hin*dIII, *Eco*RI, *Bam*HI), fractionated on an agarose gel, transferred to a nylon membrane, and hybridized to two labeled DNA probes derived from the 3' and 5' portion of M-bcr. After autoradiography, a band corresponding to the unrearranged BCR allele is visible; for patients with CML, one or two additional bands may also be present. Using this technique, a *BCR* rearrangement is detectable in about 98% of Ph-positive patients and in a significant proportion of Ph-negative cases. For routine use, *Bgl*II and *Xba*I are sufficient and are informative in almost all cases.

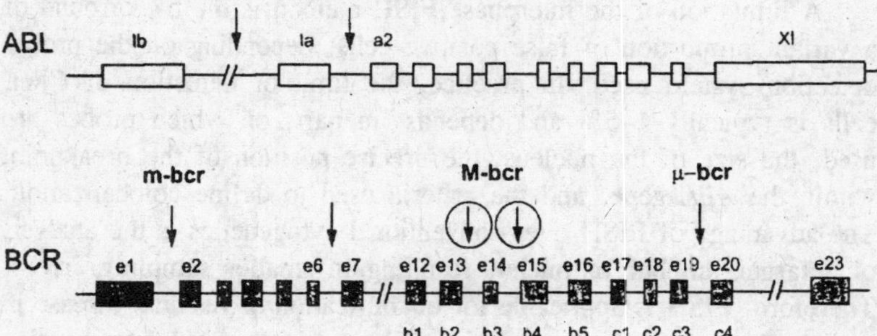

Fig. 11.2. Map of the exon-intron structure of ABL and BCR.

Because there are rare restriction site polymorphisms in the M-bcr, the finding of a rearrangement with at least two restriction enzymes is generally considered necessary to exclude a false positive result in any new patient. False negative results may arise because the rearranged band is too large, too small, or coincidentally exactly the same size as the normal allele, as a result of partial deletion of *BCR* sequences on the translocated allele or of rare variants that have breakpoints outside the M-bcr. False positive or false negative results are, however, rare.

Table 11.3. Fragment size of BCR germline allele according to restriction enzymes and probes used

Restriction enzyme	*2 kb-BglII/HindIII-5'-M-bcr-probe*	*1.2-kb-HindIII/BglII 3'-M-bcr-probe*
*Bgl*II	5.0 kbp	
*Eco*RI	18.1 kbp	
*Xba*I	8.9 kbp	
*Bam*HI	12.2 kbp	3.4 kbp
*Hind*III	10.1 kbp	4.5 kbp

Once a rearrangement is identified, it is almost always stable throughout the course of the disease. Therefore, Southern blot analysis allows quantification of the proportion of cells with *BCR* rearrangement compared to all cells investigated. The proportion of CML cells is determined by twice the intensity of the rearranged band divided by the sum of the intensities of the rearranged plus germline bands (BCR ratio); each CML cell contributes signals from one normal and one rearranged chromosome 22, whereas the normal cells contribute identical signals from two normal chromosomes. Subsequent samples from the patient after treatment are analyzed with the same restriction enzyme–probe combination to determine whether there has been a change in the proportion of malignant cells. The level of disease detected in contemporaneous peripheral blood and bone marrow samples is essentially identical, and, therefore, peripheral blood is normally used for analysis. Quantitative Southern blot allows the detection and quantification of down to 1% leukemic cells. To evaluate the response to treatment, knowledge of the initial restriction pattern and intensity of the rearranged band is mandatory. Complete cytogenetic responses are associated with the disappearance of rearranged *BCR* bands in most cases.

The BCR ratio is usually lower than the proportion of Ph-positive metaphases. The reason for this is that in Southern blotting analyses there are a large number of dividing and resting cells, including BCR-ABL-negative lymphocytes, and cytogenetics analysis provides information on a small number of dividing myeloid cells. The main advantage of Southern blotting over cytogenetics is the independence from dividing cells, which permits the use of peripheral blood instead of bone marrow.

The comparison of 235 blood and bone marrow samples analyzed by Southern blot and conventional cytogenetics showed a rank correlation between both methods of $r = 0.82$ ($p < 0.001$). The BCR ratio was significantly different among cytogenetically defined minor, partial, and complete response groups ($p < 0.001$). Empirically derived cutoff points in the BCR ratio were introduced in order to define molecular response groups: A BCR ratio of 0% was defined as a complete response; and ratios of 1–24, 25–50, and >50% were defined as partial, minor, and no molecular response, respectively. Using these cutoff points, a major cytogenetic response could be predicted or excluded in >90% of cases.

Western blot analysis

Western blotting can be used to detect BCR-ABL proteins directly in cell extracts qualitatively and quantitatively in both bone marrow and in peripheral blood. Leukocytes are lysed in the presence of potent protease inhibitors, fractionated on a polyacrylamide gel, transferred to a nylon membrane, and probed with an anti-ABL antibody. After washing, bound antibody is detected using a labeled secondary antibody. Blots are autoradiographed and a band corresponding to the normal p145 ABL is visualized; BCR-ABL, if present, is larger and therefore migrates more slowly. The limit of sensitivity is about 0.5–1%. The Western blot assay can distinguish the three major types of BCR-ABL proteins, p190, p210, and p230, and is able to detect rare types of BCR-ABL proteins, such as p200. Using a quantitative Western blot assay, a linear correlation between BCR-ABL/ABL protein ratios and contemporaneous conventional cytogenetics has been described in 392 sample pairs ($r = 0.97$; $p < 0.001$).

Reverse transcriptase PCR

In 1989, first encouraging results concerning the detection of MRD by PCR in CML patients after allogeneic bone marrow transplantation were reported. However, conflicting data from a comparative multicenter study revealed serious problems of the method with a high rate of false positive results and provoked an open discussion. Over the past 10 yr, PCR has been optimized and developed. Specificity has been increased considerably by the partial standardization of methodology and the introduction of rigorous precautions to avoid contamination. Sensitivity has been improved by using nested primer pairs and performing two consecutive PCR steps. In view of the limited value of qualitative PCR for monitoring CML patients after therapy, quantitative BCR-ABL PCR assays were developed to monitor patients after bone marrow transplantation or treatment with IFN-α, and STI571 and are now in routine clinical use.

Screening for BCR-ABL mRNA transcripts at diagnosis

For diagnostic samples, the use of multiplex PCR has been suggested to detect simultaneously several kinds of BCR-ABL and BCR transcripts as internal controls in one reaction by using three BCR and one ABL primers. This method allows the reliable detection of typical BCR-ABL transcripts, such as b2a2 or b3a2, and atypical types, such as, transcripts lacking *ABL* exon a2 (b2a3 and b3a3), or transcripts resulting from *BCR* breakpoints outside M-bcr, such as e1a2 or e6a2.

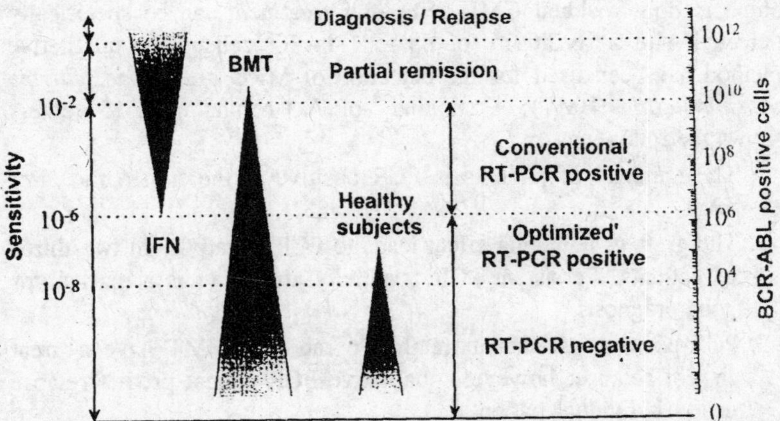

Fig. 11.3. Schematic illustration of therapeutic response of CML patients on molecular level.

Detection of MRD: nested RT-PCR

The term "*minimal residual disease*" (MRD) refers to the presence of detectable malignant cells in patients who are in conventional remission. The aim of MRD analysis is to distinguish patients who have differing levels of residual leukemic cells and who may therefore benefit from either reduced or intensified treatment regimens.

Since patients with leukemia at presentation or relapse usually have a total burden of $>10^{12}$ malignant cells, and since cytogenetics, Western blot, and conventional FISH have a maximum sensitivity of 1%, a patient with negative results may harbor as much or few as zero or as many as 10^{10} residual leukemic cells. At this point, the patient is judged to be in clinical and hematologic remission, although the term remission refers only to an arbitrary point toward one end of leukemic cell numbers.

RT-PCR for BCR-ABL mRNA is by far the most sensitive assay in this context and can detect a single leukemia cell in a background of 10^5–10^6 normal cells. Therefore, PCR is up to four orders of magnitude more sensitive than conventional methods. However, patients who have no MRD detectable by this technique may still harbor up to 1,000,000 malignant cells that could contribute to subsequent relapse. The sensitivity with which MRD can be detected will be limited by the amount of peripheral blood or bone marrow that can be analyzed.

By using nested RT-PCR with two pairs of ("*nested*") primers corresponding to appropriate *BCR* and *ABL* exons in two rounds of amplification, residual CML cells after treatment can be specifically detected with a sensitivity of up to 1 in 10^6 cells. This qualitative method has been used for the detection of MRD after *bone marrow transplantation* (BMT). A summary of 700 results from 15 centers shows the following:

1. The majority of patients is PCR positive in the first 6 mo after BMT.
2. The graft vs leukemia effect leads to PCR negativity in two-thirds of patients. Persistent PCR negativity after 1 yr is a marker for good prognosis.
3. PCR-positive patients more than 6 mo after BMT have a great risk of relapse; however, qualitative PCR cannot predict relapse in the individual patient.
4. In the majority of cases after BMT, RT-PCR, and DNA-PCR (using patient-specific primers), results are concordant; that is, that patients in remission do not generally harbor a substantial pool of CML cells that do not express BCR-ABL mRNA.

Nested PCR is essentially useless in patients after IFN-α therapy, because almost all patients are repeatedly positive.

By using an optimized RT-PCR method, BCR-ABL mRNA can be detected at a very low level of 1–10 transcripts/10^8 cells in normal individuals in an age-dependent frequency. One interpretation of this finding could be that *BCR-ABL*, and probably several other fusion genes, is being formed continuously in mitotic cells in the normal bone marrow, but only the combination of the correct *BCR-ABL* fusion in the correct primitive hematopoietic progenitor has a selective advantage and becomes functional as an expanding clone.

Quantitative PCR

In view of the very limited value of qualitative PCR, several groups have developed quantitative PCR assays to estimate the amount of MRD in positive specimens. Most groups have initially used competitive PCR strategies that can effectively control for variations in amplification efficiency and reaction kinetics.

In general, nested PCR is performed using serial dilutions of a BCR-ABL competitor construct added to the same volume of patients' cDNA. The equivalence point at which the competitor and sample band would be of equal intensity is determined by densitometry. To standardize results for both quality and quantity of blood, RNA, and cDNA, quantification of transcripts of normal housekeeping genes, such as *ABL* or *glucose-6-phosphate dehydrogenase* (*G6PD*), has been employed. The standardized results are expressed as the ratios of BCR-ABL/ABL or BCR-ABL/G6PD in a percentage. The quantification of the transcript level of control genes is of special importance if different RNA qualities are expected, i.e., particularly when samples are mailed in multicenter trials.

In patients after BMT, rising or persistently high levels of BCR-ABL mRNA can be detected prior to cytogenetic or hematologic relapse. Of 69 patients with low or falling *BCR-ABL* transcripts, 3% relapsed compared with 79% in 29 patients with high or rising BCR-ABL transcript levels. By contrast, patients who remain in remission have low, stable, or falling BCR-ABL levels.

Quantitative PCR is the method of choice to determine the best time point for therapeutic interventions in case of relapse after BMT. Quantitative PCR data have been used to determine the optimum time point to initiate donor lymphocyte transfusions and to monitor its response. The great majority of patients who respond to donor lymphocyte infusions achieve durable molecular remission (RT-PCR negativity) with a median follow-up of >2 yr.

Quantitative RT-PCR for *BCR-ABL* has been shown to be a reliable method for monitoring residual leukemia load in mobilized peripheral blood stem cells, particularly in Ph-negative collections. Quantitative RT-PCR allows selection of the best available collections for reinfusion into patients after myeloablative therapy (autografting).

For 96 Ph-positive patients after IFN-α therapy, all were positive for *BCR-ABL* transcripts. The MRD in complete responders spanned a range over four orders of magnitude. The median ratios of complete, partial, minor, and nonresponders differed significantly ($p < 0.0001$).

The results of nonresponders on IFN-α therapy and patients at diagnosis were not different.

Cytogenetic response to IFN-α (complete, partial, minor/none) was compared to molecular response by introducing cutoff points for the BCR-ABL/ABL ratio. Using optimum cutoff points of 2 and 14% (i.e., comparing a ratio up to 2% to complete cytogenetic responders, between 2 and 14% to partial responders, and >14% to minor and nonresponders), the concordance between the two methods was 82%, the χ^2 test was highly significant ($p < 0.001$).

All 54 patients investigated who had achieved *complete response* (CR) to IFN-α treatment had molecular evidence of MRD during complete remission, although 3 patients were intermittently negative by RT-PCR. In general, *BCR-ABL* transcript numbers were inversely related to the duration of CR. The median ratio of BCR-ABL to ABL at the time of maximal response for each patient was 0.045% (range 0–3.6%). During the period of observation, 14 patients relapsed, 11 cytogenetically to chronic phase disease, and 3 directly to blastic phase. The median ratio of BCR-ABL/ABL at maximal response was significantly higher in patients who relapsed than in those who remained in CR (0.49 vs 0.021%; $p < 0.0001$). The findings show that the level of MRD falls with time in patients who maintain their cytogenetic response to IFN, but molecular evidence of disease is rarely if ever eliminated. The RT-PCR analysis of colony-forming unit granulocyte macrophage colonies grown from bone marrow of eight complete cytogenetic responders demonstrated that residual disease resides in myeloid colony-forming cells, which may have the potential to repopulate the bone marrow and contribute to relapse. Therefore, it is unlikely that CML can be cured by IFN-α therapy. The actual level of MRD correlates with the probability of relapse. For patients who reach complete cytogenetic remission should be continued at least until relatively low levels of residual leukemia are achieved.

In other series, the frequency of PCR negativity in complete cytogenetic responders is higher in a long-term follow-up using an RT-PCR strategy with a lower sensitivity. However, since the actual level of residual *BCR-ABL* transcripts is related to the probability of relapse, molecular monitoring may identify a subset of patients for whom treatment may be safely withdrawn.

Rising levels of BCR-ABL mRNA in sequential samples from patients who are not in cytogenetic remission may precede disease progression.

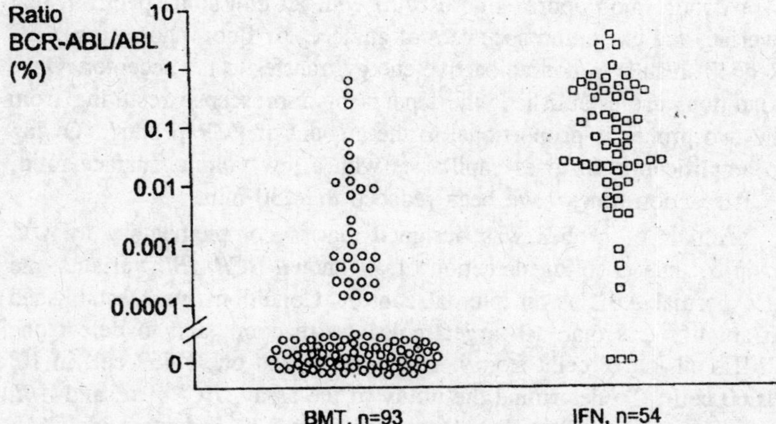

Fig. 11.4. Quantitative PCR analysis for the ratio to BCR-ABL/ABL in complete cytogenetic responders after allogeneic BMT and IFN therapy.

The low-level expression of e1a2 BCR-ABL mRNA in patients with M-bcr-positive CML is a common finding. Whether increasing levels of e1a2 mRNA transcripts correlate to disease progression is still controversial.

Recently, novel real-time PCR procedures have been developed that promise to simplify existing protocols. Several procedures for quantification of BCR-ABL mRNA using the TaqMan system have been developed. The assay is based on the use of the 5' nuclease activity of *Taq* polymerase to cleave a nonextendable hybridization probe during the extension phase of PCR. The approach uses dual-labeled fluorogenic probes. One fluorescent dye serves as a reporter and its emission spectrum is quenched by the second fluorescent dye. The nuclease degradation of the probe releases the quenching, resulting in an increase in fluorescent emission. The fluorescence is monitored by a sequence detector in real time. C_T (threshold cycle) values are calculated by determining the point at which the fluorescence exceeds a threshold limit. C_T corresponds to the amount of target transcripts in the sample.

An alternative real-time RT-PCR approach for detection and quantification of *BCR-ABL* fusion transcripts has been established using the new LightCycler technology, which combines rapid thermocycling with on-line fluorescence detection of PCR product formation as it occurs. Fluorescence monitoring of PCR amplification is based on the concept of fluorescence resonance energy transfer between two adjacent hybridization probes carrying donor and acceptor fluorophores. Excitation of a donor fluorophore (fluorescein) with an emission spectrum that overlaps the excitation spectrum of an acceptor fluorophore (e.g., LC Red640) results in nonradioactive energy transfer to the acceptor. Once conditions are established, the amount of fluorescence resulting from the two probes is proportional to the amount of PCR product. Owing to amplification in glass capillaries with a low volume/surface ratio, PCR reaction times have been reduced to <30 min.

A pair of probes was designed that is complementary to *ABL* exon 3, thus enabling detection of all known *BCR-ABL* variants and also normal ABL as an internal control. Conditions were established to amplify less than 10 target molecules/reaction, and to detect one CML cell in 10^5 cells from healthy donors and one K562 cell in 10^7 HL60 cells. To determine the utility of the assay, *BCR-ABL* and *ABL* transcripts in a series of 254 samples from 120 patients with CML after therapy were quantified. The level of MRD was expressed as the ratio of BCR-ABL/ABL. This ratio was compared to results obtained by three established methods from contemporaneous specimens. A highly significant correlation was seen among the BCR-ABL/ABL ratios determined by the LightCycler and (1) the BCR-ABL/ABL ratios obtained by nested competitive RT-PCR ($n = 201$; $r = 0.90$; $p < 0.0001$); (2) the proportion of Philadelphia chromosome positive metaphases determined by cytogenetics ($n = 81$; $p < 0.0001$), and (3) the BCR ratio determined by Southern blot analysis ($n = 122$; $p < 0.0001$).

Real-time PCR approaches with TaqMan or hybridization probes are reliable and sensitive methods to monitor CML patients after

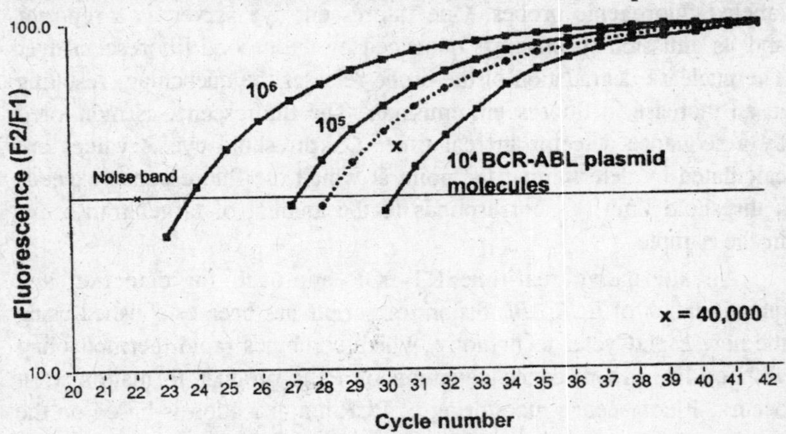

Fig. 11.5. Example of real-time PCR.

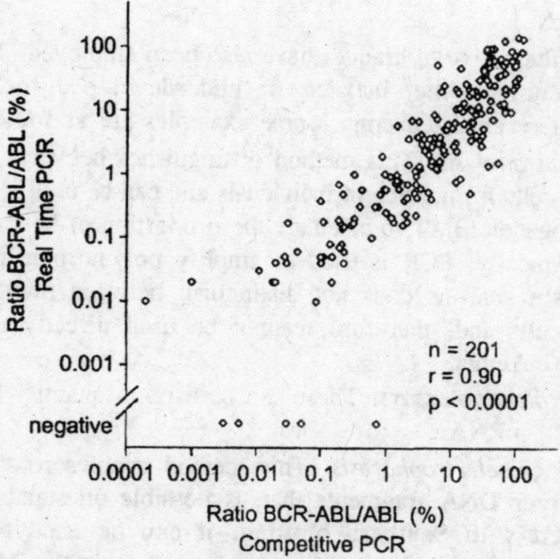

Fig. 11.6. Comparison of the quantification of the ratio of BCR-ABL/ABL with real-time PCR vs competitive PCR.

therapy. The major advantages of the methodology are that amplification and product analysis are performed in the same reaction vessel, avoiding the risk of contamination, and that the results are standardized by the quantification of housekeeping genes.

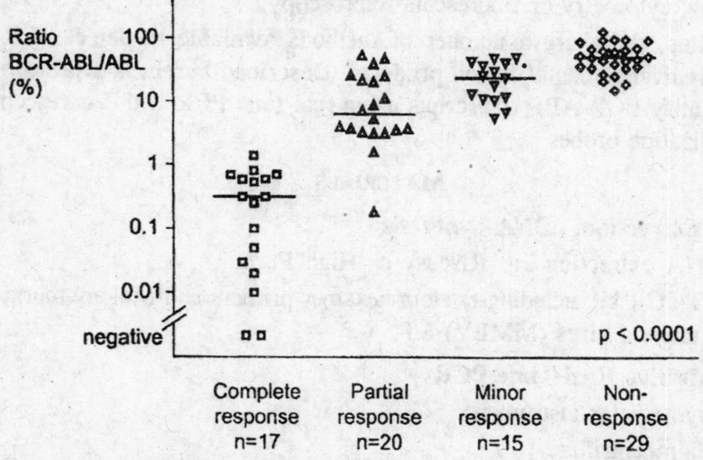

Fig. 11.7. Ratios of BCR-ABL/ABL derived from real-time PCR according to contemporaneous cytogenetic response. The ratios of BCR-ABL/ABL are significantly different among complete, partial, minor, and nonresponders ($p < 0.0001$).

Other methods

Several alternative techniques have also been employed. They are mostly too cumbersome, inexact, or underdeveloped for routine assessment of residual leukemia. Some examples are as follows:

1. *Chimerism analysis.* This method distinguishes between genomic DNA or cells from different individuals and can be used in patients after allogeneic BMT to calculate the proportion of host to donor cells. Typically, PCR is used to amplify polymorphic markers. Chimerism analysis does not distinguish between malignant or normal cells and, therefore, cannot be used directly to detect residual leukemia.
2. *RNAse protection assays.* These can be used to quantify levels of BCR-ABL mRNA.
3. *Pulsfield gel electrophoresis.* This method enables resolution of much larger DNA fragments than is possible on standard gels. Combined with Southern blotting, it can be used to detect rearrangements outside the M-bcr and also within the *ABL* gene.
4. In situ *PCR.* This method used on single cells can specifically identify cells with BCR-ABL transcripts. Its results are concordant with those of karyotyping and RT-PCR. Because of its limited sensitivity and specificity, however, it appears to have limited value in the analysis of MRD. Positive cells are enumerated by low cytometry or fluorescent microscopy.

Thus, there are a number of methods available to detect BCR-ABL rearrangements/ fusion products. Described herein is a protocol to quantify BCR-ABL transcripts using real time PCR with fluorescent hybridization probes.

Materials

RNA Extraction, cDNA Synthesis

1. RNA extraction kit: RNeasy or High Pure.
2. RT-PCR kit including random hexamer primers and Molony murine leukemia virus (MMLV) RT.

Quantitative Real-Time PCR

1. LightCycler instrument.
2. Microcentrifuge.
3. Vortex.
4. LightCycler-DNA Master Hybridization Probes.
5. dNTPplus (dATP, dUTP, dGTP, dCTP).

6. Heat-labile uracil DNA glycosylase (UDG).
7. Amplification primers (MWG).
8. Hybridization probes.

METHODS

RNA Extraction, cDNA Synthesis

1. Extract total leukocyte RNA from 10–20 mL of *peripheral blood* (PB) and/or from 1 to 5 mL of *bone marrow* (BM) aspirate after lysis of red blood cells.
2. Process the samples as soon as possible after aspiration, although some may spend 1–3 d in transit.
3. Perform RNA extraction by CsCl gradient centrifugation or by commercially available extraction kits.
4. Reverse-transcribe RNA using random hexamer priming and MMLV RT as described.
5. Store the cDNA samples at –20°C.

Quantitative Real-Time PCR

1. Perform PCR using 2 μL of master mix ([LightCycler DNA Master Hybridization Probes] containing buffer, dATP, dCTP, dGTP, dUTP, and *Taq* polymerase), 4 m*M* $MgCl_2$, 0.25 μ*M* of each 3' and 5' fluorescent hybridization probes, 0.5 μ*M* of each 3' and 5' oligonucleotide primer (highly purified salt-free grade; MWG), 1 U of heat-labile UDG, 2 μL of cDNA, and water to a final volume of 20 μL.
2. Prior to amplification, incubate the mixes for 5 min at room temperature to allow degradation of specific contaminating PCR products from previous amplifications by UDG. To improve reliability of the assay, prepare master mixes for 35 samples.
3. Deactivate heat-labile UDG by an initial denaturation step of 1 min at 95°C.
4. Amplify in a three-step cycle procedure (denaturation at 95°C, 1 s, ramp rate 20°C/s; annealing at 64°C, 10s, ramp rate 20°C/s; and extension at 72°C, 26 s, ramp rate 2°C/s) for 45 cycles. The following primers were used for amplification: b2a2, b3a2, b2a3, or b3a3 BCR-ABL, primers B2A and NA4–; e1a2 BCR-ABL, primers PE1+ and NA4–; ABL, primers A2N and NA4–.
5. Perform amplification, fluorescence detection, and postprocessing calculations using the LightCycler apparatus.

5' Hybridization probes are labeled with fluorescein, 3' probes with LC Red640. Fluorescence is measured after each annealing step

Table 11.4. Temperature profile of the PCR cycles

Parameter		*Value*	
Cycles		45	
Temperature target	Segment 1	Segment 2	Segment 3
Target temperature (°C)	95	64	72
Incubation time (s)	1	10	26
Temperatur transition rate (°C/s)	20	20	2
Acquisition mode	None	None	Single

and expressed as the ratio between fluorescence at 640 nm and at 530 nm. The fluorescence signal is plotted against the cycle number for all samples and external standards. These standards consist of serial dilutions (10^1–10^7 molecules per reaction) of plasmids pGD210 (b3a2$^{BCR\text{-}ABL}$) and pB190 (e1a2$^{BCR\text{-}ABL}$). Initially, the crossover point is determined for each standard dilution, i.e., the point at which the signal rose above the background level. The higher the initial number of starting molecules, the earlier the signal appears above the background. A standard curve for each run is constructed by plotting the crossover point against the log (number of standard molecules). The number of target molecules in each sample is then calculated automatically by reference to this curve. Results were expressed initially as the number of target molecules/2 μL of cDNA. Normalized levels of disease are calculated as the ratios (expressed as percentage) between *BCR-ABL* and *ABL* transcripts in 2 μL of cDNA.

Quantitative data on MRD may be achieved by various methods. However, no standard technique is used. Interlaboratory reproducibility needs a standardization of the method and of the interpretation of the results. The efficiency of this technology needs to be confirmed in large clinical trials. Recommendations of the European Investigators on CML group for the clinical use of quantitative PCR monitoring in CML have been published. The new real-time RT-PCR procedures promise to greatly simplify the cumbersome protocols that are currently in use. They also offer a unique opportunity to standardize the assay and to develop rigorous standards and controls. Quantitative real-time PCR soon will become a routine and robust basis for clinical decision making in leukemias with specific molecular markers.

Wilms Tumor Gene WT1 as a Tumor Marker for Leukemic Blast Cells and Its Role in Leukemogenesis

Patients with acute leukemia have a total of approx 10^{12} leukemic cells at the time of diagnosis, and still have as many as 10^{10} leukemic cells in complete remission. The most important problem in the treatment of leukemia patients is the uncertainty of whether leukemic cells have been totally eradicated when complete remission has been achieved. Through accurate assessment of a small number of leukemic cells (*minimal residual disease* [MRD]) that still remained in complete remission, individual patients will be able to be treated with different protocols based on the extent of the MRD, resulting in improvement of cure rates.

In this chapter, we focus on the clinical usefulness of the WT1 assay (quantitation of expression levels of Wilms tumor gene *WT1*) not only for the detection of MRD of leukemia but also for the diagnosis of hematopoietic malignancies. Also, I discuss an oncogenic function of the *WT1* gene in leukemogenesis and tumorigeneis rather than a tumor suppressor gene function.

Wilms Tumor Gene WT1

The *WT1* gene is a candidate gene for Wilms tumor, a childhood renal tumor that is thought to arise as a result of inactivation of both alleles of the *WT1* gene located at chromosome 11p13. The *WT1* gene has been considered to be a tumor suppressor gene on the basis of the following data: intragenic deletions or mutations in Wilms tumor, germline mutations in patients with leukemia predisposition syndromes, and WT1-mediated growth suppression of Wilms tumor cells expressing a WT1 splicing variant. The *WT1* gene encodes a zinc-finger transcription factor that represses transcription of growth factor (platelet-derived growth factor-A chain, colony-stimulating factor-1, and insulin-like growth factor-2) and growth factor receptor (IGF-IR and epidermal growth factor receptor) genes, and the other genes (RARα, c-myb, c-myc, and bcl-2).

Tumor suppressor genes such as *Rb* and *p53* are expressed ubiquitously. On the other hand, expression of the *WT1* gene is restricted to a limited set of tissues, including gonads, uterus, kidney, and mesothelial structures, but it is highest in the developing kidney, reflecting the significant role of WT1 in renal development. WT1 knockout mice were shown to have defects in the urogenital system and to die at embryonic d 3.5, probably owing to heart failure.

WT1 Gene Expression in Leukemias

Miwa et al. examined the expression of the *WT1* gene in leukemias using Northern blot analysis. The *WT1* gene expression was detected in 15 of 22 *acute myelogenous leukemias* (AMLs), in 7 of 16 *acute lymphoid leukemias* (ALLs), and in 8 of 10 *chronic myelogeneous leukemias* (CMLs) in blastic crisis. Miyagi et al. also detected the WT1 transcript in 4 of 10 AMLs, in 1 of 9 ALLs, and in 1 of 6 CMLs in accelerated-phase or blastic crisis. These two reports have shown that the *WT1* gene is expressed in some cases of myeloid or lymphoid leukemias.

Inoue et al. provided a new development for the significance of the *WT1* gene expression in leukemias by the quantitation of the expression levels of the *WT1* gene using quantitative reverse transcriptase polymerase chain reaction (RT-PCR). Forty-five patients with AML, 22 with ALL, 6 with *acute mixed lineage leukemia* (AMLL), and 23 with CML (8 chronic phase, 5 accelerated phase, and 10 blast crisis) were quantitated for the expression levels of the *WT1* gene using quantitative RT-PCR. In all the leukemia samples examined, significant levels of *WT1* gene expression were found, and the levels were approx 1000 and 100,000 times higher than those in normal bone marrow or in normal peripheral blood, respectively. In CML, the levels increased as the disease progressed.

A clear correlation between the WT1 expression levels (<0.6 vs ≥0.6) and the prognosis of acute leukemia was observed (WT1 expression level in K562 cells was defined as 1.0). Patients with levels of <0.6 had significantly higher rates of complete remission, and disease-free and overall survivals than those with levels of ≥0.6. All seven patients with levels of *WT1* gene expression of >1.0 did not achieve complete remission. Bergmann et al. also reported the correlation between the WT1 expression levels and the prognosis. Brieger et al. detected WT1 transcript in 41 of 52 (79%) AML patients, while most of the 14 patients studied in complete remission lost their WT1 expression. In three of the four patients in complete remission, the reappearance of WT1 expression preceded their relapse.

Menssen et al. also found *WT1* gene expression in 53 of 57 (93%) AML patients, 12 of 14 (86%) pre-pre-B ALL patients, 33 of 41 (80%) cALL patients, and 23 of 31 (74%) T-ALL patients. They confirmed the *WT1* gene expression in leukemic blast cells by an immunofluorescence assay using WT1-specific antibodies. Patmasiriwat et al. quantitated WT1 expression levels in 62 AML samples and found that 82% strongly expressed WT1. Im et al. studied WT1 expression in children with acute leukemia by means of RT-PCR. WT1 was detectable in all 3 AML and 7 of 10 ALL patients, but not in 2 ALL patients in remission. The expression levels were higher for AML than for ALL. These reports demonstrated that the *WT1* gene expression is a novel tumor marker for leukemic blast cells in both children and adults and a new prognostic factor for acute leukemia.

Detection of MRD of Leukemia by Quantitation of Expression Levels of WT1 Gene

The average levels of the WT1 expression in leukemic cells were approx 3 logs higher than those in normal bone marrow cells and more than 5 logs higher than those in peripheral blood cells. This striking difference in WT1 expression levels between leukemic and normal cells made it possible to detect MRD of leukemia by the quantitation of the expression levels of the *WT1* gene (WT1 assay). To determine the sensitivity of the WT1 assay, RNA from the leukemic cells (WT1 expression level = 0.58) of acute promyelocytic leukemia (APL) with the *PML/RARα* fused gene was serially diluted with RNA from normal bone marrow or peripheral blood cells, and then WT1 and PML/RARα mRNAs were quantitated by RT-PCR with the respective primers. The WT1 mRNA was quantitated in parallel with the PML/RARα mRNA along with dilutions. This meant that the amount of the WT1 mRNA directly reflected that of APL blast cells, confirming that WT1 mRNA is a tumor marker for APL blast cells. The detection limit of leukemic cells by RT-PCR with the PML/RARα primer was 10^{-4} for both bone marrow and peripheral blood samples, whereas that by RT-PCR with the WT1 primer was 10^{-3} to 10^{-4} for bone marrow samples and 10^{-5} for peripheral blood samples. Therefore, the detection sensitivity of APL blast cells was superior in the RT-PCR method with the WT1 primer to the RT-PCR method with the PML/RARα primer. Tamaki et al. found that WT1 expression levels increased at relapse and that the levels at relapse were significantly higher than those at diagnosis (mean: 0.73 ± 0.12 vs 0.38 ± 0.04; $p < 0.01$). In nine AML patients from whom paired samples were obtained at both diagnosis and relapse, the average WT1 expression level at relapse (1.05) was 4.5 times higher than that assayed at diagnosis (0.23) (maximal change: 27.7-fold increase from 0.013 to 0.360; minimal change: 1.9-fold increase from 0.44 to 0.85). Accordingly, these results should mean an increase in detection sensitivity of MRD by the WT1 assay as relapse nears.

A clean correlation existed between the MRD detected in the paired bone marrow and peripheral blood samples for various types of leukemia (AML, ALL, and CML), with MRD in peripheral blood samples being approx one-tenth of that in bone marrow samples. Since background levels of WT1 expression in peripheral blood is less than one hundredth of those in bone marrow, peripheral blood samples should be, in practice, superior to bone marrow samples for the detection of MRD.

Long-Term Follow-Up of MRD of Leukemia by WT1 Assay

Thirty-one patients (27 AML, 2 ALL, and 2 AMLL) treated with *conventional chemotherapy* (CHT) and 23 patients (13 AML, 5 ALL, and 5 CML) treated with allogeneic *bone marrow transplantation* (BMT) were monitored for WT1 expression levels in bone marrow and peripheral blood using RT-PCR over a long-term period (mean: 29 mo for CHT and 24 mo for BMT). Nineteen patients (16 CHT and 3 BMT) who achieved complete remission eventually relapsed. In 10 of these patients, WT1 expression that had returned to normal bone marrow background levels ($<10^{-3}$) at complete remission either gradually or rapidly increased again to abnormal levels 1–18 mo (mean 7 mo) before their clinical relapse. In nine patients, WT1 expression never returned to normal bone marrow background levels even during complete remission, and their subsequent relapse was accompanied by a rapid increase in WT1 expression to levels higher than 10^{-2}. On the other hand, the remaining 35 patients (15 CHT and 20 BMT) maintained their complete remission. In 29 (11 CHT and 18 BMT) of these, WT1 expression either gradually or rapidly decreased to normal bone marrow background levels, whereas in the other 6 patients (4 CHT and 2 BMT), low levels of WT1 mRNA (10^{-3}–10^{-2}) still remained detectable, but no clinical signs of relapse were evident. These results showed that clinical relapse is impending when there is a rapid or gradual increase in WT1 expression levels to or over 10^{-2} after an initial return to normal bone marrow background levels in complete remission, or when there is retention of the WT1 expression at levels near or over 10^{-2} in the bone marrow without a return to normal bone marrow background levels even during complete remission. The absolute levels of WT1 that predict with certainty that a patient will relapse are 10^{-2} levels in bone marrow and 10^{-3} levels in peripheral blood. Patients with these signs should be immediately and appropriately treated before clinical relapse becomes apparent. Bergmann et al. also found that patients achieving complete remission after chemotherapy usually lose detectable signals of WT1, and in relapse of the disease, recurrence of WT1 mRNA can be determined in almost all patients with initially detectable WT1 mRNA. Detectable levels of WT1 during follow-up in AML patients have been shown to be useful as a marker for MRD or even to predict relapse of AML.

In a patient with AML who recieved allogeneic BMT, WT1 expression levels gradually increased to 5.9×10^{-3} in bone marrow (normal range: $<1.0 \times 10^{-3}$) and 2.4×10^{-3} in peripheral blood (normal range: $<1.0 \times 10^{-5}$) on d 367 post-BMT. However, bone marrow aspiration showed no evidence of relapse (100% donor type chromosomes). Since the increase in WT1 expression levels over 10^{-2} in bone marrow or 10^{-3} in peripheral blood predicts that clinical relapse is impending, we diagnosed this patient as having molecular relapse on d 367 and performed *donor leukocyte transfusion* (DLT). Leukemic blast cells increased and reached a miximum (50%) 29 d after DLT, but thereafter rapidly decreased and became undetetable 39 d after DLT and complete remission was achieved. The patient showed no evidence of graft-vs-host disease or other complications. Note that the patient did not manifest marrow aplasia, which is a common complication of DLT. The WT1 expression levels rapidly decreased from 29 d post-DLT and returned to normal range 60 d post-DLT. The patient was in complete remission with a normal range of WT1 expression levels for more than 21 mo after DLT. This case clearly demonstrated that early application of DLT at molecular relapse is essential for the improvement of the efficacy of DLT for relapsed AML after BMT, confirming the availability of the WT1 assay for the monitoring of MRD of leukemia.

Taken together, the WT1 assay has made it possible to rapidly assess the effectiveness of treatment, to evaluate the degree of eradication of leukemic cells, and to diagnose molecular relapse in individual leukemia patients. Thus, treatment for leukemia patients can be individualized by the monitoring of MRD by the WT1 assay, resulting in the improvement of cure rates.

Continuous Assessment of Disease Progression of Myelodysplastic Syndromes by WT1 Assay

The WT1 expression levels were examined for 57 patients with *myelodysplastic syndromes* (MDS) (refractory anemia, 35; *refractory anemia with excess of blasts* [RAEB] 14; RAEB in transformation [RAEB-t]), 6; and MDS with fibrosis, 2) and 12 patients with AML evolved from MDS. These levels significantly increased in proportion to the disease progression of MDS from refractory anemia to overt AML via RAEB and RAEB-t in both bone marrow and peripheral blood, demonstrating that the WT1 expression levels directly reflect the disease progression of MDS. WT1 expression levels in peripheral blood, but not in bone marrow, significantly correlated with the evolution of RAEB or RAEB-t to overt AML within 6 mo. An increase in WT1 expression levels to 10^{-2} in peripheral blood means that disease progression to overt AML is impending within 6 mo. Thus, the WT1 expression levels in peripheral blood are superior to those in bone marrow for early prediction of the evolution to AML by the means of the WT1 assay. Furthermore, WT1 expression in peripheral blood of overt AML patients was significantly decreased by effective chemotherapy or allogeneic stem cell transplantation and became undetectable in long-term survivors. Interestingly, the WT1 expression levels in bone marrow did not correlate with the percentages of morphologically leukemic blast cells in bone marrow in RAEB or RAEB-t patients, suggesting that the WT1 expression levels reflect the amount of not only morphologically leukemic blast cells but also of abnormal, transformed cells that are undetectable morphologically as blast cells. These results showed that WT1 expression levels are a tumor marker for both morphologically leukemic blast cells and abnormal cells that are undetectable morphologically as blast cells in MDS and thus reflect the disease progression of MDS. Monitoring of WT1 expression levels has made continuous assessment of the disease progression of MDS possible, as well as the prediction of the evolution of RAEB or RAEB-t to overt AML within 6 mo. The WT1 assay is also useful for diagnosis of MRD of MDS with high sensitivity, thus making it possible to evaluate the efficacy of treatment for MDS.

Differential Diagnosis Between Reactive and Leukemic Leukocytosis by WT1 Assay

Juvenile chronic myeloid leukemia (JCML) and infantile monosomy 7 syndrome (IMo7), which belong to childhood MDS, have common clinical features such as a male predominance, prominent hepato-splenomegaly, the presence of immature precursors in peripheral blood, an excessive proliferation of myeloid progenitor cells, and poor prognosis. The etiology and classification of both diseases, however, have been the subject of controversy. Two JCML and two IMo7 patients with characteristic clinical features were examined on the WT1 expression levels in bone marrow and peripheral blood by the WT1 assay. The WT1 expression levels ($2.4 - 7.2 \times 10^{-2}$) in bone marrow of these four patients were significantly elevated in comparison with the levels ($< 10^{-3}$) in normal bone marrow and equivalent to those in bone marrow of the patients with AML, ALL, or CML at blastic crisis. In two patients who were successfully treated with allogeneic peripheral blood stem cell transplantation, the WT1 expression returned to normal background levels in bone marrow and to undetectable levels in peripheral blood. Abnormally increased WT1 expression levels, which were equivalent to those in acute leukemias, in both JCML and IMo7 strongly indicated that both the diseases are defined as an etiologically similar entity and result from leukemic transformation of hematopoietic progenitor cells. The results that the WT1 expression levels in both JCML and IMo7 were approx 10 times higher than those in CML at chronic phase are compatible with clinical findings that the clinical course of JCML is much more aggressive than that of CML at chronic phase. The WT1 assay may become a clinical test indispensable for the discrimination between JCML and CML, and between myeloproliferative disorders and reactive leukocytosis in childhood such as congenital viral infection and persistent Epstein-Barr virus infection, both of which present a picture quite similar to JCML, because WT1 expression levels significantly increase in leukemic growth, but not in reactive states.

Acute eosinophilic leukemia (AEoL) is a rare form of AML that presents with a substantially increased series of left-shifted but maturing eosinophilic precursors and an increased number of blasts in bone marrow. By contrast, the idiopathic hypereosinophilic syndrome consists of a heterogeneous group of nonmalignant myeloproliferative disorders of unknown origin that is characterized by persistent overproduction of mature and sometimes immature eosinophilic cells, leukocytosis, and eosinophilic organ infiltrations. Reactive eosinophilia usually can be discriminated from AEoL, However, the distinction between AEoL and hyperoscinophilic syndrome is known to be difficult, because clinical and hematological features do not necessarily differ between the two diseases. Menssen et al. analyzed WT1 expression levels in patients with AEoL, hyperoscinophilic syndrome, or reactive eosinophilia by means of RT-PCR. They found that the WT1 expression was restricted to AEoL patients and that isolated central nervous system–related leukemia could be diagnosed by detecting WT1 mRNA transcript in the cerebrospinal fluid in an AEoL patient. Thus, the WT1 assay is a powerful complementary diagnostic tool to distinguish AEoL from hyperoscinophilic syndrome.

WT1 Expression in Various Types of Solid Tumors

WT1 gene expression was examined in 34 solid tumor cell lines and four freshly isolated lung cancers and detected in 3 of the 4 gastric cancer cell lines, all of the 5 colon cancer cell lines, 12 of the 15 lung cancer cell lines, 2 of the 4 breast cancer cell lines, 1 germ tumor cell line, 2 ovarian cancer cell lines, 1 uterine cancer cell line, 1 thyroid cancer cell line, and 1 hepatocellular carcinoma cell line. Therefore, of the 34 solid tumor cell lines examined, 28 (82%) expressed WT1. Furthermore, WT1 expression was examined in fresh lung cancer tissues.

Tissue masses resected from lung cancer patients were separated into two parts: normal-appearing tissues and cancer cell–rich tissues. WT1 expression levels in three paired normal-appearing and cancer cell–rich tissues obtained from three lung cancer patients were $<10^{-5}$, and 3.9×10^{-3}, 4.1×10^{-4}, and 3.6×10^{-2}, and 1.4×10^{-4}, and 1.2×10^{-3}, respectively. The WT1 expression level of cancer cell-rich tissues from another lung cancer patient was 1.4×10^{-3}. These results demonstrated that WT1 expression is significantly higher in cancer cell–rich tissues than in normal-appearing tissues, suggesting abnormal expression of the *WT1* gene not only in the cultured cancer cell lines but also in fresh lung cancer cells.

WT1 Gene Exerts an Oncogenic Function in Leukemogenesis and Tumorigenesis

The *WT1* gene originally was defined as a tumor suppressor gene. However, Inoue et al. have recently proposed that the *WT1* gene has basically two functional aspects—that of a tumor suppressor gene and that of an oncogene—but that in leukemias and various types of solid tumors mentioned earlier, it performs an oncogenic rather than a tumor suppressor gene function on the basis of the following data: high levels of expression of wild-type WT1 in leukemic blast cells and various types of solid tumor cells; a clear inverse correlation between WT1 expression levels and the prognosis of leukemia; increased WT1 expression at relapse; growth inhibition not only of leukemic cells but also of various types of soiid tumor cells by treatment with WT1 antisense oligomers; and blocking of differentiation but induction of proliferation in response to granulocyte colony-stimulating factor in both 32D cl3 myeloid progenitor cells and normal myeloid progenitor cells, both of which constitutively express WT1 as a result of transfection with the *WT1* gene.

Furthermore, molecular analysis of dimethylbenz anthracene (DMBA)–induced rat leukemia by Osaka et al. has supported our hypothesis. WT1 expression was detected in 15 (71%) of 21 DMBA-induced erythroblastic leukemias, and cells with high expression levels of WT1 tended to develop into leukemia. Differences in the interactions of the WT1 protein with other regulatory proteins might determine whether the *WT1* gene acts as a tumor suppressor gene or performs an oncogenic function, because the WT1 protein does interact with regulatory proteins such as P53, par-4, and Ciao 1.

Inoue et al. examined whether the *WT1* gene overexpressing in leukemias has mutations or deletions. Samples from 12 acute leukemia patients were subjected to PCR *single-strand conformation polymorphism* (SSCP) analysis. However, no point mutations were found. Algar et al. also found no tumorigeneic point mutations or small deletions or insertions in the *WT1* gene when they examined 15 AML and 33 ALL patients. Concerning WT1 mutations in CML, Carapeti et al. examined 39 patients with CML blast crisis, and they concluded that dominant-negative mutations of the zinc-finger region of the *WT1* gene are uncommon in CML blast crisis. On the other hand, King-Underwood et al. found mutations in the *WT1* gene in 4 of 36 acute leukemias by SSCP analysis. The mutations comprised small insertions or a nonsense mutation. Furthermore, they extended their study and found that WT1 mutations occur in 14% of AML and 20% of biphenotypic leukemias, but are rare in ALL. In AML, the presence of a WT1 mutation is associated with failure to achieve complete remission and a lower survival rate. Miyagawa et al. also found WT1 mutations in 6 of 46 (13%) AMLs, but they were rare in ALL. Concerning the biologic significance of *WT1* gene mutations in leukemias, note that the majority of leukemias expressing high levels of WT1 have no mutations in the *WT1* gene, indicating that wild-type *WT1* gene expression plays an important role in leukemogenesis.

WT1 Protein is a Tumor-Specific Antigen Capable of Eliciting Cytotoxic T-Lymphocyte Responses

The *WT1* gene is expressed at high levels not only in leukemias but also in various types of solid tumors and exerts an oncogenic function in these malignancies. To determine whether the WT1 protein can serve as a target antigen for tumor-specific immunity, 9-mer WT1 peptides, which contain *major histocompatibility complex* (MHC) class I binding motifs and have a comparatively higher binding affinity for MHC class I molecules, were tested for the induction of *cytotoxic T-lymphocytes* (CTLs) against these WT1 peptides. Immunization in vivo of C57BL/6 mice (MHC class I: H-2D^b) with WT1 peptide Db126 (RMFPNAPYL) elicited CTLs against the WT1 peptide. The CTLs specifically lysed not only Db126-pulsed target cells but also WT1-expressing murine leukemic cells in an MHC class I (H-2D^b)–restricted fashion. The mice immunized with this WT1 peptide completely rejected the challenges by WT1- expressing leukemic cells and survived for a long time with no signs of organ damage by autoimmunity mediated by the CTLs. Also, in vitro stimulation of human peripheral blood mononuclear cells with the WT1 peptide Db126 elicited CTLs against the WT1 peptide. The CTLs specifically killed WT1-expressing human leukemic cells as well as WT1 peptide-pulsed target cells in an human leukocyte antigen class I–restricted manner. Therefore, the WT1 protein was identified as a novel tumor antigen of leukemia and various types of solid tumors. Immunotherapy targeting the WT1 protein should find clinical application not only for leukemias but also for solid tumors.

MATERIALS

Sample Preparation

1. Phosphate-buffered saline (PBS): Dissolve 0.2 g of KCl, 0.2 g of KH_2PO_4, and 8 g of NaCl in 800 mL water. Adjust the pH to 7.2, and make up to 1 L with water.
2. Ficol-Paque.
3. Solution D: 4 mol/L of guanidin thiocyanate, 25 mmol/L of sodium citrate, pH 7.0, 0.5% sarcosyl, 0.1 mol/L of 2-mercaptoethanol.

Reverse Transcriptase Polymerase Chain Reaction

1. Diethylpyrocarbonate (DEPC)-treated water.
2. RT buffer: 50 m*M* Tris-HCl, pH 8.3, 70 m*M* KCl, 3 m*M* $MgCl_2$, 10 m*M* dithiothreitol.
3. Moloney murine leukemia virus (MMLV) RT.
4. Deoxynucleotide triphosphates.
5. Oligo dT primers.
6. RNase inhibitor.
7. Agarose.
8. Ethidium bromide (10 mg/mL).
9. Polaroid 664 film.

METHODS

Sample Preparation

1. Mix heparinized bone marrow aspirates or peripheral blood cells with isovolumes of PBS and centrifuge on Ficol-Paque.
2. Gather mononuclear cells from the mononuclear cell layer and wash twice with PBS to remove platelets.
3. Dissolve cells (1×10^6 to 1×10^7) in 0.5 mL of solution D and store at –80°C until use.

Reverse-Transcriptase Polymerase Chain Reaction

RT-PCR was performed as described previously.

1. Isolate total RNA with the acid-guanidine-phenol-chloroform method, dissolve in DEPC-treated water, and quantitate spectrometrically with absorbance at 260 nm.
2. Heat 2 μg of total RNA in 12.5 μL of DEPC-treated water at 65°C for 5 min.
3. Mix with 17.5 μL of RT buffer containing 600 U of MMLV RT, 500 *μM* of each deoxynucleotide triphosphate, 750 ng of oligo dT primers, and 40 U of RNase inhibitor.
4. Incubate the reaction mixture at 37°C for 90 min, heat at 100°C for 5 min, and then store at –20°C until use.
5. Perform PCR on a DNA thermal cycler under the following optimized conditions: denaturation at 94°C for 1 min, primer annealing at 64°C for 1 min, and then chain elongation at 72°C for 1.5 min.
6. Separate the PCR products on 1.3% agarose gels containing 0.05 μg/mL of ethidium bromide, and photograph with Polaroid 665 film.
7. Develop the negative film at 25°C for 5 min, and measure the band density (densitometric units) with a densitometer.

Optimal conditions for PCR to quantitate WT1 expression levels were determined as follows. PCR was performed for various cycles using WT1 primers (sense primer for exon 7: 5'-GGCATCTGAGACC AGTGAGAA-3'; antisense primer for exon 10, 5'-GAGAGTCAGACT TGAAAGCAGT-3') with serial dilutions of the cDNA prepared from total RNA of K562 human leukemia.

12

APOPTOSIS IN CANCER

In normal tissues, cell proliferation is limited by terminal differentiation and counterbalanced by cell loss, often via apoptosis. Cell damage also elicits apoptosis or necrosis. Moroever, apoptosis can be induced in response to inappropriate proliferation or by cytotoxic immune cells. Replicative senescence provides a different kind of limit to cell proliferation. Cells survive, but irreversibly exit from the cell cycle, as during terminal differentiation. Replicative senescence is established after cells have undergone a large number of replicative cycles, or more rapidly as a response to '*inappropriate*' proliferation signals.

Apoptosis can be induced by two largely separate signaling pathways which converge into a common executing cascade. Signaling and execution use proteases called caspases. The intrinsic pathway elicited, e.g., by strong DNA damage signals or by activated oncogenes, generates a mitochondrial permeability transition ultimately leading to the establishment of the '*apoptosome*' protein complex that activates execution caspases. The extrinsic pathway is initiated by cell surface receptors, labelled '*death receptors*'. These are activated by cytokine ligands and surface proteins of cytotoxic immune cells. The intracellular '*death domains*' of the activated receptors associate with FADD adaptor proteins in a 'DISC' complex that puts distinct initiator caspases into action. These initiate the execution cascade, with or without support by the intrinsic pathway.

Apoptosis is regulated at several steps in both pathways. BCL2 prohibits the related pro-apoptotic proteins BAX or BAK from acting at the mitochondria. They are regulated by further members of the BCL2 family, which mediate pro- or anti-apoptotic signals. FLIP inhibits the extrinsic pathway at the receptors, whereas IAPs like survivin act at the apoptosome inhibiting caspases. They are in turn antagonized by SMAC/Diablo liberated during the mitochondrial permeability transition.

Replicative senescence was first observed in cultured human fibroblasts which undergo >50 population doublings but then stop to proliferate, with distinctive changes in morphology and gene expression. Since some evidence of replicative senescence is found in aging tissues, senescence may be related to human aging. More unequivocally, replicative senescence acts as a fail-safe mechanism against inappropriate proliferation, alternatively to apoptosis. Cancer cells must overcome the barriers presented by apoptosis and replicative senescence. The apoptotic response in cancers is inadequate or blocked. Likewise, cancer cells are in general '*immortalized*' and proliferate beyond the limits of replicative senescence.

Diminished apoptosis in tumor cells can be caused by several means. Down-regulation of death receptors or secretion of decoy receptors mutes the extrinsic pathway. Some cancers may even use death receptor ligands to counterattack the immune system. Mutational inactivation of TP53 as well as silencing or mutation of its downstream pro-apoptotic mediators diminishes the response to signals activating the intrinsic pathway. Moreover, the PI3K or NFκB pathways conferring survival signals are often overactive. Overexpression of inhibitory proteins, such as BCL2, survivin and other IAPs, occurs in almost all cancers. More rarely, inactivation of genes acting in the executing cascade is observed. Replicative senescence is induced after multiple cell doublings when telomeres lengths have reached a critical minimum size. It is established by mechanisms similar to those that activate cell cycle checkpoints as a consequence of DNA double-strand breaks.

Telomeres in humans consist of several hundred repeats of the hexanucleotide TTAGGG. They form a specialized T-loop structure which is protected by binding of several different proteins. In most somatic cells, telomeres shorten during each division. In contrast, germ cells and likely tissue precursor cells express the specialized reverse transcriptase hTERT and its RNA subunit hTR which serves as a template during telomere elongation by hTERT. Many cancers express telomerase and thereby stabilize telomere length. An alternative (hence: ALT) mechanism for the stabilization of telomere length is rarer and at present obscure. It may use DNA recombination. Induction of replicative senescence can also be mediated through activators of RB1 or TP53. Proliferating cells gradually accumulate the CDK inhibitors $p21^{CIP1}$, $p57^{KIP2}$, and particularly $p16^{INK4A}$, which induce cell cycle arrest through RB1. A more acute induction of replicative senescence is mediated by induction of $p14^{ARF1}$ and $p16^{INK4A}$ by oncogenes or viral infection and activation of TP53 as well as RB1. Therefore, defects in RB1, TP53 and CDK inhibitors in cancer cells also prevent replicative senescence. Shortened telomeres possess an increased potential for recombination and fusion with each other. If replicative senescence cannot be established, reactive telomeres contribute to chromosomal instability in cancer.

Limits to Cell Proliferation

The number of cells in normal tissues as well as in tumors is determined by the number of cells newly produced by proliferation and division and by the number of cells that die or are otherwise lost (e.g. by abrasion). Two principal modes of cell death exist, apoptosis and necrosis, with variations and intermediate forms. The overall growth rate of a tissue is additionally dependent on the proportion of cells with an active cell cycle, i.e. the proliferative fraction. Terminal differentiation and replicative senescence are two mechanisms that irreversibly remove cells from the proliferative fraction, although the cells are not destroyed, at least not in the short run.

Apoptosis is a rapid process by which cells are destroyed in a thoroughly controlled fashion within hours. Cells develop multiple blebs on their surface, lose their connections to other cells and the extracellular matrix, and round off while the nucleus and later the entire cell are fragmented into small membrane-enclosed particles. DNA is first cut into large >50 kb fragments, and later into smaller fragments corresponding to multiples of the nucleosomal units. So, free DNA ends can be labeled in apoptotic cells and cytologically detected, while isolated DNA from apoptotic cells often appears as a '*nucleosomal ladder*' on agarose gels. During uncomplicated apoptosis, all cell remnants are phagocytosed or lost from the tissue, e.g. into the lumen of an organ, without evoking an inflammatory reaction.

Apoptosis can be elicited by external or internal signals. It is employed to shape tissues during development, to eliminate superfluous or autoreactive immune cells, to maintain homeostasis of tissues with rapid or cyclic cell turnover, and to destroy cells infected by viruses. An absolute or relative decrease in the apoptotic rate or a failure to respond properly to apoptotic signals is an almost universal property of human cancers. The mechanisms of apoptosis are therefore under intense scrutiny to better understand the development and progression of cancer and to find new angles for therapy.

Necrosis is a different form of cell death elicited, e.g., by mechanical, chemical, or thermal damage as well as by some infectious agents. Necrotic cells burst, usually after swelling, releasing their content into the surrounding tissue in an uncontrolled fashion. Frequently, inflammation follows. Unlike apoptosis, necrosis may proceed in the absence of cellular energy. Thus, in a large solid tumor, hypoxic areas will typically show an enhanced rate of apoptosis, but the central core, which is almost anoxic and devoid of nutrients, will be necrotic. Theoretically, the inflammatory reaction ensuing from necrotic tumor cells could be beneficial, since it attracts immune cells. In reality, it might be a sort of double-edged sword, because inflammation may not only eliminate tumor cells but also contributes to the destruction of normal tissue structures and thereby may facilitate invasion and metastasis.

The specific functions of many tissues are exerted by cells that have once and for all exited from the cell cycle. Their formation is meant by the more precise usage of '*terminal differentiation*'. Diverse strategies of terminal differentiation are used in various tissues. In many tissues, terminally differentiated cells are polyploid and/or multinuclear, e.g. the syncytia of the skeletal muscle or, less spectacularly, polyploid (tetraploid or octoploid) hepatocytes of the liver or umbrella cells of the urothelium. Robust terminal differentiation can also be efficiently achieved in diploid cells with normal, very active nuclei, as impressively demonstrated by neurons. In some tissues, however, the nuclei of terminally differentiated cells shrink and/or are expelled or dissolved. The epidermis, the lens of the eye, and the erythrocyte lineage provide examples of this strategy. In some instances, the destruction of the nucleus resembles an apoptotic process and is indeed implemented by similar mechanisms. In fact, in some tissues terminal differentiation is a prelude to actual apoptosis, e.g. in the gut. During differentiation, enterocytes move from the crypts towards the tips of the villi, where they undergo apoptosis, their remnants being lost into the lumen.

A decreased rate of terminal differentiation is a fundamental requirement for tumor growth. Many cancers are characterized by its complete lack, while some produce terminally differentiated cells at a diminished rate. Accordingly, in many cancers, proteins that are only expressed in terminally differentiated cells are not detectable. In others, some such proteins are expressed in a fraction of the tumor cells that still differentiate, or the cancer cells express some proteins of their differentiated tissue counterparts, but do not exit from the cell cycle.

Replicative senescence is also defined by an irreversible exit from the cell cycle, after which cells survive for an extended period. This distinguishes replicative senescence from apoptosis, but the borderline towards terminal differentiation cannot always be drawn as easily. Cultured cells undergoing replicative senescence often take on a characteristic morphology with a flattened appearance, large nuclei, and many small granuli. They express some characteristic proteins, such as SAβ-GAL, a β-galactosidase with a comparatively acidic pH optimum, and high levels of CDK inhibitors like $p21^{CIP1}$ or $p16^{INK4A}$. Conversely, senescent cells express few or none of the markers that are diagnostic for terminally differentiated cells. There are overlaps, however, and senescent fibroblasts have been as well considered as terminally differentiated. In human tissues, replicative senescence is not easily ascertained, although cells with conspicuous morphologies that express SAβ-GAL have been observed.

In cultured cells, replicative senescence can be more clearly defined and is elicited in two very different instances. The '*classic*' mode of induction occurs after propagation of normal human cells over many passages. It sets in gradually. In fibroblasts, where the phenomenon was first described, it may occur after as many as 50-80 cell doublings. In cultured epithelial cells, it appears much earlier. It can be prevented by infection with certain DNA viruses, typically the SV40 papovavirus or its large T-antigen. Thus, replicative senescence presents a limit to the life-span of normal human somatic cells.

Replicative senescence can also be induced in a rapid mode, long before cells have exhausted their normal life-span, by inappropriate proliferation signals, specifically by overexpressed mutant RAS proteins. Unlike apoptosis and terminal differentiation, replicative senescence does not seem to be employed in the human body for tissue homeostasis. Rather, it appears to act as a fail-safe mechanism. Its only normal function may be setting a maximum to the human lite-span.

Evidently, cells in the germ-line must be exempt from replicative senescence. Moreover, it is plausible that tissue stem and/or early precursor cells must be subject to replicative senescence to a lower degree than more differentiated somatic cells, since during a human life-time in a continuously replicating tissue they will have to undergo many more than 100 divisions.

Replicative senescence is circumvented in many cancers. Cancer cells grown in culture or as xenografts in experimental animals can often be propagated for many more than 100 cell doublings and apparently indefinitely, without introducing T-antigen or its like. They are therefore considered '*immortalized*'. It is, of course, difficult to ascertain immortalization as such in a human cancer tissue. It is easier in vitro, but not all human cancers can be grown in culture or as xenografts. Therefore, it is not certain whether all human cancers are really immortalized. Indefinite growth is not a necessary condition for a cancer to kill its host, because 50 cells doublings can theoretically produce more cells than an entire human body holds.

However, mechanisms that allow cancer cells in vitro to circumvent replicative senescence can be shown to be also active in many cancer tissues. In other cases, tumor cells may evade replicative senescence by acquiring a kind of '*stem cell*' character. This is evident in germ-cell cancers, e.g. in the testes or ovary. In addition, some cancers originating in somatic tissues may acquire (or maintain) properties of the respective tissue stem cell or early precursor, e.g. basal cell carcinoma of the skin and colon carcinoma.

Mechanisms of Apoptosis

Apoptosis can be divided into several stages, i.e. initiation, execution and removal of the cell remnants ('*burial*'). Initiation can be performed by two separate pathways, often designated '*intrinsic*' and '*extrinsic*', which converge towards a common execution pathway. The intrinsic pathway responds to internal signals, e.g. from DNA damage, whereas the extrinsic pathway responds to external signals, e.g. by cytotoxic T-cells. In some cells, the extrinsic pathway can proceed towards execution on its own while in other cells it needs some contribution from the intrinsic pathway. All steps in these pathways are well defined and controlled. Considering apoptosis as a '*programmed cell death*' is certainly justified.

The decisive step of the intrinsic pathway takes place at the mitochondria. Its most important regulators are members of the BCL2 family. Around 20 members are known, some of which are pro-apoptotic, whereas others are antiapoptotic. They share common domains, termed BH1 to BH4. The founding member, BCL2, was discovered as the oncogene at the characteristic translocation site t(14;18) in follicular B-cell lymphoma. This translocation places the *BCL2* gene under the control of the immunoglobulin heavy chain enhancer. Overexpression of BCL2 prevents apoptosis of follicular B-cells and is the initiating event in this relatively slow-growing cancer. Induction of apoptosis by the intrinsic pathway requires inactivation of BCL2 and other anti-apoptotic proteins such as BCL-X_L. These proteins are located at the mitochondrial membrane, probably forming heterodimers with BAX and BAK, which are pro-apoptotic members of the BCL2 family. Other members of the family are distinguished by containing only a BH3 domain, and none of the other motifs. They also lack a transmembrane domain. These relay different pro-apoptotic signals to the mitochondria.

Cellular stress of various kinds can induce apoptosis. In many cases, activation of TP53 is involved, e.g. when DNA double-strand breaks are created by radiation. Activated TP53 induces transcription of one or several pro-apoptotic BCL2 signaling proteins such as NOXA or PUMA, also increasing BAX, while down-regulating BCL2. The precise mechanisms may differ according to cell type and type of cellular stress. The pro-apoptotic proteins induced by TP53 override anti-apoptotic signals to initiate the next step in the intrinsic apoptotic pathway, i.e. formation of pores in the mitochondria.

BID mediates the '*cooptation*' of the intrinsic pathway in cells in which it is needed for amplification of the extrinsic pathway. In that case, two shorter forms of BID, p15 or p13, are produced by proteolytic cleavage of an inactive precursor protein by Caspase 8 or Caspase 10. These then activate BAX or BAK, respectively.

The next step in the intrinsic pathway, mediated a.o. by BAX and BAK, consists of a change in the mitochondrial structure and function designated '*mitochondrial permeability transition*' (MPT). At the contact sites between the outer and the inner mitochondrial membrane, pores are formed by a multiprotein complex to which proteins from all mitochondrial compartments contribute. One crucial component is the adenine nucleotide translocator which otherwise exchanges ADP + P_i against ATP across the inner mitochondrial membrane. The pores let molecules <1500 D pass. This leads to a break-down of the mitochondrial transmembrane potential, since protons and other ions, including Ca^{2+}, can now move freely across the membrane. Mitochondria are thus the first organelles functionally inactivated in the intrinsic apoptotic pathway.

In conjunction with the mitochondrial permeability transition, mitochondria release several proteins, mostly from the intermembrane compartment, such as cytochrome c and the SMAC/Diablo protein. *Apoptosis-inducing factor* (AIF), a flavoprotein is released from the mitochondrial matrix. In the cytoplasm, 8 molecules of cytochrome c associate with an equal number of APAF1 proteins to form a large structure resembling the spokes of a wheel. It is therefore called '*wheel of death*' or '*apoptosome*'. The apoptosome binds a stochiometric number of the pro-protease, pro-caspase 9 and supports its autocatalytic activation in an ATP-dependent process.

Caspases are cysteine proteases which cleave the peptide bond following an Asp in the consensus sequence QAD↓RG. In man, 14 caspases are known, which are categorized in three groups, initiator caspases (including caspase 9), executor caspases (including caspase 3), and inflammatory caspases, which are not directly involved in apoptosis, but process cytokines. The prototypic enzyme of that group is caspase 1, or *interleukin-converting enzyme* (ICE). Pro-caspase 9 is a homodimer containing two 'CARD' domains by which it binds to the APAF1 adaptor proteins in the apoptosome. Following autocatalytic cleavage, the active caspase 9 is a heterotetramer of two smaller and two larger subunits each. Active Caspase 9 goes on to process and activate the executioner caspase 3 to initiate the execution phase of apoptosis.

Activation of caspases is supported by the AIF protein released from the mitochondrial matrix. The other protein liberated from this compartment, SMAC/Diablo, has a distinct function. Activation of initiator - and sometimes even executioner caspases - is not always sufficient to actually elicit apoptosis, because a number of small proteins in the cell are capable of inhibiting these proteases. They belong to a group of proteins called IAPs (inhibitors of apoptosis). IAPs are mostly small proteins characterized by one or several 'BIR' domains. XIAP and survivin inhibit the intrinsic pathway at the step of activated caspase 9 and even caspase 3. They bind caspases through their BIR domains and inhibit their protease activity. SMAC/Diablo binds and sequesters IAPs like survivin and XIAP, thereby removing a further obstacle to apoptosis. Interestingly, several viruses - oncogenic or not - express their own IAPs to prevent a cell from apoptosis while they replicate.

The extrinsic pathway is initiated when specific cell surface receptors are engaged by their specific ligands. As a rule, these '*death receptors*' belong to the TNF receptor superfamily. Tumor necrosis factor α (TNFα) is one of several cytokine ligands of this receptor superfamily. This peptide is secreted by monocytes, macrophages and other cells of the immune system during inflammatory reactions and in response to cellular stress. It elicits various reactions, including apoptosis in some cells containing the TNFRI receptor.

Other ligands of TNFRSFs are present mainly on the surface of immune cells, e.g. CD95L, and the ligand-receptor interaction is part of a cell-to-cell-interaction. CD95L is also called FAS ligand and activates TNFRSF6, alias CD95, FAS, or APO-1. The CD95/CD95L system is considered one of the most important components in killing of infected and tumor cells by cytotoxic T-cells. It is also employed in the selective elimination of auto-reactive immune cells. Defects in CD95 function occur in autoimmune diseases as well as in cancers.

In fact, the borderline between membrane-bound and soluble ligands is blurred. Some cytokines, including TNFα, are also present as a active membrane-bound form on the cell surface and CD95L is also secreted. The regulation of receptor-ligand interactions in this system is in fact very complex. For instance, at the receiving end, the response is modulated by the presence of modulating and decoy receptors. The response to TNFα is modulated by the TNFRII receptor. When present at the cell surface, the TNFRII appears to bind the cytokine and pass it on to the TNFRI which mediates the actual response. When TNFRII is sheared off the cell, it acts as a '*decoy receptor*', sequestering the ligand and preventing it from acting on TNFRI.

Similarly, in addition to the membrane-bound form of CD95 (also tmFAS), a soluble form is generated by alternative splicing (sFAS), which also acts as a decoy receptor to decrease the responsiveness to CD95L. Apoptotic responses to the TNFα-related cytokine TRAIL are also dependent on the relative expression of four different TNFRSF members, TRAIL-R1 through TRAIL-R4, two of which are true receptors and two are decoys.

Members of the TNFRSF family act through several pathways, notably the NFκB pathway. Family members that can activate the extrinsic apoptosis pathway differ from their homologues by the presence of an additional intracellular domain, called the '*death domain*'. This part of the protein is required for the activation of the extrinsic apoptotic pathway. Since the NFκB pathway as a rule counteracts apoptosis, the actual cellular response will often depend on the relative strengths of the two pathways activated in parallel. In specific cell types, cytokine receptors like TNFRI also stimulate cell proliferation.

Following ligand binding to an active TNFR, such as TNFRI or TNFRSF6, the ligand/receptor complexes trimerize and the receptor death domains bind FADD proteins by interaction with the homologous domains in this adaptor. In addition, FADD contains a death effector domain homologous to that in initiator caspases. By binding to the death receptor, this domain is exposed and binds an initiator pro-caspase, usually pro-caspase 8 or pro-caspase 10. The resulting complex appears sometimes in the literature as '*death inducing signaling complex*' (DISC). Its function in apoptosis is to bring pro-caspase molecules into close proximity to dimerize and activate one another. The activated initiator caspases 8 or 10 then activate executioner caspases like caspase 3 setting the execution phase into motion. The FLIP protein acts as an inhibitor of the extrinsic pathway by interfering with initiator caspase dimerization.

In some cells, activation of the extrinsic pathway by certain death receptor ligands is sufficient to elicit apoptosis. In such cases, the expression levels of BCL2 and $BCLX_L$ are quite irrelevant. In others, induction of apoptosis requires the participation of the intrinsic pathway. In response to external signals, this is typically stimulated via the BID protein cleaved by caspase 8. Conversely, the intrinsic pathway also influences the extrinsic pathway. For instance, TP53 induces activators of the extrinsic pathway, but also increases the expression of CD95, thereby sensitizing cells to pro-apoptotic external signals.

The multiple biochemical and morphological changes that take place during the execution phase of apoptosis are caused by proteolytic cleavage of >300 cellular proteins by caspase 3 and other executioner caspases like caspase 6. The substrates comprise regulators of the cell cycle such as RB1, DNA repair proteins such as DNA-PK and poly-ADP-ribosyl polymerase (PARP), and cytosketelal proteins such as actin, lamins, and keratin 18. The characteristic '*nucleosomal ladder*' DNA fragmentation is caused by several DNases, prominently CAD (*caspase activated DNase*) that are liberated by cleavage of inhibitory proteins to which they are normally bound. Cleavage of FAK (*focal adhesion kinase*), PAK2 (*p21-associated kinase*), and Gelsolin contributes to the loss of adhesion and the characteristic membrane changes such as blebbing and redistribution of membrane proteins and phospholipids. These redistributions create signals for the subsequent burial phase. Importantly, phosphatidylserine which is normally restricted strictly to the inner layer of the membrane phospholipid bilayer, is flipped to the outer layer and recognized by receptors on macrophages that are attracted by further chemotactic signals diffusing out from the dying cell.

Mechanisms of Diminished Apoptosis in Cancer

Diminished apoptosis of cancer cells is important for a number of reasons.

1. In some cancers decreased apoptosis is the primary cause of tumorous growth, e.g. in follicular B-cell lymphoma and perhaps in early prostate cancer. In these tumors, cells that ought to undergo apoptosis in the course of normal tissue homeostasis survive, which leads to an oversized and progressively disorganized tissue mass.
2. A diminished rate of apoptosis exacerbates hyperproliferation in many different cancers.
3. Apoptosis is a fail-safe mechanism in response to '*inappropriate*' proliferation signals (as is replicative senescence) and following pronounced DNA damage, e.g. unrepaired double-strand breaks. Therefore, a decreased response to '*internal*' pro-apoptotic signals allows cells to proliferate in spite of proliferation signals being inappropriate or in spite of persisting severe DNA damage. This occurs in many cancer types, at the latest during progression.
4. Cytotoxic T-cells from the immune system which protect against cancer and infections employ induction of apoptosis as a mechanism of cell killing. Decreased responsiveness to '*external*' pro-apoptotic signals therefore is one of the mechanisms by which tumor cells evade the immune response. This aspect becomes particularly relevant during invasion and metastasis. At an earlier stage of cancer development, some viruses, e.g. Epstein-Barr virus or HHV8, express anti-apoptotic factors which diminish apoptosis in response to both internal and external signals, thereby creating a population of cells more susceptible to carcinogenesis.
5. Many cytotoxic drugs employed in chemotherapy as well as radiotherapy act by inducing apoptosis. Decreased apoptotic responsiveness therefore contributes to primary and secondary resistance to chemo- and radiotherapy.

In human cancers, diminished apoptosis can originate from alterations in many different steps of apoptosis by a variety of mechanisms. Proteins that relay internal or external pro-apoptotic signals can be inactivated, the extrinsic or the intrinsic pathway become deactivated or desensitized, and even the execution stage can be impeded.

In one and the same cancer, several different steps can be affected. Moreover, decreased apoptosis in cancer cells is often caused by overactivity of survival signal pathways rather than by primary alterations in apoptotic pathways. Nevertheless, some degree of apoptosis does take place in human cancers, but not at the same rate as would be elicited in normal cells by comparable external and internal signals.

Typical changes that diminish the apoptotic rate in human cancer cells include the following.

Desensitization of Death Receptors

The CD95/CD95L system is inactivated or desensitized in many different human cancers, in hematological cancers as well as in carcinomas. While mutation of the *TNFRSF6* gene encoding CD95 is occasionally observed, in most cases down-regulation of receptor expression is the major mechanism responsible. In some cancers, a shift in expression from the transmembrane towards the soluble (decoy) receptor takes place.

Altered expression of FADD proteins, decreased expression of Caspase 8, and overexpression of FLIP which inhibits the activation of Caspases at the DISC have been identified as causes of post-receptor defects in some cancers. In each case, the overall consequence is a decreased response to cytotoxic immune cells, but also to chemotherapeutic agents, which induce apoptosis partly through increased expression of both CD95 and its ligand. Other members of the TNFRSF family like the TRAIL receptors are also often inactivated by similar mechanisms.

Counterattack

Additionally, decreased expression of the CD95/FAS receptor in some cancers is accompanied by increased expression of soluble CD95 ligand. It is thought that secretion of CD95L normally contributes to the establishment of '*immune-privileged*' sites in the human body. Immune-privileged sites are established in organs such as the anterior eye chamber or the testes that could not function properly in the presence of lymphocytes and therefore have to keep them out. In consequence, increased production of CD95L may help cancers to prevent immune responses and may even destroy T-cells and other cells that express CD95. This '*counterattack*' may account for some tissue damage caused by invasive cancers locally and perhaps even in distant organs like the liver.

Loss of TP53

While down-regulation or mutation of CD95 inactivate external pro-apoptotic signaling, inactivation of TP53 may be the most common alteration that compromises internal pro-apoptotic signaling. TP53 mediates induction of apoptosis in response to DNA damage as well as to hyperproliferation. Some think that loss of its pro-apoptotic function may be the most important consequence of TP53 inactivation.

Intrinsic Pathway Inactivation

The most varied assortment of alterations affect the intrinsic apoptotic pathway. BCL2 was discovered as an oncogene protein activated by the most characteristic translocation in follicular lymphoma. It is also over-expressed in a wide range of other cancers, including different types of carcinoma, prominently breast and prostate cancer. Alternatively to BCL2, cancers contain high levels of BCL-X_L, which is induced a.o. by the NFκB pathway.

Conversely, pro-apoptotic members of the BCL2 family such as BAD or NOXA are down-regulated in a variety of cancers, in some cases by promoter hypermethylation, and cannot be induced by activated TP53 or other signals. The most generally down-regulated member of the family may be BAX, perhaps due to its effector function at the mitochondria.

An even stronger block to apoptosis may ensue when APAF1 expression is down-regulated, typically by promoter hypermethylation. In summary, in almost all cancers the balance between pro-apoptotic and anti-apoptotic members of the family is tilted. The overall result of this imbalance is a decreased sensitivity towards apoptotic signals, particularly those elicited by hyperproliferation and aneuploidy, but also by chemotherapy.

IAP Overexpression

Both the intrinsic and extrinsic pathway are affected by over-expression of IAP proteins which block signaling through caspases as well as the actual execution caspases, e.g. caspase 3. Survivin, e.g., is expressed at high levels during fetal development, but almost undetectable in normal resting tissues. Some expression is found associated with normal proliferation and regenerative processes such as wound repair. However, in many human cancers the levels of this IAP protein are so strongly and consistently increased that it is being developed as a tumor marker.

IAPs may also be expressed or be induced by viruses present in a tumor cell such as EBV or HBV. The overexpression of IAPs that block the execution phase can result in chaotic situations within a cancer cell, viz. partial activation of caspases which is not sufficient for execution of cell death. Consequences of such partial activation could be altered cell morphology and adhesion as well as genomic instability. Overexpression of other IAPs or of c-FLIP impede primarily the signaling phase of the extrinsic pathway by inhibiting the signal from FADD to caspase 8 or 10.

Activation of Antiapoptotic Pathways

The defects in the actual apoptotic signaling and execution cascades occurring in cancer cells are almost regularly complemented by increased activity of pathways that convey survival signals. Perhaps the most important ones in this regard are the PI3K and the NFκB pathways. The PI3K pathway is activated in many cancers, indirectly by growth factors, oncogenic mutation of receptor tyrosine kinases, or RAS mutations, or directly by inactivation of negative regulators in the pathway like PTEN or by oncogenic overexpression of PI3Kα. The pathway does stimulate proliferation and particularly the growth of cells, but in many cancers, the main importance of its activation may lie in the ensuing inhibition of apoptosis.

This is mediated through activity of AKT/PKB which phosphorylates BAX preventing it from activating the intrinsic apoptotic pathway. The kinase also phosphorylates and activates the forkhead transcription factor FKHR-L1, which counteracts apoptosis at the level of transcription. Activation of the PI3K pathway also diminishes the effect of cancer chemotherapy. Compared to the PI3K pathway, the NFκB pathway is less frequently subject to direct activation by mutation in human cancers. However, in many cell types, it limits the extent of induction of apoptosis resulting from activation of TNFRSF death receptors. Therefore, its indirect activation in tumor cells, which can be achieved by a variety of cytokines and stress signals, contributes to the resistance towards induction of apoptosis by external signals such as TNFα or CD95L.

Replicative Senescence and its Disturbances in Human Cancers

Apoptosis is normally a rapid process, occurring within a period between one hour and one day. It is elicited likewise by rapid signals, such as the binding of cytokines to death receptors at the cell membrane or the activation of TP53 by ATM following a DNA double-strand break. Moreover, cells subjected to apoptosis vanish quite rapidly by phagocytosis. In all these respects, replicative senescence differs. It sets in slowly, it is usually elicited by signals that accumulate gradually, and cells persist, at least in the short run.

Replicative senescence can be evoked by two different signals which use overlapping pathways for execution. One type of signal emanates from short telomeres, and the second type from CDK inhibitors.

Telomeres in human cells are 5-30 kb long and made up of 1000-5000 repeats of TTAGGG hexamers. The bulk of each telomere consists of double-stranded DNA, but 75-150 nt at the ends are single-stranded. Normally, these single strands are folded back into the double strand, forming a T-loop. This is a structure similar to the D-loops occuring during DNA repair by homologous recombination. In humans, telomeric DNA is wrapped around nucleosomes. Therefore, core histones are present, but in addition an unusual assembly of further proteins. The TRF2 (*telomeric repeat binding factor* 2) protein induces and seals T-loops. It also serves as an anchor for a number of further proteins that are located to the telomere under normal circumstances, in particular the RAD50/NBS/MRE11 complex. This complex processes double-strand breaks during DNA repair.

The KU70 and KU80 proteins which mark and protect DNA double-strand breaks during repair are also present at telomeres. Thus, telomeres appear to serve as reservoirs for these proteins on one hand, but on the other the repair proteins are strategically placed for dealing with damage to the telomeres themselves. A further protein, TRF1, which is homologous to TRF2, limits telomere length, being regulated itself by tankyrase, a poly-adenosine diphosphate ribosylase and TRF1-interacting nuclear protein 2. TRF1 also helps to maintain the RAD50/NBS/MRE11 complex at the telomere.

With each DNA replication in somatic cells, telomeres shorten. This is caused in principle by the end-replication problem. The top strand.(with a 5'-end at the telomere) is replicated by elongation of an RNA primer at or near its end. When it is removed by RNase H after DNA synthesis has proceeded, the resulting gap cannot be filled, since DNA polymerases work invariably in the 5'→3' direction. This endreplication dilemma predicts a theoretical minimum loss of telomere sequences during each replication. In reality, its extent can be larger and is regulated by TRF1.

In germ-line cells, the decrease in telomere length is prevented by a specialized enzyme, telomerase. Accordingly, telomeres in germ line cells are approximately twice as long as in somatic cells. Telomerase is a specialized reverse transcriptase that uses an RNA template (AAUCCC) provided by its hTERC subunit to elongate telomeres. While the hTERC subunit is expressed in almost all human cells, the catalytic subunit hTERT is restricted to a small set of cells with high replicative potential, like germ-line cells, tissue stem cells and memory immune cells. Expression of the *TERT* gene is induced by a number of proliferation-stimulating and stem-cell maintaining factors. In particular, its promoter is a target of MYC proteins.

Shortening of telomeres to below a certain length causes replicative senescence. In cells cultured over longer periods, actually two successive steps can be distinguished, which are called M1 and M2. They are operationally defined: M1 can be bypassed by obliteration of RB1 and TP53 function. In the laboratory, this can be achieved by introduction of viral proteins such as SV40 large T antigen. After 40 - 50 further doublings, senescence sets in irreversibly at the M2 point. Circumventing the M2 point requires activation of telomerase. It is not precisely known what happens at M1 and M2.

Human telomeres are very variable. So, one idea is that M1 is triggered by the first telomere reaching a critical length. This would then activate a checkpoint response through the RB1 and TP53 pathways. At M2, further telomere shrinking has taken place. Some telomeres may have become so short that they can no longer form a T-loop. In addition, they may not be capable of storing DNA repair proteins any more. So, some sort of DNA double-strand repair response may be initiated, likely through ATM, which induces replicative senescence once and for all. While some of these ideas are not fully proven, DNA damage signaling is certainly involved in replicative senescence.

Telomere shortening leads to chromosomal instability. Of course, shortened unsealed telomeres are expected to become substrates for exonucleases which would gradually degrade a chromosome. In fact, a greater danger to genomic integrity may be recombination between different telomeres that are not protected by proteins. Recombination between the telomeres of two chromosomes can generate a dicentric chromosome.

During mitosis, this may become missegregated or be pulled to opposite sides of the spindle and disrupted. Disruption would cause two open chromosome ends which could again fuse to other chromosomes and form further dicentrics to continue the cycle. Of note, in this classical breakage-fusion-bridge sequence, the breakpoints tend to move from the telomeres towards the centromere.

In human cancers, establishment of replicative senescence as a consequence of telomere shortening is impeded, often at M1 as well as M2. Many human cancers contain defects in the RB1 and TP53 pathway. While these have many other consequences as well, loss of RB1 and TP53 function would be expected to permit the bypassing of the M1 limit. This would establish a population of cells continuing to proliferate with at least some critically shortened telomeres and therefore an enhanced potential for genomic instability. Dicentric chromosomes and a movement of chromosome breaks towards the centromere are quite common observations in carcinoma cells. Moreover, telomere instability due to telomerase dysfuntion is the cause of a human disease, dyskeratosis congenita. Patients with this rare inherited affliction do not only present with defects in skin, hair, and the hematopoetic system, but are also prone to cancer.

In addition to the defects in the RB1 and TP53 pathways, many human cancers express hTERT which can be shown to be enzymatically active in tissue extracts. In some tissues, hTERT expression or activity could therefore serve as a cancer biomarker. In cancers with hTERT expression, telomere lengths are at least stabilized at a low level, albeit they do not always rebound.

There is evidence for a different, alternative mechanism of telomere stabilization, named ALT, in some cancers and even in normal tissues, where telomeres are stabilized or even expanded in the absence of detectable telomerase activity. The unspecific designation ALT reveals that the mechanism is presently mostly based on conjecture, with hints from alternative mechanisms employed in organisms that lack telomerase. There, telomere expansion can be achieved by a kind of homologous recombination double-strand repair. Indeed, there is some evidence for such a mechanism in humans and, specifically, that the WRN helicase might be involved.

Telomere erosion is certainly to a large degree responsible for the limited life-span of cultured human cells. It can be regarded as a mechanism counting the number of cycles a cell has undergone. A second mechanism appears to rely on CDK inhibitor proteins, in particular $p16^{INK4A}$, $p21^{CIP1}$, and $p57^{KIP2}$

Among the CDK inhibitors, $p21^{CIP1}$ is strongly induced by TP53 and may be largely reponsible for the arrest of the cell cycle after telomere shortening. However, it is thought that $p21^{CIP1}$ also accumulates in cells that proliferate continuously, independently of TP53, since it is induced by many proliferative stimuli. This is certainly so for $p16^{INK4A}$ which is not regulated by TP53. In somatic human cells $p16^{INK4A}$ is induced by E2F and other transcription factors activated during cell cycle progression. Because the protein has a relatively long half-life, it accumulates when successive cell cycles follow rapidly upon each other. In some cell types that express $p57^{KIP2}$, this inhibitor behaves in a similar fashion. So, the level of certain CDK inhibitors - like telomere length - depends on the number of successive cell cycles. This may provide a second counting mechanism.

However, in this mechanism counting not only depends on the actual number of cell cycles, but more critically on how quickly they follow each other and on which signals elicit proliferation. An extreme case is hyperproliferation induced by oncogenes such as *RAS* and *MYC*. In human cells, such hyperproliferation induces not only $p14^{ARF1}$ to sensitize TP53, but also $p16^{INK4A}$. Together, these proteins lead to a rather quick arrest of the cell cycle, certainly more rapidly than the telomere shortening mechanism would. This mechanism could account for the different life-spans of different human cell types in culture, because it may be more sensitive in epithelial cells that become relatively soon senescent in culture. More generally, the involvement of both $p14^{ARF1}$ and $p16^{INK4A}$ in the response to hyperproliferation in human cells may explain why the *CDKN2A* locus is such a frequent target for inactivation in such a wide variety of human cancers. Specifically, it may solve the enigma why $p16^{INK4A}$ of all INK4 proteins is the most important tumor suppressor.

The mechanisms involved in the regulation of replicative senescence constitute one of the more important differences between humans and rodents with regard to cancer. Since these mechanisms may be related to organism aging, this is plausible. A two year old mouse is approaching old age, whereas a two year old human is a toddler and a long way from maturity. Moreover, 70 kg humans living for 70 years or so may require additional mechanisms for protection against cancer than 50 g mice living for 30 months. On a less intuitive argument, it has been observed for a long time that human cells are much more difficult to transform in vitro than rodent cells. It had been a long-standing speculation that there might be (at least) one additional mechanism that protects them from becoming cancerous. It is now established that somatic cells in rodents more generally express telomerase and telomeres in rodents are longer than in humans. Moreover, the regulation of CDK inhibitors is different, particularly that of $p16^{INK4A}$. There is good reason to believe that the long-sought difference may reside here.

INDEX